BEDSIDE CARDIAC DIAGNOSIS

BEDSIDE CARDIAC DIAGNOSIS

HENRY J. L. MARRIOTT, MD, FACP, FACC

Director, Clinical Research and Education, Rogers
Heart Foundation, St. Petersburg, Florida

Clinical Professor of Medicine (Cardiology),
Emory University School of Medicine,
Atlanta, Georgia

Clinical Professor of Pediatrics (Cardiology),
University of Florida College of Medicine,
Gainesville, Florida

Clinical Professor of Medicine,
University of South Florida,
College of Medicine,
Tampa, Florida

Formerly Head, Division of Physical Diagnosis,
University of Maryland, School of Medicine,
Baltimore, Maryland

J. B. LIPPINCOTT COMPANY
Philadelphia

Acquisitions Editor: Charles McCormick
Sponsoring Editor: Kimberley Cox
Project Editors: Virginia Barishek and Dina K. Rubin
Indexer: Anne Cope
Designer: Doug Smock
Production Manager: Caren Erlichman
Production Coordinator: Kevin P. Johnson
Compositor: Waldman Graphics, Inc.
Printer/Binder: Courier Book Company/Westford

6 5 4 3 2

Library of Congress Cataloging-in-Publication Data

Marriott, Henry J. L. (Henry Joseph Llewellyn), 1917–
    Bedside cardiac diagnosis / Henry J. L. Marriott.
        p.   cm.
    Includes bibliographical references and index.
    ISBN 0-397-51085-3
    1. Heart—Diseases—Diagnosis.   2. Physical diagnosis.   3. Heart—
Sounds.   4. Medical history taking.   I. Title.
    [DNLM: 1. Heart Diseases—diagnosis.   2. Medical History Taking.
WG 141 M359b]
RC683.M355   1993
616.1'2075—dc20
DNLM/DLC
for Library of Congress   92-6256
                                                                  CIP

The authors and publisher have exerted every effort to ensure that drug selection and dosage set forth in this text are in accord with current recommendations and practice at the time of publication. However, in view of ongoing research, changes in government regulations, and the constant flow of information relating to drug therapy and drug reactions, the reader is urged to check the package insert for each drug for any change in indications and dosage and for added warnings and precautions. This is particularly important when the recommended agent is a new or infrequently employed drug.

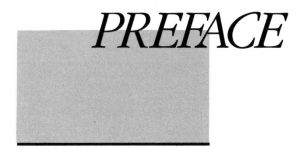

PREFACE

"In an age of complex technology, any news of a new use for a simple old physical sign is bound to quicken the pulse. It is thrilling to see little David take on Goliath."

— *Vaisrub*[1]

In an outpatient department in England—where the simple methods have always been held in high esteem—a landmark study demonstrated that, of the diagnoses finally arrived at, 82 percent were first made after taking the history.[2] Another nine percent required the physical examination to make the diagnosis (and these were all cardiovascular diagnoses), while only the remaining nine percent depended on additional laboratory investigations.

The pendular swing toward sophisticated technology, at the expense of simple and more rewarding basic explorations by history and physical, has been a mixed blessing. Technical advances are spectacular indeed, but they have been achieved at a price. Hurst[3] points to "the apparent decline in physicians' ability to analyze chest pain, perform a physical examination of the heart, and interpret electrocardiograms and chest films" and sagely comments that "the poorer the screening examination, the poorer the choice of high technology." It is impossible to overstress the fact that intelligent use of today's expensive techniques heavily depends upon a good, informed and thorough interrogation and examination of the patient. To use one of today's "in" words, the history and physical are the "infrastructure" of the quality diagnostic workup. And in this painfully cost-conscious decade

of the nineties, the prudent, unwasteful use of technology is an undeniable priority.

This book is directed at those who wish to get the most enjoyment out of the art of using these simple tools. The text encompasses the historical highlights, but the chief thrust is in the elicitation of physical signs; and it contains no information about laboratory tests. Your eyes, your hands and your ears are always with you, and the wonder is how much diagnostic information you can obtain with the skilled use of just the primary senses of sight, touch and hearing. One's sense of smell is rarely of prime importance, though it may occasionally lead one to the rapid diagnosis of diabetic or uremic coma. The use of taste has fortunately fallen into desuetude since more acceptable means of recognizing sugar in the urine have become available.

The casual peruser of the references may be surprised and disappointed to see so many "old" articles referenced and relatively few "modern" ones. This is, of course, because so much of the pioneer work in refining physical diagnosis was accomplished during the decades following the introduction of the phonocardiograph and of equipment to record pulse tracings; so the golden years of revelation were between 1950 and 1970. That is why nearly two thirds of the more than 1,200 references antedate 1970. Since

1970, the main advances in understanding physical signs have been the result of correlations with echocardiography and other sophisticated techniques.

The first observation of many physical signs was made in the 19th century, often by French physicians. It is so unlikely that the reader of this text will search out the dusty, foreign journal concerned that I have included no 19th century references in detail; yet the author and date of first descriptions are always of academic interest, and so I have supplied name and date, of the originator of many important observations made before, or soon after the turn of the century, e.g., (Kussmaul, 1873).

Pithy clinical sayings — "burrs that stick in the memory"[4] — are sprinkled throughout the text and set in italic type.

The text is divided into 40 chapters in the belief that short chapters are more inviting and more likely to be read!

Henry J. L. Marriott

References

1. Vaisrub S. Pulsus paradoxus of the airways. JAMA 1975; 232:1041.
2. Hampton JR, et al. Relative contributions of history-taking, physical examination, and laboratory investigation to diagnosis and management of medical outpatients. Br Med J 1975;2:486.
3. Hurst JW. The examination of the heart: The importance of initial screening. Emory University Journal of Medicine 1991;5:135.
4. Osler W. Aphorisms from his bedside teachings and writings. In: Bean WB, ed. New York: Henry Schuman, 1950:23.

CONTENTS

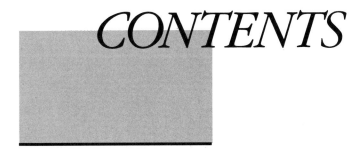

BEDSIDE CARDIAC DIAGNOSIS

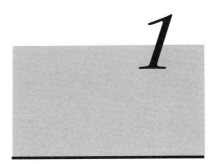

Taking the History

*A doctor who cannot take a good history and a patient who cannot
give one are in danger of giving and receiving bad treatment.*

The value of a skillfully taken history is immense. Without a good history, the remainder of the clinical work-up cannot be intelligently undertaken. Remember—as I pointed out in the Preface—that the majority of the diagnoses that will be made can be suspected from the history alone. No claim remotely approaching this can be advanced for any other part of the work-up. The physical examination and the whole battery of special investigations never enjoy such a measure of success.

The precious history-taking time, now so often replaced by an impersonal printed questionnaire, or even an inquisitorial computer, has four purposes (Table 1-1). It is not just the time for diagnostic delving—that is obviously of prime importance—but it is also the time for gaining the patient's confidence, for sizing up the individual milieu in which the disease process is enveloped, and for formulating the work-up plan.

Don't underestimate the importance of these secondary goals: There is many an answer that a person who values his or her privacy will not commit to the paper of a questionnaire or to the memory of an inquisitive computer, but will reveal to another human being who has gained their confidence after several minutes of verbal exchange and eye contact. And there is much to be gained from one's assessment of the patient, because every disease is modified to some extent by the host in which it finds itself. The time spent in listening to and interrogating the patient is the opportunity to evaluate his character and personality and assess what impact they might have on his symptoms. Is he a type A or a type B personality? This assessment is truly the first stage of the physical examination. Indeed it is axiomatic that a good work-up plan is based on a good history supplemented by the subsequent physical examination.

Clinical teachers caution students to avoid asking leading questions, that is, questions that may suggest a particular answer. And it is true that we must avoid molding the shape of our patient's reply. But it is also true that the good interrogator knows when to ask a leading question and also how to interpret the reply: "The best history-taker is he who can best interpret the answer to a leading question."[1]

One final point before addressing the specifics of history-taking: LISTEN TO THE PATIENT'S OWN IDEA OF HIS DIAGNOSIS. There is an

Table 1–1
Goals of the History-Taking Time

1. Gaining the patient's confidence.
2. Assessing the patient's personality and character.
3. Arriving at a tentative diagnosis.
4. Plotting the work-up.

Table 1–2
Symptoms of Cardiac Disease

SHORTNESS OF BREATH (dyspnea)
SWELLING OF FEET (edema)
PAIN IN CHEST (angina)
PALPITATIONS
CYANOSIS, CLUBBING
Hemoptysis
Nycturia
Loss of appetite, nausea, vomiting
Abdominal pain
Dysphagia
Dizziness, syncope
Visual disturbances
Epistaxis
Skin dry/sweating/pale/flushed

undeniable tendency for the expert to discount the opinion of the amateur; in fact the expert often seems to bridle—"I'm the doctor! How many years did you go to medical school?"—and even make every effort to disprove the amateur's suggestion. In medicine, I have seen this response repeatedly in medical students, in physicians and in nurses; and it is self-defeating. For it is remarkable how often the patient's idea is correct, or at least partly so. Always ask the patient: "Do you have your own opinion of what is wrong?" If you pleasantly "go along" with any suggestions he may make (provided they are not medically ill-advised or harmful), you will have a much happier and more cooperative patient to deal with; and he may steer you in the right diagnostic direction.

SPECIFIC SYMPTOMS

Remember the aphorism:

The greater the number of symptoms, the less the significance of each.

Patients with organic disease usually have one or two cardinal complaints; people with psychoneurosis often have a "laundry list" of symptoms. In the potential cardiac patient, there are five major and nine minor symptoms of which you should make routine inquiry (Table 1-2).

Shortness of Breath
(Aliases: Breathlessness, Dyspnea)

Breathlessness and shortness of breath are synonymous, and are both used interchangeably with dyspnea (difficulty in breathing), although there is a subtle difference between them: for example, breathlessness can certainly be used of the normal panting that overcomes the healthy youth after

running up three flights of steps, but one would never apply dyspnea to this natural state. The causes of breathlessness/dyspnea[2] are summarized in Table 1-3.

"The history is the most valuable means of establishing the etiology."[3] Dyspnea is the cardinal symptom of a "decompensating" left ventricle. As the ventricle fails to eject its normal complement of blood, the blood congests the lungs and encroaches on the airspace at the expense of breathing. You must be sure that the patient understands "shortness of breath" to mean what you mean by the term. If you ask the question, "Do you have shortness of breath?" and the answer comes back in the affirmative, be sure you ask,

Table 1–3
Causes of Breathlessness/Dyspnea

Increased Demand	Faulty Performance
Physiological	Neuromuscular
Exercise	Mechanical thoracic defects
High altitude	Abnormal lung stiffness*
Pregnancy	Obstruction to air flow*
Pathological	Impaired gas exchange*
Hyperthyroidism	
Anemia	
Metabolic acidosis	

*Operative in cardiac dyspnea

"What do you mean by shortness of breath?" It is not uncommon, for example, for the patient to reply, "Every now and then I have to take a deep breath, like this," and then heave a profound sigh typical of an anxiety state.

Having established that the "shortness of breath" is genuine dyspnea, you ascertain whether it is present only with exertion, or is present at rest as well; or if it is the sort of breathlessness that occurs when the patient is lying flat and is relieved by sitting or standing (*orthopnea*). *Paroxysmal nocturnal dyspnea* wakes the patient after an hour or two of sound sleep, and is characteristically improved if he sits up in bed, or gets out of bed and sits in a chair or stands at an open window. *Cardiac asthma* is the term applied when pulmonary congestion or edema of cardiac origin evokes wheezing.

Swelling of Feet/Ankles
(Alias: Pedal Edema)

Obviously, there are many causes of swollen feet and ankles besides congestive heart failure. Prominent among general causes are renal and hepatic disease and anemia, and among local causes, thrombophlebitis and varicose veins.

To elicit a history of edema it may be necessary to ask if shoes feel tighter towards the end of the day, or if constricting bands (garters, sock-tops, etc.) leave indentations when removed.

Several pounds of unwanted fluid will have been retained by the time swelling is obvious; *weight gain*, therefore, is an earlier index of fluid retention than demonstrable edema.

In some patients, the major subjective complaint may be an increase in abdominal girth from accumulating *ascites*; in congestive failure, however, edema always precedes ascites, and if ascites is out of proportion to the edema, one should think of restrictive cardiomyopathy or constrictive pericarditis.

Chest Pain
(Alias: Angina Pectoris)

One's inquiry after chest pain constitutes one of the most important segments of history taking. Sometimes the origin of the pain is immediately obvious; at other times it is anything but. A dangerous short-cut—and one that in the past has created many a cardiac cripple—is the hasty reflex of ordering an electrocardiogram for a patient with chest pain, without first taking a careful history. When the cause of pain is obscure, the accompanying schema provides a useful, systematic framework for interrogation. The schema is easy to remember because it is mnemonically based on the letters of the ECG (P-Q-R-S-T) with O—for the all-important ONSET[4]—tacked on in front.

The vast majority of people have some sort of chest pain, most of which is not cardiac. When lecturing to a sizeable audience, I often confirm this point by asking for a show of hands from the individuals who have *never* had chest pain: Invariably the response is only 1 or 2 percent—and it is obvious to the audience that most, if not all, of the pain experienced by the 98 or 99 percent is not of cardiac origin.

It is therefore of prime importance to separate the cardiac from the noncardiac pain, and this can be done in the large majority by simple questioning. The greater the clinical experience, however, the more one is aware that there is a significant minority in which the pain's description can be treacherous; and one must be on one's guard, keep an open mind, and be ready to delve more deeply in the doubtful case.

The spectrum of ischemic cardiac pain extends from the one or two minutes of angina of effort to hours of pain from cardiac infarction. Regardless of the clinical subset, however, the pain or sensation of discomfort is recognizably similar,

Schema for Taking History of Obscure Pain	
OP	Onset of pain
Qualitative	Is it really pain? What sort of pain is it? How severe is it?
Relative	Associated symptoms? Relieving factors? Aggravating factors?
Spatial	Where is it? Diffuse or localized? Deep or superficial? Radiation?
Temporal	How long have you had it? How long do attacks last? Special times of occurrence?

though differing in degree and duration. And we always must remember that myocardial ischemia may be completely painless ("silent ischemia").

There are three cardinal features that are so characteristic that one should always pursue them with the following questions:

1. Does the pain have maximal intensity from its onset, or is there a build-up for several seconds?
2. Can you point to the area of pain with one finger?
3. Is the pain deep inside your chest or does it feel as though it is close to the surface?

The cause of the pain is the myocardium contracting in the absence of adequate oxygen. You can reproduce the same genesis of pain by putting a cuff around your upper arm and inflating it above systolic pressure so that no pulse is palpable at the wrist; then open and close your fist repeatedly and pain will gradually develop in the muscles of the forearm. Since the causal mechanism is continuing contraction in the absence of oxygen, it follows that it requires a number of heart beats to maximize the pain; therefore, there is always a period of BUILD-UP. It may be only a matter of a few seconds, but it is impossible for anginal pain to begin with already maximal intensity.

One of the most characteristic and descriptive gestures of the patient with angina is the use of his whole hand or clenched fist pressed against his breastbone to indicate the location and quality of pain. This is so typical that Levine described it as a sign of angina. The corollary of this is that any pain that can be localized by a fingertip is unlikely to be angina.

Angina is visceral pain; and although visceral pain is often referred to superficial areas, there is virtually always a deep, internal component.

Be aware that angina is not necessarily painful; it is often better described as discomfort, pressure, squeezing, tightness, constriction, and heaviness—and these sensations may not reach the threshold of pain. Terms frequently used to describe anginal discomfort or pain are bursting, burning, and indigestion. The discomfort is generally behind the sternum, spreading to both sides; and it may radiate to one or both arms (spread to the right arm often signals inferior wall involvement), to the shoulders, neck, jaw, teeth, and back. Angina is usually brought on by physical effort or by emotional stress; and it is more likely to come on after a meal, in the cold, or walking uphill or against the wind. It is relieved rapidly by rest or nitroglycerin—important diagnostic clues.

Pain is unlikely to be anginal if it is described as superficial, sharp, stabbing, knifelike, or throbbing; or if it is associated with precordial tenderness. One must, however, keep in mind that coronary disease and chest wall syndromes are both common, and that both may be simultaneously accommodated by the same afflicted host.

Although angina is usually the product of coronary artery insufficiency, it is possible to develop genuine angina in the presence of normal coronary arteries, because of an imbalance between the cardiac workload and the oxygen supply; such an imbalance may occur in hypertension, anemia, thyrotoxicosis, and tachycardia.

Cardiovascular pains that must be differentiated from those of coronary insufficiency include those that are due to pericarditis, pulmonary embolism, dissecting aneurysm of the aorta, cardiomyopathy, and aortic valve disease.

Pericarditis

Pericarditic pain is described as sharp, and tends to be more left-sided than central.[1] It is aggravated by deep breathing, swallowing, lying down, and movement; and it is relieved by sitting up and leaning forward. The pain may radiate to the left shoulder or scapular region, and the patient may recognize that it is influenced by each heart beat.[5]

Pulmonary Embolism

The pain of pulmonary embolism is usually retrosternal and associated with simultaneous sudden shortness of breath that overshadows the pain. Tachycardia is the rule, and pallor with peripheral cyanosis and hypotension develop rapidly. If pulmonary infarction results, the pain becomes lateral and is aggravated by breathing.

Dissecting Aneurysm

The pain of dissecting aneurysm is tearing, excruciating, and maximal at the onset—no build-up. It is more inclined to the back than the anterior chest and may travel progressively down the back. Some patients may have remarkably little pain.

Cardiomyopathy

The chest pain associated with both hypertrophic and dilated cardiomyopathy may be of typical anginal type; but in the dilated type, the pain may come and go with symptoms of heart failure.

Aortic Valve Disease

The pain of aortic valve disease is due to impairment of coronary artery flow (because of obstruction to the coronary ostia or because of aortic regurgitation) and therefore is indistinguishable from classical angina.

Many more causes of chest pain are listed in Table 33-2.

Palpitations
(Alias: Heart Awareness or Consciousness)

Palpitations are the abnormal awareness of one's beating heart; the awareness may be of the rate, the rhythm, or the vigor of the cardiac contractions. Although most people are not conscious of the beating of their heart, a few normal individuals—if they sit quietly and concentrate—can appreciate each heart beat as a rhythmical thud within the thorax. It is therefore not invariably abnormal to be aware of your heart's beating, but it is unusual.

Now if the rhythm is irregular and you are aware of it, that indeed is palpitations, and the clinical utility of the symptom is mainly to draw attention to arrhythmias, and particularly the tachycardias. The patient may be painfully aware of the sudden onset and abrupt ending of a paroxysm of tachycardia, or of the tumultuous irregularity of atrial fibrillation with rapid ventricular response. Isolated extrasystoles are usually recognized more from the forceful postectopic beat or from the cannon wave in the neck; the patient may describe his sensation as the heart "turning over," or "skipping a beat," or temporarily "stopping." Of course, cannon waves may be obtrusive during tachycardias, but they are usually overshadowed by the intrathoracic tumult.

Awareness of the heart's contractions also results from hyperdynamic states, such as anemia and thyrotoxicosis, and in cardiac diseases with high stroke volume, such as aortic regurgitation and complete heart block.

Cyanosis and Clubbing

Cyanosis and clubbing are both more objective signs than subjective symptoms, and their genesis and recognition are described in Chapter 7. But the mother of an infant with congenital heart disease may be the first to notice the baby's diagnostic duskiness; and the older patient may volunteer the information that his lips grow unnaturally dusky with exertion.

An occasional patient may note the earliest change in contour of his fingers—bulbous tips, or beaked nails—before it is obvious to the detached observer.

Hemoptysis
(Aliases: Bloodspitting, Pulmonary Apoplexy)

In response to an affirmative answer to the question, "Have you ever coughed up blood?" one should always inquire as to the form of bloodspitting[6]: bloodstreaked, or pink, frothy sputum, or frank blood (dark or bright red).

In the cardiac patient, the spitting up of blood usually indicates pulmonary embolism or mitral stenosis. Frank but small hemoptysis may be the first symptom of *mitral stenosis*, and is due to engorgement of pulmonary venules secondary to the increased left atrial pressure. This form of hemoptysis tends to cease when the venous walls thicken in response to the chronically raised pressure within them. *Pulmonary embolism with infarction* is usually a complication of congestive heart failure and therefore a late manifestation of heart disease. Bloodstained sputum may characterize the pulmonary congestion of *left ventricular failure* or mitral stenosis; pink, frothy sputum is typical of the resulting *pulmonary edema. Disseminated lupus* or *arteriovenous aneurysm* may be the cause of arterial rupture with frank hemoptysis; and of course noncardiovascular diseases that are coincidentally present may be the source of bleeding that complicates heart disease.

Nycturia
(Alias: Nocturia)

Although getting up at night to urinate can be caused by any of a number of genitourinary diseases, it may also be a useful index of early congestive heart failure. The failing heart, during daytime activity, may deny adequate perfusion to the kidneys and so reduce their output. But with the muscular inactivity of bed rest, the kidneys may be favored with a more adequate blood flow and consequently increase their production of urine.

Loss of Appetite (Alias: Anorexia)/ Nausea/Vomiting

In the cardiac patient, anorexia may result from congestive failure alone, or it may be caused by the treatment, especially digitalis. Nausea and vomiting may complicate acute myocardial infarction; they are common manifestations of digitalis intoxication.

Abdominal Pain

Although abdominal pain is not a common finding in heart disease, there are several circumstances that may afflict the cardiac patient with pain below the diaphragm. Most important is the fact that anginal pain can be entirely epigastric; many a patient with myocardial ischemia or infarction has been discharged from emergency rooms with the diagnosis of indigestion or dyspepsia. In fact, angina is no respecter of boundaries, and the pain of infarction may be felt anywhere from the teeth to the rectum, or in any area of "lowered resistance" such as an old abdominal or renal incisional scar.

The congested liver of heart failure is tender and may evoke a spontaneous soreness—a source that can readily be recognized by palpation of the sensitive organ.

In a patient with infective endocarditis, embolization of the spleen or mesenteric artery may produce intense abdominal pain simulating an acute abdomen; and if surgery is mistakenly attempted, the cardiac disaster is compounded.

Example   A 26-year-old man in evident acute distress was being trundled along the hospital corridor on a stretcher by two operating room orderlies. A passing physician observed his "café-au-lait" pallor and vigorous carotid pulsations, stopped the orderlies, and ascertained that he was on his way to the operating room for surgery for an "acute abdomen." She applied her stethoscope to

the patient's precordium, confirmed the aortic regurgitation, and made the correct diagnosis of infective endocarditis with embolus to the mesenteric artery.

Dysphagia (Alias: Difficulty with Swallowing)

Dysphagia is an uncommon symptom of cardiac disease, and usually implies external pressure on the esophagus; it can result from a greatly enlarged left atrium in mitral disease compressing the esophagus, or from pressure by an aortic aneurysm (usually associated with hoarseness), or by encircling vascular rings. Scleroderma, as well as affecting the skin, the lungs, and the heart, may involve the esophagus and so produce dysphagia.

Dizziness; Syncope (Alias: Fainting)

In cardiac disease, dizziness and syncope usually signal inadequate perfusion of the brain such as may occur during periods of asystole from heart block, or from marked bradycardias or tachycardias. They sometimes complicate aortic stenosis.

Dizziness, lightheadedness, syncope, and convulsions can result from inadequate cerebral perfusion. Morgagni (1761), and later Adams (1826) and Stokes (1846), noted that these disturbing cerebral symptoms could result from bradyarrhythmias (Adams-Stokes attacks). But of course they can result from any mechanism that fails to supply the brain with adequate blood, and therefore disabling tachycardias may engender similar symptoms.

Visual Disturbances

The initial symptom of infective endocarditis may be sudden blindness in one eye—thanks to an embolus to the central retinal artery. The other important disturbances of vision are related to digitalis intoxication: the patient may complain that everything looks yellowish or greenish, or that he seems to be "seeing through a snowstorm." There are usually other evidences of the drug's toxicity, but the visual aberration may stand alone.

Epistaxis
(Alias: Nosebleed)

Clinicians used to regard nosebleed in youth as a manifestation of the rheumatic state, but the connection is dubious. It may occur in a few young patients with coarctation of the aorta[1]; in the older patient, hypertension is an important cause of severe epistaxis.

Skin: Dry/Sweating/Pale/Flushed

Although the skin certainly does not play a major role in cardiac diagnosis, there are times when it may afford the first clue: The hypothyroid patient may complain of her dry skin, and the thyrotoxic of excessive sweating. Pallor is associated with aortic regurgitation and flushed malar eminences with mitral stenosis.

THE PAST HISTORY

In an infant or young child, one is interested in the mother's pregnancy: Did she have rubella or some other viral infection during her first trimester? Was the infant a "blue baby?"

In the older patient, you are interested in any previous serious illnesses, especially rheumatic fever, pneumonia, tuberculosis, thrombophlebitis, pulmonary embolism, or chest injury. Does the patient have diabetes, thyroid disease, or any other metabolic disorder?

Has the patient's occupation or travels exposed him to any cardiotoxic materials? Has he taken a digitalis preparation or any other cardiac drugs? What is the coffee, tea, tobacco, and alcohol history? Has he or she been a cocaine user? Has she been taking "the pill?"

You should get a good idea of the patient's diet and how much physical exercise he or she gets. Has the patient's weight remained steady over the past several months or years? Does he get adequate vacation time? Or is he a "workaholic?"

THE FAMILY HISTORY

You are interested to know if any close member of the family has congenital heart disease or has had rheumatic fever; or whether diabetes, tuberculosis, hypertension, or coronary disease runs in the family; and especially if any family members have died of hypertension or ischemic disease at an early age. Always record the age of family members, living and dead—a record of longevity is reassuring.[7]

Details of the marriage may be of great import; one should delicately ascertain the number of marriages, inquire the age and health of spouse and children, and try to obtain a feel for the home atmosphere. Domestic stress is usually more important than occupational.

REFERENCES

1. Wood P. Diseases of the heart and circulation, ed 3. Philadelphia: JB Lippincott, 1968:1–25.
2. Ogilvie C. Dyspnoea. Br Med J 1983;287:160.
3. Braunwald E. Heart disease: a textbook of cardiovascular medicine, ed 3. Philadelphia: WB Saunders, 1988:2.
4. White PD. Heart disease, ed 4. New York: Macmillan, 1951:41–51.
5. Silverman ME. Examination of the heart: I. the clinical history. New York: American Heart Association, 1975.
6. Hurst JW, et al. The history: symptoms and past events related to cardiovascular disease. In: Hurst JW, ed. The heart, ed 7. New York: McGraw-Hill, 1990:122–134.
7. Sprague HB. Examination of the heart: I. history taking. New York: American Heart Association, 1967.

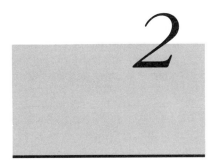

General Appearance

The examination does not wait the removal of the shirt!
Waring

The history doesn't end when the physical examination begins—observations during the examination often lead to further lines of questioning; nor does the physical examination begin only after the history has been taken.

As the patient enters your presence, or as you approach the bed (or chair), the examination begins; this chapter deals with physical findings that may be observed as you are taking the history while the patient is still fully clad; you may cull invaluable clues from your first impressions. You take note of his general demeanor, his posture, his gait. You note facial expression, complexion, and any superficial detail of eyes, ears, skin, and hands. Although these individual parts will be examined in detail later, keen observation as you take the history may be richly rewarded.

GENERAL BEARING AND GAIT

The experienced physician quickly gets a feeling for his patient's general affect. An air of self-confidence, or of anxiety, or of defeat, is readily communicated. Although the seriously ill patient can sometimes look remarkably well, more often the sickness leaves an indelible stamp upon his appearance, and one may get an immediate and accurate impression of "toxicity."

If the patient has had a stroke, it may be immediately apparent in face, limb, or gait—and a cardiac patient with a stroke suggests a number of possibilities: In the acute context one is alerted to atrial fibrillation, myocardial infarction, or infective endocarditis; in the younger patient, to mitral valve prolapse, mitral stenosis, atrial myxoma, or lupus erythematosus; and in the older age group, hypertensive heart disease, infective endocarditis, and prosthetic valves are considerations.

Gross obesity brings to mind the possibility of a Pickwickian syndrome with right ventricular failure secondary to chronic hypoventilation.[1]

If the patient's approach reveals a wide-based gait and slapping feet, tabes dorsalis is suggested, and you are alerted to the possibility of aortic disease.

The habitus of the individual with Marfan's syndrome is recognizable at a glance: The height, the long arms producing a span greater than the height, the arachnodactyly, the sometimes visibly tremulous iris. Aortic regurgitation and dissecting aneurysm are the most likely cardiac complications.

As you approach the patient who, in bed, is not particularly dyspneic but is sitting and leaning forward over his bedside table, you make a provisional diagnosis of pericarditis.

THE HEAD

The head that shakes perceptibly with each heart beat makes the diagnosis of aortic regurgitation easy (de Musset's sign, after the French poet whose head displayed it).

The enlarged skull of Paget's disease is a signal to look for an increased pulse pressure and the possibility of high-output heart failure secondary to the arteriovenous fistulae in affected bones.

Premature frontal baldness is not infrequently an outward and visible clue to coronary disease.

THE FACE

The coarse, puffy face of myxedema, with dry, sallow skin and sparse eyebrows, is sometimes recognizable at a glance; and the exophthalmos and lid-lag of thyrotoxicosis are equally apparent. In myxedema, you may find pericardial effusion or congestive heart failure, and you are alerted to the increased likelihood of coronary artery disease and mild hypertension; although pump failure is unlikely to result from uncomplicated hypothyroidism, its overzealous treatment with replacement therapy may precipitate heart failure. In thyrotoxicosis, atrial fibrillation and high-output failure are common complications, and there is an increased incidence of mitral valve prolapse.

Cyanosis may be immediately apparent and require one to differentiate the central form (due to a right-to-left shunt, lung disease, etc.) from the peripheral variety (resulting from obstruction to venous return) (see Chapter 7).

The freckle-faced, red-haired woman seems to attract the unwanted attentions of acute rheumatism (rheumatic fever), with the consequent development of mitral valve disease; if her pedigree is Irish, the rheumatic plot thickens. The so-called "mitral facies" implies rosy malar prominences tainted with mild peripheral cyanosis.

The "butterfly rash" of disseminated lupus[2] may alert one to the possibility of pericarditis, myocarditis, or verrucous endocarditis (Libman and Sacks, 1924).

Another cause of vivid coloration is the rare carcinoid syndrome. Perhaps best described as "brick-red cyanosis," it points to the possibility of damage to the right-sided valves, usually pulmonic stenosis and tricuspid regurgitation, owing to the ravages of circulating serotonin. The high color is intensified by paroxysmal flushing.

The hint of jaundice in a cardiac patient suggests tricuspid valve disease, perhaps associated with the development of cardiac cirrhosis; mild cyanosis may conspire with jaundice to produce a faintly greenish hue. Other possibilities are pulmonary infarction and hemolysis caused by a prosthetic valve.

Three other color changes that may inform the observant eye are the bronzed skin of hemochromatosis, which is associated with a secondary, usually dilated, cardiomyopathy; the slaty-blue discoloration from prolonged ingestion of the drug amiodarone; and the "coffee-with-cream" (café-au-lait) tint to the face in infective endocarditis, which is quite characteristic but nowadays seldom seen because it is a relatively late manifestation developing in the untreated case.[3]

Two facies are commonly associated with congenital cardiac anomalies. The mongoloid face with slanting eyes and heavy epicanthic folds suggests the possibility of Down's syndrome, the cardiac lesion usually being an atrial septal or endocardial cushion defect. The puckish face with poorly developed lower jaw, thick lips, wide-set eyes, low-set ears, and a somewhat retarded but impish expression betrays an associated supravalvar aortic stenosis.

THE EYES

Drooping of the eyelids (ptosis) may result from neurosyphilis. To compensate for the ptosis, the forehead muscles elevate and produce horizontal furrows, together producing the features of the tabetic facies. To diagnose tabes is to diagnose syphilis, a disease that is enjoying an impressive comeback in this AIDS-ridden era, which in turn points to aortic root disease including coronary ostial obstruction, with consequent anginal syndromes, aortic regurgitation, or aneurysm of the ascending aorta.

Arcus senilis—more considerately known as corneal arcus—is of little significance in the elderly, but in white people under the age of 50 years may be a sign of hyperlipidemia and precocious atherosclerosis. The yellow plaques of xanthelasma in the eyelids have comparable significance.

The presence of a cataract can sometimes be seen without the use of instruments and immediately suggests the possibility of diabetes, with its attendant implications. Cataracts are also part of the rubella syndrome[4] and, therefore, in the infant or young child alert you to the likelihood of a patent ductus arteriosus.

THE EARS

The lobe of the ear may yield a clue: If it visibly pulsates, tricuspid regurgitation is likely; and if there is a diagonal crease running across it, one is reminded that there may be an association with coronary disease,[5] although this does not apply to native American Indians.

THE NECK

Vigorous arterial (carotid) pulsation may be evident in the neck without close inspection, and this suggests aortic regurgitation, coarctation of the aorta, thyrotoxicosis, or anxiety.

Obviously distended veins alert you to right ventricular failure, tricuspid valve disease, or a superior vena caval syndrome.

Example A 65-year-old man had a cardiac arrest, and a permanent pacemaker was implanted. Two years later he felt that something in his body was "changing for the worse"; he was troubled by "congestion in the head" if he exerted himself, or bent over, and he also developed progressive shortness of breath. Apart from these symptoms, he made a point of stating that he felt strong and vigorous. Two cardiologists diagnosed heart failure. On casual inspection there was evident distention of his jugular veins, especially on the right side; when he bent over, as if to tie his shoes, his head and neck became suffused and the jugulars greatly distended. Computed tomography scan showed thrombotic occlusion of the superior vena cava and left innominate vein, presumably secondary to the indwelling pacemaker leads.

The webbed neck is found in at least two congenital syndromes,[6,7] Turner's (infantilism, webbed neck, and cubitus valgus in females), which makes an associated coarctation of the aorta likely; and Noonan's (short stature, webbed neck, hypertelorism, mental and sexual retardation in either sex), which is usually attended by pulmonic stenosis, often with an associated atrial septal defect.

THE CHEST

It is not difficult to recognize the increased anteroposterior diameter of the emphysematous chest when it is still encased in clothing; you may be able to go one step further and discriminate between the "pink puffer," who maintains normocarbia by hyperventilating, and the "blue bloater," who ignores the hypercarbia and is prone to the development of right ventricular failure.[8] Kyphoscoliosis (if sufficiently marked) can be recognized through the clothing and may be responsible for an associated cor pulmonale.

Cheyne-Stokes respiration (spells of noisy waxing and waning hyperpnea separated by periods of apnea) in the bedridden patient is easily recognized and identifies serious cardiovascular or cerebrovascular disease[6]; it is usually associated with left ventricular failure, and it may be precipitated or aggravated by too much sedation.

THE HANDS

The initial clue may be the warm, sweaty palm of hyperthyroidism noted in the greeting handshake (as opposed to the cool sweat of anxiety), or the rough, dry skin of the hypothyroid state.

Clubbing of the fingers may be noticed immediately and alert you to congenital cardiac or pulmonary disease—its recognition and causes are detailed in Chapter 7.

"Splinter" hemorrhages (linear petechiae under the nail) may be grossly noticeable and deserve special comment. They have long enjoyed an association with infective endocarditis, but they are far from diagnostic, as they can be found in many other diseases and, indeed, are not uncommon in normal people in whom they appear to develop as the result of repeated minor traumata—including exposure to the bristles of a nailbrush. They are perhaps more commonly seen in individuals who live at high altitudes.[9] Nevertheless, in certain circumstances, for example in a patient with fever of uncertain origin, splinter hemorrhages may be the first clue to an underlying infective endocarditis.

The polydactyly of the Ellis Van Creveld dwarfism or the "fingerized thumb" of the Holt-Oram (atrio-digital) syndrome will indicate that the most likely associated cardiac lesion is an atrial septal defect, although other defects may less often be found.[10,11]

The tight, shiny skin of scleroderma may be obvious on the hands (sclerodactylia) and alert you to the possibility of myocardial fibrosis and necrosis secondary to coronary involvement.

REFERENCES

1. Rochester DF, Enson Y. Current concepts in the pathogenesis of the obesity-hypoventilation syndrome. Am J Med 1974;57:402.

2. Doherty NE, Seigel RJ. Cardiovascular manifestations of systemic lupus erythematosus. Am Heart J 1985;110:1257.

3. Proudfit WL. Skin signs of infective endocarditis. Am Heart J 1983;106:1451.

4. Scott AW. Examination of the eye in cardiovascular disease. Prog Cardiovasc Dis 1968;10:353.

5. Elliott WJ. Ear lobe crease and coronary artery disease: 1,000 patients and review of the literature. Am J Med 1983;75:1024.

6. Turner RWD. General observation of the patient. Prog Cardiovasc Dis 1967;10:144.

7. Perloff JK: The clinical recognition of congenital heart disease, ed 3. Philadelphia: WB Saunders, 1987:134.

8. Johnson MA, et al. Are "pink puffers" more breathless than "blue bloaters"? Br Med J 1983;286:179.

9. Heath D, Williams DR. Nail hemorrhages. Br Heart J 1978;40:1300.

10. Sternberg MA, Neufeld HN. Physical diagnosis in syndromes with cardiovascular disease. Prog Cardiovasc Dis 1968;10:385.

11. Silverman ME. Inspection of the patient. In: Hurst JW, ed. The heart. New York: McGraw Hill, 1990:135–149.

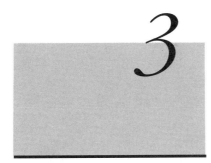

The Jugular Veins

The neck is a vantage point for studying the flow of traffic to and from the citadel of the heart. Yet this important information center is often overlooked, and the declarative veins are especially ignored. The jugulars reflect the traffic pattern entering the heart, the arterial pulse the issuing pattern; both should be evaluated in conjunction with the impulses and sounds of the heart itself.

Modesty, false or otherwise, should not prevent you from examining the chest and neck in one piece. You should be able to see the pulsations in the neck, unobstructed by a coy towel, at the same time that you are inspecting, palpating, or listening to the heart.

Before focusing on the veins, it is imperative that one thoroughly understands the time relationships between cardiac, arterial, and venous events. To this end, Figure 3-1 depicts a simultaneous recording of heart sounds, carotid pulse, and jugular venous pulse—recorded respectively as phonocardiogram (PCG), carotid pulse tracing (CPT), and jugular pulse tracing (JPT). Master their time re-lationships: The carotid pulse reaches its peak just after the first heart sound,[1] whereas the first venous wave (a) peaks just before the first sound; the second venous wave (v) peaks just after the second sound (A-P). At this cardiac rate of 64/minute, note that the ''v'' wave is nearer to the next ''a'' wave than to the preceding one. If the rate accelerated, the ''v'' wave would draw closer to the next ''a'' wave until, at a rate of about 110/minute, the two waves would be superimposed.

The jugular veins have three spheres of diagnostic usefulness:

1. Representing a direct pipeline to the right atrium, they serve as built-in manometers for gauging right atrial and venous pressures,
2. Changes in the amplitude of their pulse waves serve as indicators of structural or dynamic disease of the right heart and lesser circulation, and
3. Changes in wave form and the identification of ''a'' waves contribute to the diagnosis of arrhythmias.

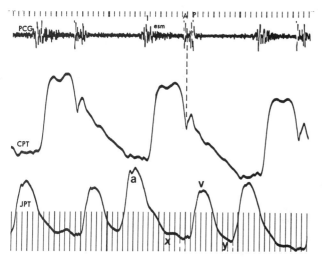

Figure 3–1. Simultaneous recording of phonocardiogram (PCG), carotid pulse tracing (CPT), and jugular venous pulse tracing (JPT). 1, first heart sound; A, aortic component of second heart sound; P, pulmonic component of second heart sound; a, x, v, y, venous waves.

POSITIONING AND LIGHTING

For best results in all three uses, the patient's position is of supreme importance—although it differs for different purposes. For all purposes, head and trunk should be in a straight line without significant flexion of the neck, the body bending at the hips (Fig. 3-2A). For gauging venous pressure we need a posture in which any visible distention or pulsation in the neck veins is abnormal, and this is usually at an inclination of about 45° (Fig. 3-2**B**). Since the normal venous pressure is slightly positive (ie, above atmospheric), the neck veins are normally distended when they are at the same level as the right atrium (ie, when the subject is lying flat). On the other hand, when the patient is sitting bolt upright, the veins above the clavicle may appear empty even in the presence of a raised venous pressure—because the root of the neck is now several centimeters above the right atrium. The most convenient guide for gauging venous pressure is the sternal angle (angle of Louis), above which the veins should not fill more than a perpendicular centimeter or two.

At an angle of about 45°, the root of the neck is conveniently 1 to 2 cm above the sternal angle, so that any filling or pulsation now seen in the neck is above normal. If the veins are engorged to the ears in this position, the patient should sit upright or stand erect to see if a level of filling

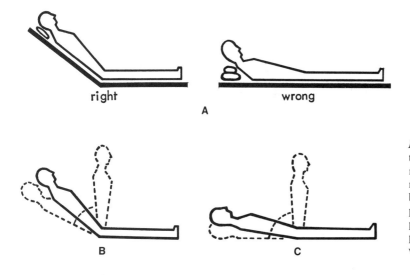

Figure 3–2. Positions of patient for venous viewing. **(A)** Correct: head and trunk in line, neck not flexed. Wrong: Neck flexed by pillows. **(B)** Range of possible positions for assessing venous pressure/distention. **(C)** Range of possible positions for studying venous pulsations.

can then be determined. When the veins are filled "to the brim," their pulsation often moves the earlobes.

For analysis of venous pulsation, on the other hand, we need the position in which the pulsations are of greatest magnitude, and this may vary considerably (Fig. 3-2**C**): In the normal person it is usually optimal with the head and trunk raised slightly above horizontal, but it may range from horizontal in some normal subjects to sitting upright in patients with marked elevation of venous pressure.

When you have the patient in the right position, use a TANGENTIAL light; and be sure to look for pulsations of the DEEP jugular veins on BOTH sides. If proper positioning and lighting are not attended to, you may miss the venous messages.

VENOUS CONGESTION

Numerous influences and lesions raise the venous pressure, and it is important to be aware of all of them (Table 3-1). It is particularly important to keep in mind that diseases (such as pleural effusion and acute nephritis), physiologic alterations in the

---

Table 3–1
Causes of Venous Distention

---

1. CONGESTIVE HEART FAILURE
2. SVC OBSTRUCTION
3. PERICARDIAL EFFUSION, CHRONIC CONSTRICTIVE PERICARDITIS, restrictive cardiomyopathy
4. Tricuspid stenosis
5. Space-occupying lesions of the right heart (thrombus or tumor of right atrium; aneurysm of ventricular septum; Bernheim's syndrome)
6. Increased intrathoracic pressure
   PLEURAL EFFUSION; obstructive airway disease; straining (Valsalva)
7. Increased intra-abdominal pressure (tight clothes, obesity, pregnancy, straining)
8. Increased blood volume
   premenstrual, pregnancy; acute nephritis; saline infusions; salt-retaining hormones
9. Hyperkinetic states
   heat, fever, pregnancy; anemia, A-V aneurysms, thyrotoxicosis, Paget's disease, severe liver disease; vasodilators
10. Bradycardia; physical effort

---

circulation (as in pregnancy, premenstrual states and bradycardia), and unphysiologic impedimenta (such as tight clothing and obesity) can produce visible distention of the neck veins without implying that the heart is compromised. With significant respiratory obstruction, as in bronchial asthma, the veins are abnormally distended in expiration but are sucked empty with inspiration. Engorgement of the left jugular vein alone may result from pressure on the left innominate vein ("kinked innominate vein")[1] by a dilated or dissected aortic arch, or by a lymphoma or other tumor.

If the level to which the veins fill is obscure, milk the vein empty with the finger and then observe the level to which it *re*fills. With the patient raised to the prescribed critical angle, the deep jugulars normally fill only from above, but in congestive heart failure they fill from below as well.

THE HEPATOJUGULAR REFLUX
(RENAMED ABDOMINOJUGULAR TEST)

Normally the jugular venous pressure rises with expiration and falls with inspiration as the negative intrathoracic pressure increases. If the veins fill with inspiration and empty with exhalation, it is known as paradoxical venous filling, or Kussmaul's sign. An allied phenomenon is the positive hepatojugular reflux, described by Pasteur in 1885, in which the neck veins fill in response to abdominal compression while the patient continues to breathe normally—naturally, if he resists your pressure, the resulting Valsalva maneuver will produce a false positive. Pressure with the palm of the hand, which need not be concentrated on the liver, is arbitrarily maintained for 30 to 60 seconds.[2–5] Both inspiration and abdominal compression increase the venous return, to which the normal, unrestricted heart responds by obeying Starling's law and accommodating to the increased return by increasing its output so that the neck veins do not become and remain engorged during the period of compression. In congestive heart failure[6] or in "restrictive disease" (see below), abdominal compression or inspiration may cause abnormal filling of the neck veins since the laboring or constricted heart cannot so accommodate. Hypervolemic states (eg, polycythemia vera) can be responsible for a temporarily positive hepatojugular test even in the presence of a normal heart.

Because (1) pressure need not be focussed on the liver, and (2) the venous distention is not due to simple reflux, a more appropriate term is abdominojugular test.[7]

Restrictive disease is a term used to embrace all diseases that mechanically prevent adequate diastolic relaxation of the ventricle, including pericardial effusion, constrictive pericarditis, and restrictive cardiomyopathy—whether its outer wrapping constricts the heart, or the unyielding texture of its endomyocardium restricts its expansion, the hemodynamic effects are the same.

The effects of abdominal compression or inspiration are similar in superior vena caval (SVC) obstruction (at or below the level of the azygos vein), but for a different reason. In SVC obstruction, venous blood from the head and upper limbs reaches the heart circuitously via the inferior vena cava (Fig. 3-3). Both inspiration and abdominal compression raise intra-abdominal pressure, impede the circuitous venous return, and so produce relative engorgement of the neck veins. Kussmaul's sign may also be seen in massive pulmonary embolism,[8] and may provide a valuable clue to the presence of right ventricular infarction.[9]

JUGULAR PULSATIONS

The beginner frequently mistakes venous pulsation for arterial, though the distinction is seldom difficult if the following characteristics—summarized in Table 3-2—are kept in mind:

1. Instead of a hard thrust, the venous pulse is relatively soft and "welling," and cannot be felt except in unusual circumstances; it is invariably easier to see than to feel,
2. It is usually best seen at the root of the neck just above the clavicle, unlike arterial pulsation, which is best seen halfway up the neck where the carotid is most superficial,
3. Instead of a single pulse wave, there are at least two positive and two negative venous waves per cardiac cycle—if any positive wave is seen in diastole, it must necessarily be venous,
4. The jugular pulse moves cephalad with expiration, abdominal compression or a Valsalva maneuver, and on lying down; it moves caudad with inspiration, release of abdominal pressure, and on sitting, and
5. Venous pulsation ceases if you compress with a finger at the root of the neck.

Although the art of venous viewing is a partially lost one, its value has not decreased since Potain in 1867 recognized the presystolic wave reflecting atrial contraction, and Mackenzie in 1892 saw, recorded, and labeled the three venous waves "a," "c" and "v." The "a" wave (Fig. 3-4) is produced by right atrial contraction, and the "v" wave by progressive filling of the right atrium and venous system while the tricuspid valve remains closed; the summit of the "v" wave signals the opening of the tricuspid valve. The origin of the "c" wave is twofold: the upward bulging of the tricuspid valve with right ventricular systole, and in the neck transmitted pulsation from the adjacent carotid artery.

But the most striking feature of the jugular pulse on inspection is usually not one of these positive waves but rather the negative systolic trough

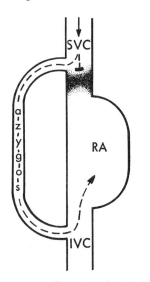

Figure 3–3. Diagram illustrating the circuitous path of blood returning from head to heart in the presence of superior vena caval obstruction. SVC, superior vena cava; IVC, inferior vena cava; RA, right atrium.

Table 3–2
Characteristics of Venous Pulse

Inspection
  At root of neck
  Multiphasic
  Welling
  Movable

Palpation
  Impalpable
  Compressible

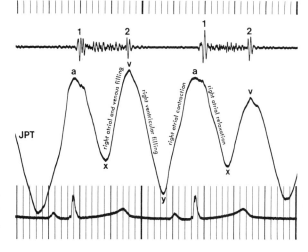

Figure 3–4. The two positive (a,v) and two negative (x,y) waves in the venous pulse (JPT) illustrating their relationship to the heart sounds and the ECG. 1, first heart sound; 2, second sound; a, x, v, y, venous waves.

following the "a" wave and separating it from the "v" wave. This negative wave is the "x" descent and is caused by diastolic relaxation of the right atrium and descent of the tricuspid diaphragm with right ventricular contraction. Following the "v" wave is a second negative wave, the "y" descent, usually not as deep as "x," due to emptying of the venous reservoir and right atrium through the now open tricuspid valve into the right ventricle.

In general, then, the most effective means of recognizing venous (and therefore right heart) events, is to look for the conspicuous negative wave or trough ("x"), confirm that it is systolic by simultaneous palpation of the carotid or auscultation of the heart, and then line up the positive "a" and "v" crests on either side of the trough. There are three practical ways of identifying the "a" wave: by inspection, it immediately precedes the major venous trough and the arterial pulse; by palpation, it just precedes the arterial pulse; by auscultation, it just precedes the first heart sound.

DISTURBANCES OF THE VENOUS PULSE (EXCLUDING ARRHYTHMIAS)

The various abnormalities of the venous pulse, with their mechanisms and causes, are listed in Table 3-3.

The "a" wave is our best index of the time and force of right atrial contraction. When the systolic workload of the right atrium is increased, as in tricuspid stenosis or atresia, right ventricular failure, pulmonic stenosis, or pulmonary hypertension, the amplitude of the "a" wave increases and it often becomes palpable—*giant "a" wave*. One must distinguish this from the *cannon "a" wave*, which results when an arrhythmia disturbs the normal A-V sequence of contraction so that the atria contract during ventricular systole against closed A-V valves.

When the tricuspid valve is incompetent, the right ventricle ejects some of its blood backwards into the right atrium and produces a prominent "c" wave (systolic venous wave) in the neck that can easily be felt. This was the first disturbance of the jugular pulse to be noticed clinically (Lancisi, 1728), and is known as *Lancisi's sign* or the *positive venous pulse*—as distinct from the normal systolic trough. The positive venous pulse can be vigorous enough to shake the whole head—de Musset's sign of venous origin.

When there is a sizeable left-to-right shunt at the atrial level (atrial septal defect or anomalous pulmonary venous return), the right atrium during its diastole fills simultaneously from two directions and this diastolic overloading may result in an unduly prominent "v" wave—*giant "v" wave*.

In restrictive disease, the high venous pressure drops abruptly when the tricuspid valve opens, resulting in an exaggerated "y" descent; the "x" trough also is sometimes exaggerated.

When the jugulars are tightly engorged, or when there is obstruction between the right atrium and the neck, as in the SVC syndrome, all evidence of venous pulsation in the neck may be lost.

Table 3–3
Clinical Disturbances of the Venous Pulse (Excluding Arrhythmias)

Disturbance	Hemodynamic Mechanism	Condition in Which Seen
Giant "a" wave	Systolic overloading of right atrium	Tricuspid stenosis Pulmonic stenosis Pulmonic hypertension Right ventricular failure
Systolic pulsation	Retrograde right ventricular ejection	Tricuspid regurgitation
Prominent "v" wave	Diastolic overloading of right atrium	Atrial septal defect Anomalous pulmonary venous drainage
Exaggerated "y" trough	High early diastolic gradient	Restrictive disease
Absent venous pulse	Tightly engorged veins; block between heart and veins	Congestive heart failure Cardiac tamponade SVC obstruction
Paradoxical venous filling (Kussmaul's sign)	Diaphragmatic traction on tensely filled pericardial sac; increased intra-abdominal pressure	Congestive heart failure Restrictive disease SVC obstruction Pulmonary embolism

REFERENCES

1. Smith KS. The kinked innominate vein. Br Heart J 1960;22:110.
2. Bryant JM. The hepatojugular reflux. JAMA 1957;165:281.
3. Constant J, Lippschutz EJ. The one-minute abdominal compression test or "the hepatojugular reflux," a useful bedside test. Am Heart J 1964;67:701.
4. Fowler NO: Examination of the heart: Part 2. inspection and palpation of venous and arterial pulses. New York: American Heart Association, 1965.
5. O'Rourke RA: The measurement of systolic blood pressure: normal and abnormal pulsations of the arteries and veins. In: Hurst JW, ed. The heart. 7th ed. New York: McGraw Hill, 1990:157–160.
6. Ducas J, et al. Validity of the hepatojugular reflux as a clinical test for congestive heart failure. Am J Cardiol 1983;52:1299.
7. Ewy GA. The abdominojugular test: technique and hemodynamic correlates. Ann Intern Med 1988;109:456.
8. Burdine JA, Wallace JM. Pulsus paradoxus and Kussmaul's sign in massive pulmonary embolism. Am J Cardiol 1965;15:413.
9. Dell'Italia I, et al. Physical examination for exclusion of hemodynamically important right ventricular infarction. Ann Intern Med 1983;99:608.

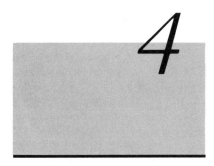

The Arterial Pulse

Feel the pulse with two hands and ten fingers.
                                        Osler

The fingers should be kept on the pulse at least until the hundredth beat.

                                        Archimathaeus

The importance of the matter that persuaded Archimathaeus and Osler to these picturesque hyperboles has not grown less with time: The pulse is the voice of the left ventricle speaking to perceptive fingers.

In every patient, at least when first seen, you should examine with care both carotid, both radial, both femoral, both dorsalis pedis, and both posterior tibial pulses. Paul Wood[1] advised the routine palpation of the patient's right artery with the thumb of the right hand. And indeed the thumb is a much neglected but most efficient digit for palpating pulses—neglected probably because of the Nightingalian superstition that it has a distracting, obtrusive pulse of its own.

CAROTID PULSE

The carotid is the closest accessible conduit from the heart and offers the most accurate peripheral picture of cardiac behavior. A finger on the carotid is an excellent referee in timing jugular events. If you are otherwise destitute (see Chapter 8) you may use it—but not without risk—as a reference for timing cardiac events. The slight lag in the pulse wave reaching even the carotid may be misleading, especially at rapid cardiac rates where small discrepancies in timing represent a larger proportion of the cardiac cycle. Inspection of the carotids may give you your first clue to aortic regurgitation or coarctation, and their palpation may provide the initial clue to aortic stenosis.

An abnormally vigorous carotid pulse is classically seen in aortic regurgitation (Corrigan, 1832); it is also present in coarctation of the aorta, and appropriately termed the carotid "swell"; in patent ductus arteriosus and other significant arteriovenous fistulas, including pregnancy and Paget's disease of bone; in thyrotoxicosis, severe anemia, and other high output states; and with the systolic hypertension and high pulse pressure of atherosclerosis. Anxiety is also a common cause, frequently precipitated in the consulting room by

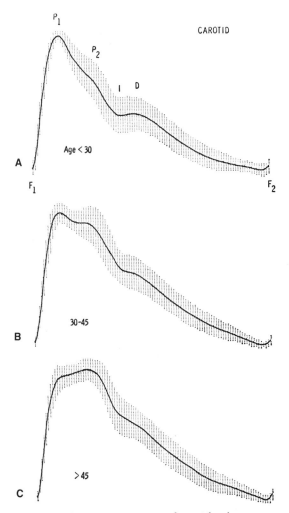

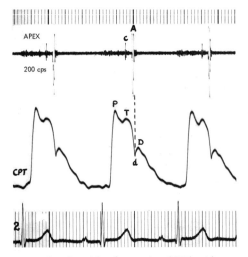

Figure 4–2. Carotid pulse tracing (CPT) with percussion (P), tidal (T) and dicrotic (D) waves labeled. Note that the aortic component of the second sound (A) just precedes the dicrotic notch (d). There is a late systolic click (c). (From a 23-year-old woman with mild mitral regurgitation.)

Figure 4–1. Average patterns of arterial pulses at various ages. **(A)** Under 30, **(B)** age 30–45 years, and **(C)** over 45 years. (Reproduced with permission from Freis and Kyle[2]).

advancing age the tidal wave tends to surpass the percussion wave (Fig. 4-1c).[2] One of the practical uses of the carotid pulse tracing is to identify the aortic component of the second sound: A2 always slightly precedes the dicrotic notch in the CPT (see dashed line in Figure 4-2).

DICROTIC AND BISFERIENS PULSES

Although the arterial pulse is described as a single thrust, the sensitive finger or thumb can often appreciate a slight rebound—the dicrotic wave (Fig. 4-2)—just after the second sound. It is much easier to feel in some normal subjects than in others, and when it is particularly exaggerated, it is called a *dicrotic pulse* or *dicrotism*. For this to develop, elastic arterial walls and a competent aortic valve are necessary (note the diminutive dicrotic wave in the presence of an incompetent aortic valve in Fig. 4-4). A dicrotic pulse occurs in feverish states, the much-quoted prototype of which is typhoid; other factors that favor its development are youth, increased cardiac rate, and myocardial failure.[3] It is particularly common in heart failure due to a cardiomyopathy,[3,4] and its presence may indeed afford a clue to that diagnosis. A significant proportion of patients with dicrotism had a low

endogenous adrenaline. A sharp, "flicking" carotid pulse is characteristic of hypertrophic cardiomyopathy with muscular subaortic stenosis.

The Carotid Pulse Tracing

There are three recognizable positive waves in the arterial pulse: the first impact of left ventricular ejection is the "percussion" wave; next, in systole, there is a so-called "tidal" wave; and then in diastole there is a sometimes palpable rebound wave known as the "dicrotic" wave. In youth, the percussion wave is dominant (Fig. 4-1a), but with

cardiac output, low stroke volume, increased pulmonary artery wedge pressure, and elevated total systemic resistance.[4]

Hypotensive states, the low pressure beats of an arrhythmia, and those during inspiration, favor its development. A prominent dicrotic pulse has been reported occasionally in a variety of conditions, including hypertensive and ischemic heart disease, acute myocardial infarction, primary pulmonary hypertension, pericardial tamponade, and constrictive pericarditis; and in some high-output states such as anemia and thyrotoxicosis. In patients with aortic or mitral regurgitation, the development of a persistent dicrotic pulse after open heart surgery for valve replacement signals a poor prognosis.[5]

Palpability of the dicrotic wave may depend not so much on its absolute amplitude as on its relative size compared with the antecedent percussion/tidal wave. Just as in auscultation a loud preceding sound may prevent recognition of a softer succeeding event ("auditory fatigue"), so a vigorous percussion/tidal wave may preclude recognition of the smaller dicrotic rebound ("palpatory fatigue"), whereas the reduced percussion/tidal wave of low-output states may permit recognition of the modest dicrotic rebound.[6]

Figure 4-3 shows unusually prominent dicrotic waves in both carotid (CPT) and radial (RPT) pulses, both of which could be easily felt, in a 12-year-old black boy with severe mitral regurgitation.

Di-crotos and *bis-feriens* are, respectively, the Greek and Latin for "twice-striking"; the time of

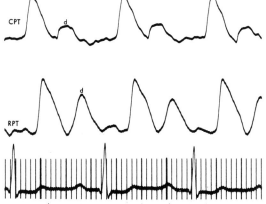

Figure 4–3. From a youngster with severe mitral regurgitation whose carotid (CPT) and radial (RPT) pulse tracings show unusually large dicrotic waves (d).

the second stroke, however, is different in the two. In Figure 4-2, the three arterial waves—percussion, tidal and dicrotic—are labeled "P," "T," and "D." The exaggerated separation of percussion and tidal waves is seen in *pulsus bisferiens* (Fig. 4-4), where the second palpable impact is the tidal wave and both palpable peaks occur well before the second sound; this gives a useful clue to the presence of aortic stenosis and regurgitation. Although usually evidence of a "two-way" aortic lesion, it is sometimes seen in pure aortic regurgitation.

The terms percussion wave, tidal wave, dicrotic

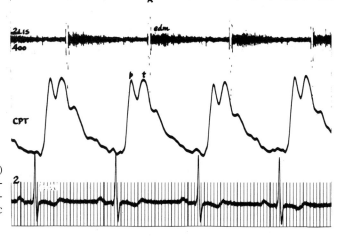

Figure 4–4. Carotid pulse tracing (CPT) from a patient with aortic stenosis and regurgitation showing pulsus bisferiens. p, percussion wave; t, tidal wave; edm, early diastolic murmur (of aortic regurgitation).

wave and pulse, and bisferiens pulse are well entrenched in clinical and cardiographic terminology; but O'Rourke[7] has pointed out that the arterial pulse is one of the topics in cardiology where definitions are inconsistent, terms meaningless (eg, "tidal"), and confusion consequently rife. He recommends that the three positive waves be simply and accurately described as "early systolic," "late systolic," and "diastolic."

OTHER ABNORMAL PULSES

The rapidly rising and falling pulse of aortic regurgitation, otherwise known as a *"waterhammer" pulse* (Watson, 1843), after the sensation imparted to the hand by swinging the Victorian toy (containing a bolus of water in a vacuum), is best felt by holding the patient's arm vertically and grasping the forearm 2 or 3 inches above the wrist with the palm of your hand pressed flat and firmly against the volar surface of his forearm. The typical pulse imparts a slapping sensation to the palpating fingers and palm, abrupt not only in its impact but in its recoil; hence the alternative term, *collapsing pulse*.

The small arterial pulse of severe aortic stenosis, *pulsus parvus*, can also result from severe stenosis of any of the heart's valves. It may be found in severe hypotension, myocardial infarction, and other states of shock, restrictive disease, myocardiopathy, and any form of low-output failure. Severe aortic stenosis also produces a slow-rising pulse (*pulsus tardus, anacrotic pulse*), which is better felt in the larger arteries (carotid or femoral) than in the radial. With practice, the slow, deliberate ascent of the percussion wave can be readily appreciated. When such a pulse feels sustained and "flat-topped," the term *plateau pulse* is applicable; and if the pulse is not only slow-rising but weak as well, it is *pulsus tardus et parvus*.

In advanced stenosis of the valve itself, the degree of obstruction remains constant throughout systole, and consequently the rise of the pulse wave is steady though diminished and retarded. In hypertrophic cardiomyopathy with subaortic stenosis, on the other hand, the obstruction increases as systolic contraction proceeds; the escaping blood makes a speedy getaway while it can in early systole, producing a quick, early upstroke to the pulse wave.

Inequality of both the radial and carotid pulses,

with the right-sided pulses stronger, is sometimes found in supravalvular aortic stenosis. Other causes of inequality—due to unilateral decrease—include dissecting aneurysm, aortic arch syndromes (atherosclerotic, syphilitic, or arteritic), thoracic outlet syndromes (cervical rib, scalenus anticus), and local occlusive disease of the peripheral artery concerned. It is important to be aware of the possibility of asymmetry and to look for it.

Example   A middle-aged man, admitted to the hospital after an automobile accident, was treated energetically for "shock" because his blood pressure was 80/45 in the left arm. Therapy produced no "improvement" in pressure; it was then discovered that the pressure in the other arm was 160/90.

A vigorous pulsating mass at the root of the neck, usually on the right and often giving the impression of an arterial aneurysm, is due to benign arteriosclerotic "buckling" of the right common carotid or innominate artery. It is seen almost exclusively in women. Less commonly, the right subclavian or left common carotid is involved.[8]

CERVICAL THRILLS

A palpable arterial thrill in the neck is most often due to aortic stenosis, but loud murmurs of coarctation, pulmonic stenosis, ventricular septal defect, and patent ductus may be transmitted into the neck to the accompaniment of a thrill. High-output states can also produce thrills, as of course can localized disease of the carotid arteries themselves. Bruits (and thrills) of aortic origin become less intense as you ascend the neck; those arising in the carotids themselves are usually louder higher in the neck. The innocent supraclavicular bruit is sometimes gross enough to produce a palpable thrill.

PULSUS PARADOXUS

Pulsus paradoxus (Kussmaul, 1873) is anything but paradoxical; it is, in fact, an exaggeration of the normal changes in arterial pressure with the phases of respiration, increasing with expiration and decreasing with inspiration. It is classically associated with pericardial effusion but it is also seen in any restrictive cardiac syndrome, in congestive heart failure—especially when acute and severe—in pulmonary embolism,[9] and in obstructive airway disease.[10] It can occur as a benign result of rhythmic compression of the subclavian artery by the shoulder-girdle. Presumably so caused it can appear as a disturbing but benign finding in patients with heart disease.

Example   In a young woman with mitral stenosis, the right brachial pulse caused much consternation on the day before valvotomy because it showed persistent pulsus paradoxus while the left did not. At surgery, no anatomic explanation was found.

Example   A middle-aged woman under treatment for hypertension, month after month at her clinic visits, showed pulsus paradoxus, sometimes extreme. At times her systolic pressure during natural breathing ranged from 180 at the depth of expiration to 130 a moment later at the height of the next inspiration.

In an occasional patient, the arterial blood pressure may increase with inspiration and decrease with expiration.[11] This truly paradoxical behavior has been given the name "reversed pulsus paradoxus," but has not been explained.

Pulsus Alternans

Pulsus alternans (Traube, 1872) is the alternation of stronger and weaker beats in regular rhythm (Fig. 4-5). In normal hearts it is sometimes seen during paroxysmal tachycardia, and then its prognosis is that of the arrhythmia. In both normal and diseased hearts it may put in an appearance for a few beats only following a premature beat. With these exceptions, it is an ominous sign when it occurs at normal heart rates, usually presaging death within a year or two. It is known as one of the two death rattles of the left ventricle—the other being an S3 gallop—and should always be looked for in persons with suspected disease of that ventricle, that is, patients with hypertension, aortic valve disease, ischemic heart disease, or cardiomyopathy.

When pulsus alternans is present at rest, the patient usually has frank signs of heart failure or of myocardial disease. In some patients, digitalis eliminates the alternans; in others it disappears with progressing congestive heart failure. The alternans may be exaggerated by measures that diminish venous return (tourniquets, phlebotomy) and may be diminished by measures that increase venous return (exercise, leg-raising). In other patients not in heart failure, alternans may appear only after exercise, and then probably indicates latent myocardial insufficiency.[12] In yet others, alternans is present only when they are sitting or standing.[13] Sublingual nitroglycerin has precipitated alternans in some individuals.[14]

Thus, the behavior and significance of pulsus alternans varies greatly in different patients. Meticulous measurement shows that the rhythm, which to all intents and purposes is regular, sometimes shows slight alternation of the cycle length.[15]

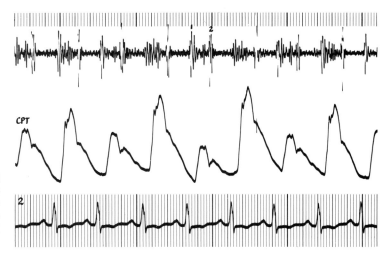

Figure 4–5. Carotid pulse tracing (CPT) from a 52-year-old woman with hypertension and mitral regurgitation. Note the marked alternation in amplitude in the carotid pulse—pulsus alternans.

The difference in arterial pressure between alternate beats is usually a matter of a few millimeters, and such alternation can only exceptionally be recognized with the palpating finger. To exclude alternation, one must employ the sphygmomanometer: Having inflated the cuff above systolic pressure, you gingerly reduce pressure until the first sound appears. You hold at this point and listen to see whether every beat is audible. If you do not hear every beat, it may be because of the usual respiratory variation—readily recognized by correlation with the breathing. If the rhythm is regular and you hear only every other beat, pulsus alternans is present and you then reduce the pressure gradually to determine at what level the missing sounds appear; this difference should be recorded as a measure of the alternation.

Pulsus alternans, though most commonly seen in patients with obvious stigmata of serious heart disease and failure, occasionally appears as the only clinical evidence of a diseased myocardium.

Example   An elderly man, admitted to the hospital for urinary retention, had no symptoms or other signs of heart disease; but he had persistent pulsus alternans, alternate beats registering the following presures: 180/80, 150/90.

REFERENCES

1. Wood P. Diseases of the heart and circulation, ed 2. Philadelphia: JB Lippincott, 1956:26–32.
2. Freis ED, Kyle MC. Computer analysis of carotid and brachial pulse waves: effect of age in normal subjects. Am J Cardiol 1968;22:691.
3. Meadows WR, et al. Dicrotism in heart disease. Am Heart J 1971;82:596.
4. Ewy GA, et al. The dicrotic arterial pulse. Circulation 1969;39:655.
5. Orchard RC, Craige E. Dicrotic pulse after open heart surgery. Circulation 1980;62:1107.
6. Smith D, Craige E. Mechanism of the dicrotic pulse. Br Heart J 1986;56:531.
7. O'Rourke MF. The arterial pulse in health and disease. Am Heart J 1971;82:687.
8. Hsu I, Kistin AD. Buckling of the great vessels. Arch Intern Med 1956;98:712.
9. Burdine JA, Wallace JM. Pulsus paradoxus and Kussmaul's sign in massive pulmonary embolism. Am J Cardiol 1965;15:413.
10. Dock W. Some paradoxes in the history of pulsus paradoxus. Am J Cardiol 1963;11:569.
11. Massumi RA, et al. Reversed pulsus paradoxus. N Engl J Med 1973;289:1272.
12. Ryan JM, et al. Experiences with pulsus alternans, ventricular alternation and the state of heart failure. Circulation 1956;14:1099.
13. Friedman B, et al. Orthostatic factors in pulsus alternans. Circulation 1953;8:864.
14. Ferrer MI, et al. Some effects of nitroglycerine upon the splanchnic, pulmonary, and systemic circulations. Circulation 1966;33:357.
15. Friedman B. Alternation of cycle length in pulsus alternans. Am Heart J 1956;51:701.

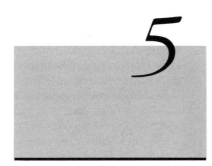

Arterial Blood Pressure

Although a cynical psychologist has said that the introduction of the sphygmomanometer is a disaster from which the human race is unlikely to recover, measuring the blood pressure (BP) is an integral part of the physical examination; and so, every practicing physician should be familiar with five methods for measuring it: Auscultatory, palpatory, oscillometric, flush, and subjective.

There are several clinical situations in which the auscultatory standby lets you down and you need other methods to fall back on. Whatever method is used, the occluding cuff should be at the level of the patient's heart, and both patient and observer should be warm and comfortable and relaxed. Readings recorded in doctor's office, clinic, or laboratory are usually higher than those taken at home by spouse or friend, or recorded by an automated ambulatory system—a phenomenon that has been called "white coat hypertension."

Anyone who assumes the responsibility of taking blood pressures should be familiar with the numerous sources of error (Table 5-1), including speed of releasing cuff pressure, dimensions of cuff, and malfunctioning equipment. The mercury manometer is more reliable than the aneroid model—it is estimated that about one in three aneroids is inaccurate.

Although there appears to be little difference in blood pressure norms between various races, in the Bogalusa study the blood pressure of black children was significantly higher than that of white children.[1]

THE AUSCULTATORY METHOD

Virtually everyone is familiar with the auscultatory method introduced by Korotkoff in 1905 (Table 5-2), but there are some practical points that are widely disregarded.

1. Always keep your finger on the pulse while you are inflating the cuff for the first time. Reasons: (1) You know immediately when you have reached systolic pressure (the moment the pulse disappears), and so you save yourself time and

Table 5–1
Common Causes of Inaccurate Blood Pressure Readings

Reading Too Low	Reading Too High
Cuff too wide	Cuff too narrow
Cuff bladder too short	Unusually fat arm
Unusually thin arm	Patient discomfort
Too rapid deflation	Repeated readings
Overlooking auscultatory gap	Distended urinary bladder
Too firm pressure with stethoscope	

your patient discomfort by not pumping the pressure unnecessarily high. (2) You ensure you will not miss an auscultatory gap (see below). (3) It will sometimes enable you to detect an otherwise overlooked pulsus bisferiens or pulsus alternans (see Chapter 4).

2. You may get an artificially high reading if the cuff is too narrow, and an artificially low reading if it is too wide.[2,3] The ideal width of cuff is 40% to 50% of the limb's (arm or leg) circumference, or 125% to 155% of its diameter.[3] If the bladder is too short for the patient's arm—its length should be 80% to 100% of the limb's circumference—again the reading may be artificially low. Recommended dimensions of the cuff ''bladder'' for average adults are 13 × 35 cm;[4] If the patient's arm is unusually fat you will likely obtain too high a reading, and if it is exceptionally thin, the reading will be too low. You may also produce an artificially high reading if you cause the patient discomfort by pumping the pressure unnecessarily high or repeatedly; or too low if you let the pressure down precipitously—for accurate readings the pressure in the cuff should be reduced not more than 2 mm per beat.

3. Do not press too firmly with the bell of your

stethoscope. If you press hard enough, you can produce Korotkoff sounds over any artery and so obtain an artificially low diastolic pressure.

The *auscultatory gap* is of no clinical importance—except that if you miss its existence, you may report a normal systolic BP when in fact hypertension is present. The way to avoid missing the gap is to keep your finger on the pulsing artery as you inflate the cuff until the pulse disappears—then you know you are above systolic pressure. With an auscultatory gap, there is complete silence for 10 to 50 mm, and if you start listening somewhere during the gap, you will record the point at which the sound returns as the systolic pressure, whereas the true pressure may be as much as 100 mm higher. Auscultatory gaps have been reported in patients with hypertension, aortic valve disease, marked bradycardia, and heart failure.

Example   A patient with syphilitic aortic regurgitation had a BP of 235/85. In a cardiac clinic affiliated with a medical school, her pressure was recorded week after week as 150/85—she had an auscultatory gap between 190 and 150. Her physicians, obviously failing to keep a finger on the pulse, each time happened to pump the cuff pressure to somewhere between 150 and 190 before they started listening.

There is still dispute concerning the proper index of diastolic pressure; adult advocates favor phase 5,[5] pediatricians phase 4.[6] Until the argument is finally settled, the point of disappearance of the sounds should always be recorded,[7] and, when the point of abrupt attenuation (phase 4) is also evident, it should be noted as well.

THE PALPATORY METHOD

This technique provides somewhat lower readings than other methods. After pumping the cuff up to

Table 5–2
Phases of Korotkoff Sounds

	Auditory Signal	Significance
Phase 1	First audible sounds as cuff deflates	Systolic pressure
Phase 2	Murmur-like, swishing sounds	Several mm Hg below systolic peak
Phase 3	Clear, well heard, tapping sounds	Several mm Hg below phase 2 sounds
Phase 4	Sudden muffling of sounds	Previously regarded as diastolic level
Phase 5	Disappearance of all sounds	Diastolic pressure; 5–10 mm Hg below phase 4

above systolic pressure, the first palpable pulsation as the cuff is slowly deflated gives one the level of systolic pressure. This method (Riva-Rocci, 1896) is of great value in, for example, the patient in shock requiring frequent BP checks. In these circumstances, serial readings of *systolic* pressure are generally enough. With the deflated cuff left in place, all one needs is access to the rubber bulb of the sphygmomanometer; then, with minimal disturbance to the patient, a finger on the pulse tells you all you need to know. Saving in nurses' time and disturbance to the patient can be considerable.

Many physicians and nurses are unaware that diastolic pressures can also be taken by palpation, and this can sometimes be accomplished more easily on the way up than on the way down. If the cuff is slowly inflated while the finger rests attentively on the brachial pulse, the point at which it assumes a tapping quality signals the diastolic level; conversely, when deflating the cuff, the end point is the first moment that the pulse regains its original quality.

THE OSCILLOMETRIC METHOD

By this method, introduced by Pachon in 1909, systolic pressure is indicated when, as the cuff is deflated, small oscillations abruptly become larger; diastolic pressure is signalled when the waning oscillations abruptly decrease or disappear. This method also affords a means of measuring the mean arterial pressure—the point at which oscillation of the column of mercury or needle is maximal. These readings can also be made—much more expensively!—by an automated oscillometric device.[3]

THE FLUSH METHOD

This technique, introduced by Gaertner is 1903, is invaluable in infants and is of use in pulseless limbs (eg, arms in aortic arch syndromes, legs in coarctation of the aorta). The cuff is applied and the limb elevated until it blanches; the cuff is then inflated and the limb restored to heart level. The cuff is slowly deflated until the first flush appears, which indicates the *mean* arterial pressure.

THE SUBJECTIVE METHOD

This method may be useful if Korotkoff sounds are not heard, yet a pulse is palpable. A conscious, relatively alert patient is essential, since the measurements depend on the patient's subjective sensations as the cuff is deflated. At the level of systolic pressure, the subject feels pulsations beneath the cuff; these become more intense until, at the diastolic level, they abruptly cease.

For those who enjoy gadgetry for simple jobs, sophisticated techniques—including Doppler and infrasound methods—are available. Doppler devices recognize systolic but not diastolic pressures.[3]

REFERENCES

1. Voors AW, et al. Studies of blood pressure in children, ages 5–14 years, in a total biracial community: The Bogalusa Heart Study. Circulation 1976;54:319.
2. Geddes LA, Whistler SJ. The error in indirect blood pressure measurement with the incorrect size of cuff. Am Heart J 1978;96:4.
3. Park MK, Guntheroth WG. Accurate blood pressure measurement in children. American Journal of Noninvasive Cardiology 1989;3:297.
4. Petrie JC, et al. Recommendations on blood pressure measurement. Br Med J 1986;293:611.
5. Frohlich ED, et al. Recommendations for human blood pressure determination by sphygmomanometers. Report of a special task force appointed by the steering committee, American Heart Association. Circulation 1988;77:501A.
6. Moss AJ. Criteria for diastolic pressure: revolution, counterrevolution, and now a compromise. Pediatrics 1983; 71:854.
7. O'Brien E, et al. Blood pressure measurement: current practice and future trends. Br Med J 1985;290:729.

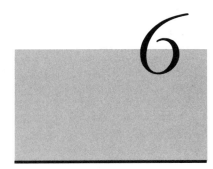

Inspection and Palpation of the Precordium

The eye often misses what is not in the observer's mind, but sees what it looks for.

Thrusts are abnormally pronounced precordial pulsations.
Shocks are abnormally palpable heart sounds.
Thrills are palpable murmurs.

INSPECTION AND PALPATION

The best feeler and analyzer of pulsations is the fingertip; the best for feeling shocks and thrills is usually the most distal part of the palm—at the base of the fingers. If you are right-handed, you may find that your left hand, being slightly less calloused and cornified, makes a more sensitive feeler. For most effective inspection and palpation of the precordium, equip yourself with a *movable light* that can be shone tangentially, and *make yourself comfortable*. It is no luxury—it is a downright necessity—for the examiner to be at ease. Be sure your hands are warm: it is not only kinder to the patient, but they themselves are more sensitive. Don't be in a hurry—remember the importance of "warm-up."

For the bulk of your inspection and palpation the patient should be lying flat or with the trunk slightly elevated. But to bring certain features to light you must sometimes change the patient's position; for example, to bring out the presence and character of a left ventricular impulse you may have to turn him on to his left side; or to bring out aortic thrills it may help to have him sit and lean forward.

Probably the most valuable single maneuver for bringing out otherwise obscure pulsations and thrills is to shrink the bulk of dampening lung by having the patient fully exhale and stop breathing. But remember that some impulses (eg, the right ventricular heave of tricuspid regurgitation) may be more conspicuous with inspiration than with expiration. In solid chests, firm, even forceful, pressure with the palpating hand may be necessary to identify the location and character of subjacent impulses.[1]

Inspection and palpation cannot and should not be separated into watertight compartments: They are an interwoven pair and every competent examiner at times looks at an area, then feels it, then looks again and feels it again before passing on to the next. He often interjects a "listen" to confirm or clarify a point; in fact, it is a good rule to double-check the timing of all precordial pulsations by auscultation.

As you begin a systematic exploration of the precordium with your eyes and hands, always keep before you the importance of "warm-up"; it is often astonishing what you can see and feel—and hear—after 15 or 20 seconds that you could not appreciate in the first 5 or 10. And while you are warming up, here's an important caveat:

Every lift is not systolic.

One tends to take it for granted that when the chest wall is being pushed outward, it must be a systolic push. But, in most enlarged hearts, there is a reciprocal see-saw motion, and whenever a part of the chest wall is being lifted, another part is receding, and vice versa. Therefore be sure that the lift you are feeling is truly a systolic impulse and not a diastolic rebound. The real apex beat is an excellent referee for timing auscultatory events, but it can be a deluding snare unless you bear this common trap in mind—you must be certain which end of the see-saw you are watching. It is particularly common in the presence of left ventricular hypertrophy to see the left parasternal region rise and fall with each beat; and you are likely to interpret this as evidence of associated right ventricular hypertrophy unless you time the movements carefully with the left ventricular impulse and see that the parasternal lift corresponds with recession of the apex beat, and is therefore diastolic. In some cases of left ventricular hypertrophy the only visible and palpable movement with the patient supine may be the parasternal rise and fall; only when he is turned toward his left may the true left ventricular impulse declare itself. In fact, examining the patient in the left lateral position should be a routine part of every examination, because palpability and audibility of third and fourth heart sounds are greatly enhanced in this position.[2]

Example   A 9-year-old child, *in extremis* with a ventricular septal defect and aortic regurgitation,

had the expected to-and-fro murmurs with systole and diastole of about equal length, making it virtually impossible to distinguish systole from diastole. One sound was muffled, but the other was extremely loud and sharp. Was it the accentuated P2 of her pulmonary hypertension? Or was it a loud aortic ejection sound? The hand placed around the child's thorax at about the level of the usual left ventricular impulse could feel a sustained outward thrust in the 5th and 6th interspaces in the midaxillary line. The sharp sound followed this lift and was therefore interpreted as a loud S2. But a later, more thorough search for an apex beat revealed a more localized impulse in the 9th interspace in the posterior axillary line; and this, the true apex beat, receded as the higher area bulged. The sharp sound, therefore, was then properly interpreted as an ejection sound, with which indeed its tone and timbre were more in keeping.

Although in practice we generally examine for pulsations, palpable sounds, and thrills in the same area before passing on to the next, for convenience of presentation, we shall here take each phenomenon in turn, beginning with precordial pulsations.

PULSATIONS

The apexcardiogram (ACG) provides a satisfactory record of the precordial impulse as you see and feel it (Fig. 6-1). Its component phases are labeled, and it is excellent practice to draw the waveform of the impulse on paper as it looks and feels to you before you actually record the ACG. Figure 6-2 is a normal ACG.

You will get the best results if you establish a routine. Haphazard exploration may strike oil, but it is amazing and chastening how often, if your examination does not follow a set pattern, you will overlook the obvious. In your methodical search, there are at least seven areas that should receive attention. A good system, often recommended, is to begin at one area and work methodically through them all in a preordained sequence; but most of us in practice probably obey Sutton's law and start with the most obvious pulsation, if there is one, and then turn our attention to the remaining areas.

Precordial "areas" (mitral, aortic, etc.) have their limitations, a point that will be enlarged upon when we discuss auscultation (Chapter 8). The

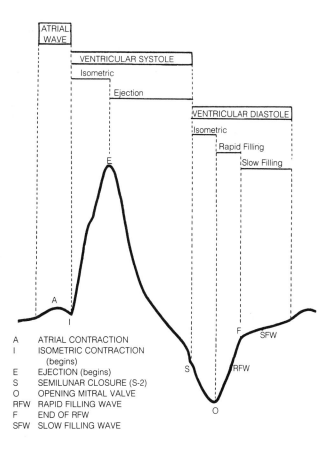

A   ATRIAL CONTRACTION
I   ISOMETRIC CONTRACTION
     (begins)
E   EJECTION (begins)
S   SEMILUNAR CLOSURE (S-2)
O   OPENING MITRAL VALVE
RFW RAPID FILLING WAVE
F   END OF RFW
SFW SLOW FILLING WAVE

Figure 6–1. Diagram of an apexcardiogram (ACG) dissected and labeled.

seven general regions (Fig. 6-3) used in this discussion, the borders of which are necessarily ill-defined, with their approximate equivalents added in parentheses, are as follows:

APICAL AREA (apex, mitral area: a vaguely de-

fined area, dependent on the size of the heart, extending downward and outward toward the axilla from about the midclavicular line at the 5th interspace),

LOWER STERNAL AREA, subdivided into:

1. Left lower sternal border (LLSB, tricuspid

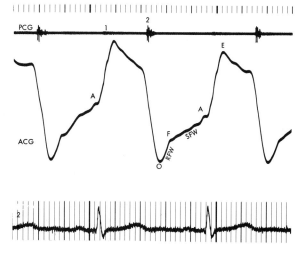

Figure 6–2. A normal apexcardiogram (ACG).

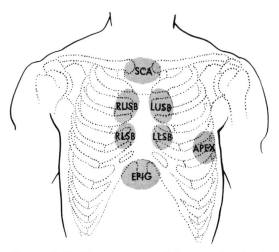

Figure 6–3. The seven precordial areas referred to in text.

area; 4th and 5th left interspaces near sternum),
  2. Right lower sternal border (RLSB; 4th and 5th right interspaces near sternum),
UPPER STERNAL AREA, subdivided into:
  1. Left upper sternal border (LUSB, pulmonic area; 2nd and 3rd left interspaces near sternum),
  2. Right upper sternal border (RUSB, aortic area; 2nd and 3rd right interspaces near sternum),
STERNOCLAVICULAR AREA (SCA), and EPIGASTRIC AREA (EPIG).

Apical Area

The apical area contains the apex beat which, by definition, is the furthest point leftward and downward at which you can see or feel cardiac pulsation. It is the best guide we have to the heart's left border and hence its overall size. Inspection and palpation are often the most sensitive techniques we have for detecting minor degrees of cardiac enlargement; better than electrocardiogram or chest x-ray,[3] and rivalled only by the echocardiogram. The point of maximal impulse (PMI) does not necessarily correspond with the apex beat; it is an unsatisfactory term, serves no useful purpose, and should be abandoned.

The normal apical impulse, caused by impact of the left ventricular apex against the chest wall, is localized in the 5th, or rarely the 4th, interspace at or medial to the midclavicular line (MCL). Be-

cause this line is not easily drawn with precision, it is well to check the distance of the apex beat from the midline (midsternal line), which should not be more than 10 cm or 3.5 to 4 inches. Even the normal impulse may be outside the MCL when a high diaphragm (pregnancy, obesity, ascites, etc.) or other noncardiac cause displaces a normal heart to the left; in normal young children, the apex beat is often found in the 4th interspace just outside the MCL.

The normal impulse lifts an area of the chest wall no larger than a nickel. It is not sustained, but consists of a single, short-lived lift ending within the first two-thirds of systole. An apical impulse may or may not be palpable in the normal person, depending on thickness of the chest wall and other factors. It may not be apparent in some normal subjects when they are lying flat, but may become readily seen and felt if they turn on to their left side.

Slight systolic retraction at the left sternal border may be seen in normal thin-chested subjects in the absence of a palpable apical impulse. On the other hand, such parasternal retraction may furnish the first clue to left ventricular enlargement. In either case the apical impulse may not be palpable until the patient has turned on to his left side. In severe aortic stenosis, the sustained apical impulse is often accompanied by a gentle parasternal retraction.[4] Constrictive pericarditis produces systolic retraction of the precordium, whereas restrictive cardiomyopathy produces a palpable systolic thrust.[4]

The abnormal impulse of left ventricular enlargement may remain relatively circumscribed but with its lift sustained—the finger is raised and held aloft up to or beyond the second sound. In fact, its sustained quality is the most important feature of left ventricular hypertrophy; probably half such impulses are not displaced leftward, but virtually all are abnormally sustained.[5] It may involve a much greater area than the normal impulse—even larger than a 50-cent piece; when the impulse involves an area greater than 3 cm in diameter, it is excellent evidence of left ventricular enlargement.[6] The palpable lift often contains more than one positive component; the additional component may be a systolic rebound, or may occur in early or late diastole, corresponding respectively to abnormal third and fourth heart sounds.

Systolic retraction—with no outward movement at all in systole—may be seen in constrictive pericarditis, pleuropericardial adhesions, and tricuspid regurgitation.[7] Abnormal apical, or near-apical, pulsations are also seen in myocardial infarction[8,9]; cardiac aneurysm[10]; and in right ventricular hypertrophy (when the right ventricle enlarges greatly and occupies the entire anterior chest, displacing the left ventricle posteriorly). Transient abnormal pulsations may develop, or be exaggerated, only during attacks of angina.[9]

Various forms of apex impulses (ACGs) are illustrated in Figure 6-4. A prominent A wave in late diastole, corresponding with an audible fourth heart sound, occurs in conditions producing systolic overloading of the ventricle (Fig. 6-4**A**). A prominent F point in early diastole due to rapid ventricular filling characterizes diastolic overloading (Fig. 6-4**B**). A prominent systolic rebound occurs in an assortment of conditions, including left bundle-branch block (LBBB) and hypertrophic cardiomyopathy with muscular subaortic stenosis (Fig. 6-4**C**); its significance is not always clear.

Associated Lags of Note

In mitral stenosis, a metallic tap (the "mitral hammer") interrupts the apical pulsation—there is a perceptible interval between the onset of the outward lift and the palpable (and audible) tap.[11] In severe aortic stenosis the carotid pulse, instead of seeming synchronous with the apex impulse, lags slightly behind it.[12] In mitral regurgitation the early apical hyperdynamic impulse is followed in late systole by a more diffuse parasternal heave.[4]

Lower Sternal Areas

This is the region in which the right ventricle makes itself felt, and any considerable outward movement in this area is almost always due to right ventricular enlargement. If the sternum itself is normal and not depressed (as in pectus excavatum), any actual forward lift by the underlying impulse is virtually diagnostic of right ventricular hypertrophy.

In the normal child or thin-chested adult there may be a slight but definite right ventricular impulse at the left sternal border, but such impulses are momentary—coinciding with the first sound and rapidly receding in the first third of systole.[13] A similar but more vigorous lift occurs in patients enjoying hyperdynamic states, such as pregnancy, anxiety, anemia, fever, and thyrotoxicosis. An exaggerated, but still brief, thrust accompanies diastolic overloading of the right ventricle (atrial septal defect, etc.), whereas right ventricular hypertrophy secondary to systolic overloading (pulmonic stenosis, etc.) produces a sustained lift lasting up to the second sound.[14] A presystolic component to the impulse, signifying right atrial hypertrophy as well, can sometimes be seen and felt. A giant presystolic impulse, overshadowing the systolic, is characteristic of hypertrophic cardiomyopathy affecting the right heart.[15]

An important exception to an otherwise rather specific sign of right ventricular hypertrophy occurs in free mitral regurgitation, in which the left atrium balloons with regurgitated blood; this lifts

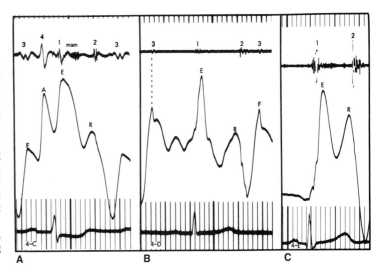

Figure 6–4. The several components of each of these three ACGs were visible or palpable on careful bedside examination. (**A**) Note prominent presystolic impulse coinciding with extremely loud S4 (from a patient with rheumatic heart disease). (**B**) Note how the early diastolic filling wave (F) points like a finger at S3 (from a patient with mitral regurgitation). (**C**) Note the systolic rebound occurring before S2 (from a patient with pectus excavatum). 1 = S1, 2 = S2, etc; msm, midsystolic murmur; A, atrial wave; E, ejection wave; F, filling wave; R, systolic rebound.

the whole heart forward and with it the chest wall. Meticulous timing shows that this forward lift begins later in systole than a true right ventricular thrust. Again, in tricuspid atresia the right ventricle may be dwarfed by a left ventricle rotated anteriorly so that the left ventricular impulse may be well seen and felt in the midprecordium.

An analysis of the sites of maximal pulsation (Fig. 6-5) in patients with known left and right ventricular overloading revealed significant overlap[16]: Although most patients with right ventricular overloading showed maximal impulses at the left sternal border, 22% were maximal to the right of the sternum, and, more important, 21% had their largest pulsations in areas further to the left. Of patients with left ventricular overloading, 75% had maximal impulses in or near the left MCL, an area shared by 6% of right ventricular impulses. Twelve percent of left and 15% of right ventricular impulses overlapped in the midzone between sternal edge and MCL, and only 13% of left ventricular impulses enjoyed an axillary area immune from encroachment by right ventricular impulses.

The right ventricular impulse of mitral stenosis tends to be more medial than those of other genesis, and often lifts the sternum maximally, whereas the right ventricular impulse of pulmonic stenosis is often situated in the left MCL.[17]

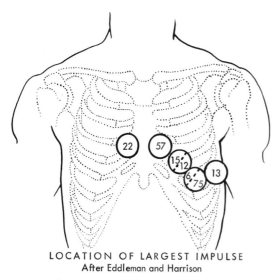

LOCATION OF LARGEST IMPULSE
After Eddleman and Harrison

Figure 6–5. Location of maximal impulses (after Eddleman and Harrison). Note that the midprecordial zones are shared by both left and right impulses (see text).

Upper Sternal Areas

At the left upper sternal border (LUSB; "pulmonary" area) pulsation may be seen and felt normally in children and in thin-chested adults. Abnormal pulsation in this area is seen when the pulmonary artery is enlarged by idiopathic dilation, poststenotic dilation (valvular pulmonic stenosis), by increased pulmonary flow (atrial septal defect, ventricular septal defect), or by pulmonary hypertension (left ventricular failure, mitral stenosis, primary pulmonary hypertension, etc.). Pulsation due to increased flow is quick and active; that due to pulmonary hypertension, more sustained and forceful.

The right upper sternal border (RUSB; "aortic" area) seldom presents obvious pulsation. When it does, it indicates dilation of the ascending aorta, as from atherosclerosis, poststenotic dilation, aortic regurgitation, dissecting aneurysm, or syphilitic aneurysm.

Sternoclavicular Area

The sternoclavicular joints rarely pulsate, but when they do it is a sign of aortic disease. Dissecting aneurysm,[18] a tortuous innominate artery, or a right-sided aorta—most often associated with a tetralogy of Fallot—may cause pulsation of the right sternoclavicular joint alone. Aortic regurgitation, or any form of aortic aneurysm, may cause pulsation of this whole region.

Epigastrium

Pulsation in the epigastrium is usually aortic, hepatic, or right ventricular. Transmitted aortic pulsations are normally visible in thin people or may become apparent in hyperdynamic states such as fever and anxiety. Abnormal pulsations may be due to aneurysm of the abdominal aorta or of one of its epigastric branches, or to aortic regurgitation. The liver may pulsate in systole with tricuspid regurgitation, and late in diastole with tricuspid stenosis, severe right ventricular failure, or pulmonary hypertension. In emphysema, right ventricular pulsations are more likely to be seen and felt in the epigastrium than over the precordium.

The following points are helpful in distinguishing these three sources of pulsation: Hepatic pulsation is as well—or better—felt in the right hypochondrium as in the epigastrium; it is better felt over a wider area; and it has the characteristics of venous rather than arterial pulsation, that is, its expansion and retreat are more gradual than the aortic or ventricular beat. A hand pressed flat against the epigastrium, with fingers insinuated upward just under the xiphocostal margin, feels aortic pulsations striking forward against the palmar surface of the fingers, whereas right ventricular pulsations strike downward against the fingertips.

Unusual Areas

Finally, pulsations may involve unexpected areas. On the right side of the chest, the apex beat will be found in the right MCL or outside it in dextrocardia—and if you don't think of dextrocardia you will probably miss it. A systolic heave in the same neighborhood may be seen in mitral regurgitation with huge left atrium extending to the right axilla. In severe tricuspid regurgitation, the whole right half of the chest may be lifted. We have already mentioned the ectopic pulsation of myocardial infarction or cardiac aneurysm so often centered above and medial to the position of the normal apex impulse.

REFERENCES

1. Dressler W. Pulsations of the chest wall as diagnostic signs. Modern Concepts of Cardiovascular Disease 1957; 26:421.
2. Bethel HJN, Nixon PGF. Examination of the heart in supine and left lateral positions. Br Heart J 1973;35:902.
3. Conn RD, Cole JS. The cardiac apex impulse. Ann Intern Med 1971;75:185.
4. Basta IL, Bettinger JJ. The cardiac impulse: a new look at an old art. Am Heart J 1979;97:96.
5. Beilin L, Mounsey P. The left ventricular impulse in hypertensive heart disease. Br Heart J 1962;24:409.
6. Eilen SD, et al. Accuracy of precordial palpation for detecting increased left ventricular volume. Ann Intern Med 1983;99:628.
7. Mounsey JPD. The cardiac impulse during ventricular systole. Am Heart J 1965;70:279.
8. Vakil RJ. Transitory precordial pulsation in coronary occlusion. Br Heart J 1956;18:248.
9. Eddleman EE, Langley JO. Paradoxical pulsation of the precordium in myocardial infarction and angina pectoris. Am Heart J 1962;63:579.
10. Vakil RJ. Ventricular aneurysm of the heart: preliminary report on some new clinical signs. Am Heart J 1955; 49:934.
11. Floyd J, et al. The apex impulse in mitral stenosis: graphic explanation of the palpable movements at the cardiac apex. Am J Cardiol 1983;51:311.
12. Chun PKC, Dunn BE. Clinical clue of severe aortic stenosis. Arch Intern Med 1982;142:2284.
13. Craige E, Schmidt RE. Precordial movements over the right ventricle in normal children. Circulation 1965; 32:232.
14. Schmidt RE, Craige E. Precordial movements over the right ventricle in children with pulmonic stenosis. Circulation 1965;32:241.
15. Gillam PMS, et al. The left parasternal impulse. Br Heart J 1964;26:726.
16. Eddleman EE, Harrison TR. The kinetocardiogram in patients with ischemic heart disease. Prog Cardiovasc Dis 1963;6:189.
17. Stapleton JF, Groves BM. Precordial palpation. Am Heart J 1971;81:409.
18. Logue RB, Sikes C. A new sign in dissecting aneurysm of aorta. JAMA 1952;148:1209.

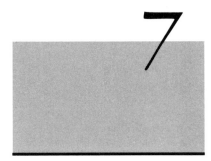

7

Inspection and Palpation Elsewhere

Apart from the pulses and the precordium, there are a few other territories in which inspection and palpation may play a major role in cardiac diagnosis. This chapter deals with physical findings that generally require closer inspection than those in Chapter 2.

CYANOSIS

Cyanosis may be evident at the first glance, or it may require intense scrutiny in good daylight. One pays special attention to lips, ears, tongue, fingers, and toes.

Cyanosis is *central* when it results from reduced oxygen content of arterial blood (''desaturation''), as when venous blood mixes with arterial (right-to-left shunt, arteriovenous fistula); or when there is inadequate oxygen uptake by diseased lungs (cor pulmonale, pneumonia). Cyanosis is *peripheral* when over-reduction of oxyhemoglobin in the capillaries results from sluggish circulation (obstruction to venous return, cold, etc.). Some conditions operate both centrally and peripherally. Heart failure, for instance, hinders venous return and produces peripheral congestion, but by also congesting the lungs interferes with pulmonary oxygenation.

Peripheral cyanosis naturally tends to be concentrated in the extremities and protrusions: Hands, feet, nose, ears, lips. Central cyanosis is more evenly distributed, importantly including mucous membranes. A warm bath makes central cyanosis worse (by bringing more of the desaturated blood to the surface) and improves peripheral cyanosis (by accelerating the sluggish flow).

There are two rare—but important, because they are so pathognomonic—uneven distributions of central cyanosis. If pulmonary hypertension forces the flow through a patent ductus to reverse, venous blood from the pulmonary artery enters the aorta below the origin of the arteries to head and arms, and this blue blood therefore mainly feeds the lower reaches of the body. The feet are therefore more cyanosed than the hands, which may not show cyanosis at all. However, the left subclavian arises close to the ductus and some venous blood is likely to enter it, causing some degree of cy-

Table 7–1
Main Causes of Cyanosis

Central

Mixing of Venous with Arterial Blood
  Congenital heart disease with right-to-left shunt
  Pulmonary A-V fistula
Inadequate Pulmonary Oxygenation
  Severe lung disease
  Pulmonary edema

Peripheral

Sluggish Capillary Circulation
Obstruction to venous return
Cold

anosis of the left upper limb. Thus, cyanosed feet, with less or no cyanosis of the hands (but, if cyanosed, the left hand more so than the right) is *differential cyanosis*, and is diagnostic of patent ductus with reversed flow. In the newborn, "reversed ductus" may result from hyaline membrane disease; it is also sometimes seen as a syndrome that spontaneously clears in babies born of diabetic mothers.

Again, if the great vessels are transposed so that the aorta receives venous blood from the right ventricle; and if the aortic arch is narrowed (coarctation) or completely interrupted so that this venous blood cannot reach the descending aorta (which receives its blood through a patent ductus from the pulmonary artery opening out of the left ventricle), the head and arms will be cyanosed, but the legs less so: *Reversed differential cyanosis.*[1] To appraise differential cyanosis, it is essential to place hands and feet side by side for simultaneous inspection.

In these two admittedly rare situations, simple bedside observation makes as accurate a diagnosis of the disturbed anatomy as the most sophisticated hemodynamic studies. The main causes of cyanosis may be grouped in a somewhat oversimplified way, as in Table 7-1, and a sampling of cyanosed states is presented in Table 7-2.

THE EYES

The Argyll-Robertson pupil (small and unreactive to light but reactive to accommodation), like the tabetic gait, points to luetic involvement and alerts you to the possibility of aortic root disease with coronary ostial obstruction or aortic regurgitation.

Cataract in a child suggests the postrubella syndrome and warns you to look for a patent ductus.

Hypertensive retinopathy (papilledema, "cotton wool" exudates, copper-wire or silver-wire arteries, and arteriovenous "nicking") informs you that the hypertension is malignant and forewarns you of the imminent threat of stroke or congestive heart failure.

Table 7–2
Selected Causes and Mechanisms of Cyanosis

Lesion	Type	Mechanism
VSD with reversed (R-to-L) shunt	Central	Veno-arterial shunt
Emphysema	Central	Inadequate pulmonary oxygenation
Recurrent pulmonary emboli	Central	Inadequate pulmonary oxygenation; if RV failure ensues, peripheral is added
Pulmonary edema	Central	Inadequate pulmonary oxygenation
Superior vena caval obstruction	Peripheral	Obstructed venous return; over-reduction of capillary oxyhemoglobin
Rupture of sinus of Valsalva aneurysm into RA	Peripheral	Venous return obstructed by raised RA pressure
Severe RV failure	Both	Congestion of limbs; congestion of lung
Longstanding MS	Both	Changes in lungs; RV failure

RV, right ventricular; VSD, ventricular septal defect; RA, right atrium; MS, mitral stenosis.

THE MOUTH

Telangiectasia of the lips may be associated with a pulmonary arteriovenous fistula, whereas the tongue is an excellent site to confirm central cyanosis or the pallor of anemia.

An enlarged, bulky tongue suggests the possibility of amyloidosis, which in turn alerts you to exclude an amyloid cardiomyopathy.

SKIN LESIONS

The *subcutaneous nodules of rheumatic fever* are painless, not tender and not attached to the skin, usually pea-sized, though they may range from the size of a pinhead to 2 cm in diameter,[2] and they are located over bony prominences such as the elbow, wrist, ankle, spine, and skull. They are usually found in the company of severe cardiac involvement by the rheumatic process.

The six skin lesions of infective endocarditis "are more useful in diagnosis than are cardiac signs."[3] The *café-au-lait complexion*, already cited (Chapters 1 and 2), is a late sign and therefore seldom seen in our antibiotic era. *Petechiae*, including splinter hemorrhages under the nail,[4] are nonspecific and are diagnostically most helpful when found in protected areas such as the conjunctivae. *Purpura and ecchymoses* are especially seen in acute endocarditis. *Osler's nodes*, much talked about but seldom seen, are diagnostic if found. They are painful, tender, and slightly raised circular, reddish lesions with a white center and a diameter of 3 to 15 mm.[5] They favor palms, soles, and the pads of fingers and toes. *Janeway lesions*, on the other hand, are common; they develop early in the disease and are painless, circular or oval macules with an average diameter of about half a

centimeter; neither raised nor tender, they change from pink to a darker hue and then to tan before fading in a week or two. They are usually multiple and also appear on soles, plantar surfaces of toes, palms, and fingers. *Gangrene of the fingertip* is probably due to arteriolar embolism; the lesion is single, tender, and painful, and complicates acute endocarditis.

CLUBBING

Clubbing of the fingers and toes may be innocently idiopathic and sometimes familiar. More often it is a sign of serious disease. Cardiologic causes include:

1. Cyanotic congenital heart disease,
2. Infective endocarditis,
3. Chronic cor pulmonale, and
4. Left atrial tumors, especially myxoma[6] and primary sarcoma.[7]

In congenital heart disease, clubbing is never present at birth. When it develops, the ends of the fingers are bulbous and blue, in contrast with those of infective endocarditis, which are characteristically bulbous and pink. The border of skin flanking the nail is likely to become reddened and shiny.

The earliest sign of clubbing is a lifting of the root of the nail off its bed. You detect this by depressing with your own thumbnail (Fig. 7-1A) the proximal subcutaneous edge of the patient's nail—the nail can be "rocked." As clubbing progresses, the nail curves longitudinally ("parrot-beaking"); the "profile sign" appears, that is, disappearance of the normal "lunular" angle between nail and skin so that they form a continuous line (Fig. 7-1B); and the terminal phalanx enlarges in all diameters ("drumstick fingers"). In infective

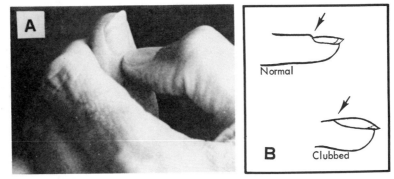

Figure 7–1. **(A)** Method of testing for early clubbing: The examiner's thumbnail presses at root of patient's nail to detect elevation above nailbed. **(B)** Profiles of normal and clubbed finger and nail; note lunular angle (arrow) in normal, and loss of lunular angle (arrow) in clubbed digit with increased curvature of nail and increased anteroposterior diameter of finger-pad.

endocarditis the clubbing may consist, at least for some time, of longitudinal curving of the nails with obliteration of the lunular angle and some increase in anteroposterior depth of the finger pad.

Noncardiac causes of clubbing, of which one must be aware, include[8]:

1. Pulmonary—especially bronchiectasis, abscess, cyst, empyema, tuberculosis, or carcinoma. Note (1) carcinoma of the lung is the most common cause of *painful* clubbing, and (2) clubbing plus cyanosis in the absence of demonstrable heart disease makes the diagnosis of pulmonary arteriovenous fistula probable,
2. Endocrine—thyroid, ovarian and pituitary disease,
3. Alimentary—cirrhosis of the liver, ulcerative colitis, regional enteritis,
4. Methemoglobinemia and sulphemoglobinemia,
5. Carcinoma of esophagus, stomach, or thymus, and
6. Prolonged residence at high altitude.

Unilateral clubbing may be associated with the differential cyanosis of a "reversed ductus," with absence of the aortic arch,[9] with subclavian or aortic aneurysm (sometimes proximal to a coarctation of the aorta), arteriovenous aneurysm, carcinoma of an upper lobe bronchus or a superior sulcus tumor, scapulohumeral subluxation, median nerve injury, or obstruction of the axillary vein.[10]

INSPECTING THE THORAX

Both the straight-back syndrome "pancaking" the heart and the funnel chest (pectus excavatum) displacing it may lead to the misdiagnosis of cardiac enlargement.

Evidence of ankylosing spondylitis should alert you to the possibility of aortic regurgitation. Marked kyphoscoliosis may be associated with cor pulmonale.

Tortuous, visibly pulsating intercostal vessels are virtually diagnostic of coarctation of the aorta, whereas a pulsating sternoclavicular joint indicates an aneurysm of the ascending aorta.

PALPATING THE LIVER

Normally, the liver edge cannot be felt. Its normally sharp edge is blunted and palpable in congestive heart failure, and the organ is tender. When cardiac cirrhosis develops, the edge is firm. Standing on the patient's right, you place your hand just below his right costal margin and ask him to take a deep breath. It is customary to describe its palpable descent in finger-breadths, and its movements should be described precisely (eg, "liver edge felt two finger-breadths below right costal margin in midclavicular line at height of inspiration").

In tricuspid stenosis, a presystolic hepatic pulsation may be felt; in tricuspid regurgitation, there may be a palpable systolic hepatic heave.

PALPATING THE SPLEEN

Feeling for the spleen is often undertaken casually, yet there is no maneuver in which the proper technique of careful palpation is more rewarding. The patient should be lying comfortably on his back while you stand on his right. Place your right hand on the left hypochondrium, the edge of the forefinger just below the edge of the ribs. *Do not depress the skin of the abdominal wall far: It is only necessary for the fingers to attain a depth equivalent to the thickness of the ribs.* Many a spleen is missed by palpating too deeply—while one's fingers are flirting with the patient's backbone, the spleen creeps out beneath the costal margin anteriorly, thumbs its nose, and returns to its bed. Gentle palpation is kinder to the patient and much more productive.

The next most important detail is to be sure that the patient takes the deepest possible breath—the exhortation "DEEP" just as he is nearing the peak of inspiration insures an ultimate inspiratory effort that may be important in bringing a lagging spleen to light. Turning the patient on his right side, placing him in a warm bath to relax the abdominal muscles, and placing a pillow or the patient's own left arm behind his lower thoracic cage, are all helpful at times, but none is nearly so important as the two pointers outlined above.

When the spleen cannot be felt, minor degrees of enlargement may be suspected by careful percussion—its dullness should not encroach beyond a line drawn from the left anterior axillary fold to the umbilicus (Gairdner's line).

REFERENCES

1. Buckley MJ, et al. Reversed differential cyanosis with equal desaturation of the upper limbs. Am J Cardiol 1965;15:111.
2. Friedberg CK. Diseases of the heart, ed 3. Philadelphia: WB Saunders, 1966:1338.
3. Proudfit WL. Skin signs of infective endocarditis. Am Heart J 1983;106:1451.
4. Heath D, Williams DR. Nail hemorrhages. Br Heart J 1978;40:1300.
5. Farrior JB, Silverman ME. A consideration of the differences between a Janeway lesion and an Osler's node in infective endocarditis. Chest 1976;70:239.
6. Goodwin JR. Diagnosis of left atrial myxoma. Lancet 1963;1:464.
7. Raftery EB, et al. Primary sarcoma of the left atrium. Br Heart J 1966;28:287.
8. Fischer DS, et al. Clubbing, a review, with emphasis on hereditary acropachy. Medicine 1964;43:459.
9. Dorney ER, et al. Unilateral clubbing of the fingers due to absence of the aortic arch. Am J Med 1955;18:150.
10. Ridot S. Unilateral clubbing following traumatic obstruction of the axillary vein. Arch Intern Med 1956;98:482.

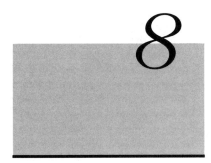

8

Auscultation

As the simplest methods of examination—history, physical examination, electrocardiogram, and chest x-ray—have to some extent been elbowed aside by sophisticated technology, so the stethoscope, as the first clinical *instrument*, tends to supersede use of our unaided senses; and inspection and palpation are glossed over in one's haste to "take a listen."

But we should not hastily produce our stethoscopes or any other instruments. The general disregard for inspection and palpation, and comparative preoccupation with auscultation, are typified by the widespread use of "listen" as a substitute for "examine": "Have you *listened* to the patient in bed seven?"

We should always "hear" as much as we can with our eyes and fingers before we tune in with our ears, and it is an excellent exercise to insist that students make a cardiac diagnosis with their eyes and hands while their stethoscopes are still reposing in their pockets. This increases the acuity of their eyes and the sensitivity of their hands, and

it often surprises them how far along the diagnostic trail they can travel by simply looking and feeling.

THE THINGS WE HEAR

The sounds we listen for are "transients" and "murmurs." A transient is a brief sound, lasting at most only a few hundredths of a second. The term serves to exclude murmurs when "sound," because of its everyday meaning, may be ambiguous. All the heart sounds (first, second, third, and fourth), clicks, and snaps are transients; indeed, the individual components of each sound are themselves transients. First and second sounds are conventionally represented by the monosyllables "lubb" and "dup."

Murmurs, on the other hand, have appreciable duration: The shortest may last only 0.12 to 0.15 second, whereas a pansystolic murmur usually has a duration of approximately 0.25 second, and the long, diminuendo diastolic murmur of aortic regurgitation may last 0.75 second. Murmurs can be simulated by making a blowing noise or clearing one's throat.

STETHOSCOPES

Laennec introduced the primitive stethoscope in 1826, and for many years all the stethoscopes in existence were made by his hand. Nowadays, good listening can be achieved with any of the standard descendants of his prototype; a comparative study of six available models found no advantage in the two-tube versus the single-tube model, and found no make to be "obviously superior."[1] But certain features are absolutely essential in the model you choose: The earpieces must be snug but comfortable, and there must be both bell and diaphragm chest pieces easily interchangeable. Acoustically, the shorter and thicker the tubing the better, but there is obviously a limit to practicality, and suitable compromise dictates tubing of about a foot long with a ⅛-inch bore and about the same wall thickness. Regardless of these necessary specifications, however, always remember that:

The most important part of every stethoscope fits between the earpieces.

The diaphragm, which should be firmly enough applied to the chest wall to leave the imprint of its rim behind it, has two advantages over the bell: It picks up higher frequencies and it gathers sound from a larger area. It is therefore better for detecting soft, high-frequency sounds and murmurs, such as the quiet, high-frequency murmur of mild aortic regurgitation, the soft P2 of pulmonic stenosis, or the faint opening snap of mitral stenosis; it is the better piece for evaluating splitting of the second sound (S2) and systolic clicks; and it is convenient for quickly screening heart and lungs.

The bell has three virtues: It is better for more accurate localization, such as points of maximal intensity; *when lightly applied* it is better for detecting low-pitched tones, such as third heart sounds and the murmur of mitral stenosis; and on bony chests, being smaller, it can sometimes be snugly bedded where the diaphragm rocks unsteadily on ribs. When firmly pressed against the chest wall, the stretched skin converts the bell into a small diaphragm, and it can therefore be used as a filtering device: For example, at first applied lightly, the low-pitched rumble of mitral stenosis may dominate diastole; then, without moving its site, firm pressure turns skin into diaphragm, attenuates the murmur, and may bring to light a previously inaudible opening snap.

PRECORDIAL AREAS

Precordial "areas,"—"mitral," "aortic," etc.— are useful but at times misleading labels. They suggest exclusivity, as though all that is heard at the mitral area is of mitral origin, and all that is of mitral origin is heard at this area. The assignment of surface regions to subjacent heart valves is an oversimplification, and one should embark on auscultation in the full realization that they are useful, geographically descriptive labels—no more.

Some examples of their lack of specificity: All acoustic aortic phenomena—ejection sound and murmur, the aortic component of S2, and the aortic diastolic murmur—may be maximal at the "pulmonic" area; the murmur of aortic regurgitation is *usually* best heard near the "tricuspid" area; the ejection sound and murmur of aortic stenosis may be best heard at the "mitral" area; the thrill and murmur of mitral regurgitation may be maximal at or near the "pulmonic" area; the murmur of tricuspid regurgitation may be well heard at the "mitral" area; and so on.

It is more realistic to partition the precordial surface as seen in Figure 6-3. Nevertheless, the valvular assignments are in common use, and, provided reservations regarding their specificity are kept in mind, they make convenient handles: "aortic area" is well entrenched and is handier than "right upper sternal border" or "second right interspace parasternally."

SYSTEMATIC AUSCULTATION

Auscultation of the heart should be compulsively systematic. It is often recommended that one begin at the apex ("mitral" area) or base—according to individual preference—and methodically listen at all "areas," not ignoring points in between; and that one concentrate first on the first sound at all areas, then systole at all areas, then on the second sound at all areas, and then diastole at all areas. This may perhaps be regarded as conventional wisdom or a counsel of perfection, but in fact it is rather impractical and certainly not what most experienced auscultators do.

It is important that the novice realize that auscultation is just as much an exercise in self-discipline as it is an examination of the patient. And it seems much more logical, and certainly an easier discipline, to listen carefully at each auscultation point to all of the four events in turn (S1, systole, S2, and diastole) before moving on, rather than listening to one phase, say, systole, to the exclusion of other phases, at each listening point in succession. Certainly this is what most experienced clinicians do.

The required self-discipline consists in interrogating oneself as one listens. As, for example, you listen to the first heart sound, you ask yourself: Is it single or split? Is it of normal intensity? Or louder or softer than normal? Is its quality normal? Is it constant from beat to beat?

Then you move on to systole: Are there any clicks? If so, early, mid, or late? Are they affected by respiration? Is there any murmur? If so, what grade is it? When does it begin? What shape is it? What is its duration? Quality? How does respiration affect it?

The second sound: Is it single or split? If split, is the splitting physiologic, persistent, paradoxical, or fixed? Is either component louder or softer than normal?

And finally, diastole: Are there any abnormal transients? Opening snap? Third heart sound? Fourth heart sound? Are there any murmurs? If so, early, mid, or late? What grade is it? Pitch? Duration? Shape?

AUSCULTATORY AIDS

Posture

No physical examination of the heart is complete unless the patient has been examined in at least three positions: Lying supine, turned on the left side, and sitting upright. *Turning to the left* throws the heart against the chest wall and accentuates many left-sided events. The opening snap and diastolic rumble of mitral stenosis, the third and fourth heart sound of left ventricular stress or distress may be audible only in this position. The faint, early diastolic murmur of aortic regurgitation, or the hard-to-hear pericardial rub may be audible only when the patient *sits up and leans slightly forward.*

Squatting causes an increase in peripheral arterial resistance and in venous return; it has no effect on most systolic murmurs[2] but usually decreases the systolic murmur of hypertrophic cardiomyopathy. On the other hand, the diastolic murmur of aortic regurgitation is made louder by squatting, and in fact a virtually inaudible early diastolic murmur may be rendered audible by this maneuver.[3]

Rising from supine to *standing*, either actively or by passive tilt, causes venous pooling and a consequent reduction in stroke volume; in mitral valve prolapse, the decrease in left ventricular volume exaggerates the leaflet prolapse, making the click earlier, and the systolic murmur longer and often louder.[4,5] The reduced stroke volume results in softening of the murmurs of semilunar valve stenosis and A-V valve regurgitation.

Respiratory Maneuvers

Another maneuver that can be invaluable is to have the patient *fully exhale*; at times it is only when respiratory noises are stilled and lung volume reduced to a minimum that faint cardiac murmurs and transients can be appreciated. Thus, although most auscultation can be satisfactorily accomplished during quiet, normal respiration, when listening for a difficult-to-hear event, always ask the patient to exhale fully and leave the breath out while you listen attentively.

Deep inspiration increases venous return to the right heart and may be helpful in distinguishing between murmurs originating in right and left sides of the heart: It has no effect on or diminishes left-sided murmurs, but usually augments those arising on the right. Thus the systolic murmur of tricuspid regurgitation and the diastolic murmur of tricuspid stenosis[6–8] become louder during inspiration, though paradoxically the murmur of pulmonic stenosis gets softer.

The effect of inspiration on the murmur of ventricular septal defect depends on where you are listening: If you listen at the point of maximal intensity (usually the 3rd or 4th left interspace) it becomes softer with inspiration; but if you listen at the left lower sternal border in the 5th or 6th interspace, the murmur gets louder during inspiration (Fig. 8-1) and may, therefore, be confused with tricuspid regurgitation.

Müller's maneuver (forced inspiration against a closed glottis) is seldom used but usually diminishes the murmur of hypertrophic cardiomyopathy.[9] The *Valsalva maneuver* usually decreases the intensity of both right- and left-sided murmurs; its value, therefore, depends on noting how long it

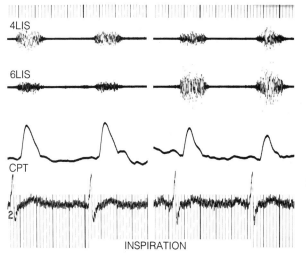

Figure 8–1. From a patient with a ventricular septal defect. Note that with inspiration the pansystolic murmur gets softer in the 4th left interspace (4LIS) but gets louder in the 6th interspace (6LIS). (A single cardiac cycle has been excised from the middle of the strip.)

takes, after cessation of the strain, for the murmur to resume its original intensity. Left-sided murmurs usually require four to 12 heart beats to regain their former intensity, whereas the right-sided murmur regains it in one or two beats.[10] The maneuver has an inconstant effect on the murmur of mitral valve prolapse.

Isometric Exertion

Isometric exercise raises the blood pressure, increases cardiac output, and is usually applied in the form of standardized handgrip. It increases the murmur of mitral regurgitation and softens those of aortic stenosis and hypertrophic cardiomyopathy[11]; thus it is another way of differentiating the murmur of aortic stenosis from that of mitral regurgitation. Handgrip also intensifies the diastolic murmurs of mitral stenosis and aortic regurgitation.

Changes in Cycle Length

When available, the effect of cycle-length changes on the intensity of the murmur affords the simplest of the ancillary bedside clues in differentiating aortic stenosis from mitral regurgitation. In the presence of extrasystoles or atrial fibrillation, a variety of cycle lengths greets the listener. Careful attention to the loudness of the murmur after longer and shorter cycles may be diagnostically rewarding because regurgitant murmurs are usually unaffected

by the preceding cycle, whereas the intensity of ejection murmurs tends to be directly proportional to the preceding cycle's length—the longer the cycle, the louder the ensuing murmur. In Figure 8-2 **(A)**, you see the intensifying effect of the post-extrasystolic cycle on the ejection murmur of aortic stenosis. Contrast this with the lack of intensification of the regurgitant murmur of mitral incompetence at the end of a lengthened cycle during atrial fibrillation (Fig. 8-2**B**). In the congenital realm, the unaffected regurgitant murmur of a ventricular septal defect contrasts with the cycle-influenced ejection murmur of aortic coarctation.

Pharmacologic Interventions

The only drug that has achieved diagnostic popularity is amyl nitrite (Table 8-1). The inhalation of a crushed, standard perle causes a reduction in vascular resistance in both systemic and pulmonary circulations, and an increased cardiac output. Ventricular ejection is therefore more effective, and the ejection murmurs of aortic and pulmonic stenosis are intensified[12]; and so are the murmurs of hypertrophic cardiomyopathy and tricuspid regurgitation. On the other hand, the murmurs of mitral regurgitation, tetralogy of Fallot, and small ventricular septal defects are unaffected or diminished.[13] Paradoxically, amyl nitrite seems to increase the murmur of a large septal defect.[14] The drug therefore provides yet another means of distinguishing between the ejection murmur of aortic

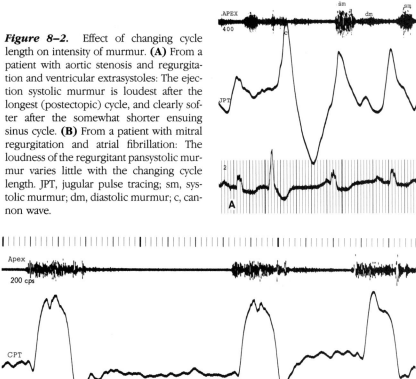

Figure 8–2. Effect of changing cycle length on intensity of murmur. **(A)** From a patient with aortic stenosis and regurgitation and ventricular extrasystoles: The ejection systolic murmur is loudest after the longest (postectopic) cycle, and clearly softer after the somewhat shorter ensuing sinus cycle. **(B)** From a patient with mitral regurgitation and atrial fibrillation: The loudness of the regurgitant pansystolic murmur varies little with the changing cycle length. JPT, jugular pulse tracing; sm, systolic murmur; dm, diastolic murmur; c, cannon wave.

Table 8–1
Usual Effect of Amyl Nitrate on Murmurs

Intensifies Murmur of	Diminishes Murmur of
Aortic stenosis	Mitral regurgitation
Tricuspid regurgitation	
Pulmonic stenosis	Tetralogy of Fallot
Hypertrophic cardiomyopathy	
Large ventricular septal defect	Small ventricular septal defect
Mitral stenosis	Austin Flint
Pulmonic regurgitation	Aortic regurgitation

stenosis and the regurgitant murmur of mitral incompetence.[11,15,16]

Amyl nitrite may also be an important aid in differentiating some diastolic murmurs: It increases the murmur of mitral stenosis[13,17] but decreases that of the Austin Flint murmur[16,18,19]; and it intensifies the murmur of pulmonic regurgitation whereas it diminishes that of aortic regurgitation.

TIMING

Audible events must be placed accurately in systole or diastole. The experienced listener times without effort, subconsciously guided by two signposts: (1) At normal rates, systole is shorter than diastole, and (2) the first heart sound (S1) is lower pitched and longer ("lubb") than S2, which is shorter and sharper ("dup"). When normal relationships are upset, as by tachycardia, he must make a conscious effort to time.

Feeling a peripheral pulse as a timer for cardiac events can mislead and is a refuge only when you are otherwise destitute. It should be resorted to only when the following precordial efforts have failed to satisfy: (1) Look for a systolic precordial impulse; if one is visible or palpable, *use it!* One often sees the student making a valiant but unnecessary effort to time: Eyes closed and finger on carotid, while his stethoscope bounces up and down on an eloquent apex impulse that is signalling "systole" to him, if only he had seeing eyes! (2) Listen at the base where the sharper and louder S2 is usually recognizable; then, keeping S2 in focus, "inch" your way towards the phenomenon to be timed and note where it falls in relation to S2.

Only when both of these methods have been tried and found wanting should you fall back on the carotid pulse.

AUSCULTATORY INTERVALS

Cobbs[20] devised an ingenious system for gauging brief intervals. Pronounce aloud as fast as you possibly can:

PA-PA interval between P and P = 0.10 second,
BUTTER interval between B and T = 0.07 second,
BLAH interval between B and L = 0.04 second, and
TH interval between T and H = 0.02 second.

Note that the time lines in all of the tracings used in this text are the same as in the conventional ECG, that is, the interval between two thick lines = 0.20 second, between two thinner lines = 0.04 second.

REFERENCES

1. Kindig JR, et al. Acoustical performance of the stethoscope: a comparative analysis. Am Heart J 1982;106:269.
2. Nellen M, et al. Effects of prompt squatting on the systolic murmur of idiopathic hypertrophic obstructive cardiomyopathy. Br Med J 1967;3:140.
3. Vogelpoel L, et al. The value of squatting in the diagnosis of mild aortic regurgitation. Am Heart J 1969;77:709.
4. Barlow JB, et al. Late systolic murmurs and non-ejection ("mid-late") systolic clicks: An analysis of ninety patients. Br Heart J 1968;30:203.
5. Fontana ME, et al. Postural changes in left ventricular and mitral valve dynamics in the systolic click-late systolic murmur syndrome. Circulation 1975;51:165.
6. Salazar E, Levine HD. Rheumatic tricuspid regurgitation: the clinical spectrum. Am J Med 1962;33:111.
7. Bousvaros GA, Stubington D. Some auscultatory and phonocardiographic features of tricuspid stenosis. Circulation 1964;29:26.
8. Kitchin A, Turner R. Diagnosis and treatment of tricuspid stenosis. 1964;26:354.
9. Bartall H, et al. Normalization of the external carotid pulse tracing of hypertrophic subaortic stenosis during Muller's maneuver. Chest 1978;74:77.
10. Rothman A, Goldberger AL. Aids to cardiac auscultation. Ann Intern Med 1983;99:346.
11. McCraw DB, et al. Response of heart murmur intensity to isometric (handgrip) exercise. Br Heart J 1972;34:605.
12. Vogelpoel L, et al. The use of amyl nitrite in the differentiation of Fallot's tetralogy and pulmonic stenosis with intact ventricular septum. Am Heart J 1959;57:803.
13. Schrire V, et al. The effects of amyl nitrite and phenylephrine on the intracardiac murmurs of small ventricular septal defects. Am Heart J 1961;62:225.
14. Vogelpoel L, et al. Variations in the response of the systolic murmur to vasoactive drugs in ventricular septal defect, with special reference to the paradoxical response in large defects with pulmonary hypertension. Am Heart J 1962;64:169.
15. Barlow J, Shillingford J. The use of amyl nitrite in differentiating mitral and aortic systolic murmurs. Br Heart J 1958;20:162.
16. Luisada AA, Madoery RJ. Functional tests as an aid to cardiac auscultation. Med Clin North Am 1966;50:73.
17. Nasser W, et al. Austin-Flint murmur versus the murmur of organic mitral stenosis. N Engl J Med 1966;275:1007.
18. Suh SK. Differentiation of the murmur of aortic regurgitation and pulmonary regurgitation with amyl nitrite. Circulation 1960;22:820.
19. Endrys J, Bartova A. Pharmacological methods in the phonocardiographic diagnosis of regurgitant murmurs. Br Heart J 1962;24:207.
20. Cobbs BW. In: Hurst JW, Logue RB, eds. The heart, ed 2. New York: McGraw Hill, 1966:788.

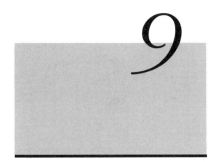

The First Heart Sound

Though less important diagnostically than the second sound, the first sound (S1) has many clues to offer. Sophisticated analysis reveals four components to S1, but for practical purposes we can regard it as having two main components: M1, related to closure of the mitral, and T1, related to closure of the tricuspid valve.

GENESIS

No doubt many tissues and structures vibrate at the time of the first sound, but there is little doubt that the main contributors to the sound are the two atrioventricular valves. The old concept that it was the closing of the valves that made the sound—analogous to slamming a door—is now outmoded; echocardiographic and hemodynamic correlations with the phonocardiogram have conclusively demonstrated that the main sound occurs *after* the leaflets have coapted and at the time of maximal tensing of the entire valvular apparatus, as earlier workers had concluded.[1,2] Others have demonstrated that blood continues to cross the mitral valve into the left ventricle after ventricular contraction has started.[3] For practical purposes we can certainly consider the sound to be produced by valve closure, even though the sound develops a split second after the leaflets meet.

SPLITTING

The mitral valve normally closes slightly before the tricuspid, and, because tricuspid closure generates the softer sound, splitting is best appreciated at the LLSB where the tricuspid component is maximal, but normal splitting is often quite well heard at the apex. Wide splitting of S1 characterizes Ebstein's anomaly of the tricuspid valve, and is also encountered in other causes of right bundle-branch block (RBBB), which, of course, delays tricuspid closure.[4,5] Left bundle-branch block (LBBB) mysteriously fails to produce splitting of S1.[6]

Splitting of S1 can also be of value in distinguishing between supraventricular and ventricular arrhythmias at the bedside. In supraventricular rhythms, not associated with aberrant ventricular conduction, S1 is single, whereas in ventricular arrhythmias it is split. The same, of course, also holds true for S2, but splitting is sometimes apparent only in S1. For example, in some ventricular premature beats, when they interrupt diastole so early that there has been no time for adequate ventricular filling and the ventricles do not contain enough blood to lift the semilunar valves, there is no second sound. Wide splitting of the heart sounds is characteristic of ventricular tachycardia, but unfortunately the same is true of supraventricular tachycardia with aberration, so that splitting is of little assistance in distinguishing between this notoriously imitative pair.

INTENSITY

Several factors influence the intensity of S1, of which the most important is probably the position of the A-V valves at the moment ventricular contraction begins. Even if the actual closure of the A-V valves is not the immediate cause of the first sound, there is an undeniable correlation between the velocity at which the valves close and the intensity of the sound; and the wider open the valves are at the moment of ventricular contraction, the greater is the velocity of their closing. Events that tend to hold the valves open and so favor a loud S1 are tabulated in Table 9-1.

Other influences that affect the loudness of S1 include the texture of the A-V valve leaflets—in mitral stenosis S1 may be deafening (Fig. 9-1); the rate and force of ventricular contraction; and the amount of tissue intervening between stethoscope and heart. Situations in which S1 is unduly loud are tabulated in Table 9-2. A consistently loud S1

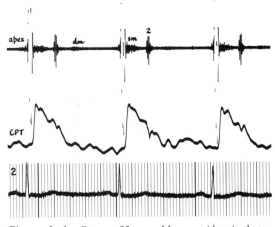

Figure 9–1. From a 55-year-old man with mitral stenosis, illustrating an extremely loud first sound (1). Soft systolic (sm) and diastolic (dm) murmurs are faintly recorded.

in an otherwise apparently normal heart suggests a constantly short P-R interval, and may therefore alert the observer to the presence of a Lown-Ganong-Levine syndrome.[7]

Conditions in which the first sound is unusually soft are listed in Table 9-3. A subdued S1, associated with a cannon wave in the neck, suggests that atrial contraction immediately follows ventricular, and identifies a junctional or ventricular rhythm with retrograde conduction to the atria (Fig. 9-2), or possibly sinus rhythm with first de-

---

Table 9–1
Events Tending to Hold A-V Valves Open

Recent atrial contraction	Effective when P-R is short (0.08–0.12 second)
Early rapid diastolic filling of ventricles	Effective when cycle length is short, eg, tachycardia
Prolonged diastolic ventricular filling	Effective in stenosis of A-V valve or sizeable L-to-R shunt

---

Table 9–2
Causes of Loud First Sound

Short P-R (0.08–0.12 second)	Valve wide open from recent atrial contraction
Premature beats, tachycardia	Valves wide open from rapid early diastolic filling
Mitral stenosis, tricuspid stenosis, atrial myxoma	Texture of valve; valve maximally open from prolonged ventricular filling
Left-to-right shunts	Prolonged ventricular filling
Exercise, fever, anemia, hyperthyroidism, epinephrine, anxiety, pregnancy, A-V fistula	Forcible ventricular contraction (plus tachycardia)
Thin chest wall, child	Minimal damping effects

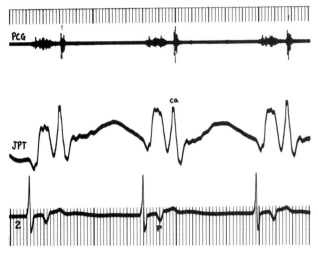

Figure 9–2. Junctional rhythm with retrograde atrial activation (P) following ventricular, and producing cannon waves (ca). Note that the first sound is subdued and unrecognizable at the onset of the systolic murmur.

gree A-V block and an exceptionally long P-R interval. A soft first sound in the presence of a normally loud S2 suggests first degree A-V block.

In assessing variation in the intensity of S1, it is most important to have the patient hold his breath, since respiratory movements themselves may cause appreciable variation in the intensity of heart sounds. The causes of varied intensity of S1 are summarized in Table 9-4, and an example of beat-to-beat variation in the loudness of S1, owing to changing atrioventricular relationships, is illustrated in Figure 9-3.

At the apex, the first component (M1) is normally louder than the second (T1). If T1 is louder than M1, it may provide a useful clue to an atrial septal defect.[8] Other causes of this sign—tricuspid stenosis, right atrial myxoma—are rare.

The comparative intensity of S1 at different areas is sometimes important. If the supposed first sound is louder at the base than at the apex, it is probably an ejection sound (see Chapter 10) rather than S1. If it is louder at the LLSB than at the apex, it suggests an atrial septal defect or tricuspid stenosis.

Table 9–3
Causes of Soft First Sound

Long P-R interval (0.20 + second)	Valves have time to float partly closed since atrial contraction
Mitral regurgitation, tricuspid regurgitation	Normal tensing impossible because of leak
Severe aortic regurgitation	Rapid diastolic filling of ventricle closes mitral valve prematurely
Severe hypertension	Noncompliant ventricle → mitral valve closes prematurely
Shock, heart failure, myocardial infarction, myocarditis, myxedema, infusion of beta blocker	Enfeebled ventricular contraction
Thick chest, emphysema, pericardial effusion	Major damping effects

QUALITY

The quality of S1 may be all-important in recognizing mitral stenosis, whose sharp, tapping, and accentuated first sound (''closing snap'') is often

Table 9–4
Causes of Varying Intensity of First Sound

A-V dissociation: Complete A-V block, ventricular tachycardia; Wenckebach phenomenon	Varying relationship of atrial to ventricular contraction → varying position of A-V valves
Atrial fibrillation	Varying cycle lengths → varying positions of A-V valves; early beats find valves open in rapid filling phase

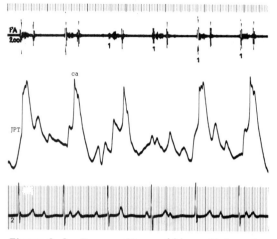

Figure 9–3.   From an 11-year-old boy with inversion of the ventricles, congenital heart block, and consequent A-V dissociation. Note the marked variation in intensity of the four consecutive, labeled (1) first sounds as the atrial to ventricular (P to QRS) relationship changes.

unmistakable. It is best heard at the apex, whereas the closing snap of tricuspid stenosis is better heard at the LLSB. The closing snap is usually preceded by a late diastolic (presystolic) murmur that rises in a crescendo until it is abruptly halted by the sharp impact of the accentuated snap. But the murmur may be inapparent or difficult to elicit, and

then the typical S1 snap is a vital but often unheeded clue.

In circulatory collapse, as from severe infection, hemorrhage, or shock from any cause, the first and second sounds may assume strikingly similar intensity and quality. Combined with tachycardia, which tends to equalize the duration of systole and diastole, the two sounds may be quite indistinguishable and closely simulate the fetal heartbeat (tic-tac rhythm, embryocardia). Embryocardia is a grave sign unless the underlying cause of the circulatory failure can soon be remedied.

REFERENCES

1. Dock W. Heart sounds from Starr-Edwards valves. Circulation 1965;31:801.
2. Leatham A. Splitting of the first and second sounds. Lancet 1954;2:607.
3. Laniado S, et al. Temporal relation of the first heart sound to closure of the mitral valve. Circulation 1973;47:1006.
4. Leatham A, Gray I. Auscultatory and phonocardiographic signs of atrial septal defect. Br Heart J 1956;18:193.
5. Braunwald E, Morrow AG. Sequence of ventricular contraction in human bundle branch block. Am J Med 1957; 23:205.
6. Braunwald E, et al. Effective closure of the mitral valve without atrial systole. Circulation 1966;33:404.
7. Lown B, et al. The syndrome of short P-R interval, normal QRS complex and paroxysmal rapid heart action. Circulation 1952;5:693.
8. Lopez JF, et al. The apical first sound as an aid in the diagnosis of atrial septal defect. Circulation 1962;26:1296.

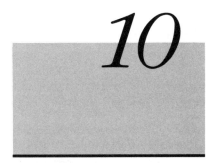

Systolic Sounds (Clicks)

EJECTION CLICKS

If the first sound seems louder at the base than at the apex, it probably isn't the first sound.

Genesis

The ejection sound (or click) is due either to the snappy opening of an abnormal semilunar valve,[1,2] or to the sudden distention of a dilated great artery. That it is not always due to the opening of a valve is proved by its occurrence in the absence of valve leaflets.[3]

The great arteries dilate when there is either distant or proximal obstruction, when they accommodate increased flow, or when there is an intrinsic abnormality of the vessel wall. The causes of great artery dilation are summarized in Table 10-1.

Timing

Correlation of the ejection sound with valve movements both by cinematography[1,2] and echocardiography[4–7] demonstrates that the ejection sound occurs at the moment of maximal semilunar valve opening—at the moment that the opening motion is checked.

The sound occurs within a few hundredths of a second of the beginning of S1, averaging 0.03 to 0.04 second in pulmonic stenosis and idiopathic dilation of the pulmonary artery[8,9]; 0.05 to 0.06 second in aortic stenosis[9,10]; and 0.06 to 0.07 second in severe pulmonary hypertension and persistent truncus.[9,11] The sound approximately coincides with the beginning of the upstroke of the carotid tracing (Fig. 10-1) and with the E point of the ACG.

Table 10–1
Causes of Great Artery Dilation

Mechanism	Aortic Dilation with Ejection Sound	Pulmonary Artery Dilation with Ejection Sound
Distal obstruction	Systemic hypertension Coarctation of aorta	Pulmonary hypertension Segmental pulmonary artery stenosis
Proximal obstruction	Aortic stenosis	Pulmonic stenosis
Increased flow	Aortic regurgitation Tetralogy of Fallot Persistent truncus Eisenmenger syndrome	Atrial septal defect Total anomalous pulmonary venous return
Abnormal wall	Aneurysm of aorta	Idiopathic dilation of pulmonary artery

Clinical Features

The deformed semilunar valve, in the absence of associated arterial dilation—as in mild valve stenosis and bicuspid aortic valve—is frequently associated with an ejection click. The loudness of the sound is clearly related to the mobility of the valve cusps and not to the severity of the valvar stenosis. The bicuspid aortic valve, with no stenosis, may be associated with a loud ejection click that is widely separated from S1.[12] At the base, the click may be considerably louder than the first sound, for which it is readily mistaken; thus clicks may either simulate the second component of a split S1, or, since they can be louder than S1, overshadow it and be mistaken for S1 itself.

The aortic ejection sound (AES) is usually best heard at the apex, but, like all other aortic phenomena, is sometimes better heard to the left of the sternum.[9] The pulmonic ejection sound (PES) is always best heard at the left sternal border, usually in the second interspace; if the associated ejection murmur is loud, the click may be better heard an interspace or two below the site of maximal murmur. The AES usually varies little in intensity with respiration, whereas the PES fades or disappears with inspiration—but there are occasional exceptions to both these generalizations.

Ejection clicks are common in mild stenosis of the semilunar valves,[13,14] and are the rule in congenital aortic stenosis, Eisenmenger syndrome, severe pulmonary hypertension, total anomalous

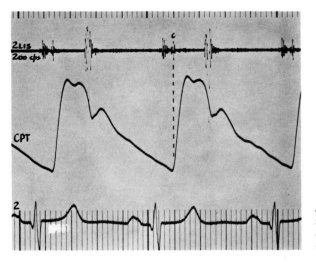

Figure 10–1. From a patient with mitral stenosis, aortic regurgitation, and an ejection click (c). Note coincidence of the ejection click with the start-up of the carotid upstroke.

venous return, idiopathic dilation of the pulmonary artery, and persistent truncus[9]; they are much less common in severe semilunar stenosis (less mobile leaflets), in atrial septal defect, and in the tetralogy of Fallot.[14] On the other hand, the presence of an ejection sound does not rule out severe stenosis being more related to mobility of cusps than to size of orifice.[2] Since the AES is not common in uncomplicated coarctation of the aorta, but is often found with bicuspid aortic valves, the presence of a click in association with coarctation is good evidence of an associated bicuspid valve.

The main importance of ejection sounds is in alerting one to look for causes of semilunar valve disease and/or great artery dilation. In the context of outflow obstruction the presence of a click identifies its level as valvular and verifies leaflet mobility.

MID–LATE SYSTOLIC CLICKS

Later systolic sounds have in the past been ascribed to a variety of cardiac and extracardiac causes, such as pleuropericardial, including adhesive pericarditis, calcific pericardial plaques, and left-sided pneumothorax; systolic expansion of a ventricular aneurysm; aneurysm of the membranous septum; incompetent heterograft valve; atrial myxoma; and costochondral or chondrosternal motion. Nowadays, one accepts a mid–late systolic click as evidence of mitral valve prolapse[15] until it is proved otherwise, especially if it moves with a typical response to some of the maneuvers listed below. Such clicks, however, are sometimes heard in individuals in whom there is no suspicion of any disease.

The late systolic click has assumed greater importance since its recognition as a sign of prolapsing mitral leaflet.[16,17] It may or may not be followed by a late systolic murmur of mitral regurgitation extending up to S2 (Fig. 10-2). Its genesis is uncertain, but it is probably caused by the tautening of the mitral apparatus as the leaflet billows back into the left atrium—an assumption consonant with Reid's original ''chordal snap.''[18] At a critical left ventricular volume, elements of the mitral apparatus become redundant and one or both leaflets prolapse into the left atrium.[19] Some late clicks have appeared only after mitral valvotomy.[16]

Most mid–late clicks are rather faint and high-

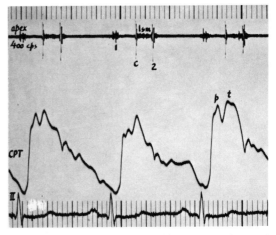

Figure 10–2. From a man in his fifties with mild mitral regurgitation secondary to ischemic myocardial disease. His mid-systolic click (c) is followed by a late systolic murmur (lsm). 1, first heart sound; 2, second heart sound; p, percussion wave, t, tidal wave.

pitched, but an occasional midsystolic sound may be louder than the other heart sounds and even be palpable. Sometimes a cluster of two or three discrete clicks can be distinguished (Figs. 10-3, 10-4).

Mid–late clicks and their associated murmurs may be influenced by a variety of agents and maneuvers (Table 10-2).[19–21] The probable mechanism is related to changes in left ventricular volume: Activities that reduce left ventricular

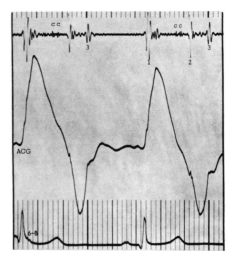

Figure 10–3. A pair of mid-late clicks (c,c) and a loud third sound (3) in a 25-year-old woman with mitral regurgitation.

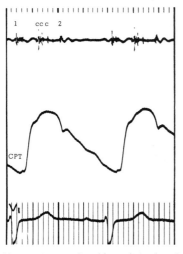

Figure 10–4. A trio of mid-late clicks (c,c,c) in a 48-year-old woman with no evidence of heart disease.

volume, such as standing and the Valsalva maneuver, decrease the time needed to reach the critical volume that determines redundancy, and both the click and the regurgitant murmur occur earlier. Conversely, agents that increase left ventricular volume, such as squatting and phenylephrine, delay the click and onset of murmur.

Table 10–2

Maneuvers/Agents Affecting Mid–Late Click/Murmur

Makes Them Earlier	Makes Them Later
Inspiration	Handgrip
Tilting to 45°	Squatting
Standing	Propranolol
Valsalva maneuver	Phenylephrine
Amyl nitrite	
Isoproterenol	

REFERENCES

1. Ross RS, Criley JM. Cineangiocardiographic studies of the origin of cardiovascular physical signs. Circulation 1964;30:255.
2. Epstein EJ, et al. Cineradiographic studies of the early systolic click in aortic valve stenosis. Circulation 1965;31:842.
3. Ahuja SP, Coles JC. Further observations on the genesis of early systolic clicks. Am J Cardiol 1966;17:291.
4. Mills PG, et al. Echophonocardiographic studies of the contribution of the atrioventricular valves to the first heart sound. Circulation 1976;54:944.
5. Mills P, Craige E. Echophonocardiography. Prog Cardiovasc Dis 1978;20:337.
6. Waider W, Craige E. First heart sound and ejection sounds: echocardiographic and phonocardiographic correlation with valvular events. Am J Cardiol 1975;35:346.
7. Weyman AE, et al. Echocardiographic patterns of pulmonary valve motion in valvular pulmonary stenosis. Am J Cardiol 1974;34:644.
8. Leatham A, Weitzman D. Auscultatory and phonocardiographic signs of pulmonary stenosis. Br Heart J 1957;19:303.
9. Minhas K, Gasul BM. Systolic clicks: a clinical, phonocardiographic, and hemodynamic evaluation. Am Heart J 1959;57:49.
10. Reinhold J, et al. Heart sounds and arterial pulse in congenital aortic stenosis. Br Heart J 1955;17:357.
11. Leatham A, Vogelpoel L. The early systolic sound in dilatation of the pulmonary artery. Br Heart J 1954;16:21.
12. Leech G, et al. Mechanical influence of P-R interval on loudness of first heart sound. Am Heart J 1980;43:138.
13. Wood P. Aortic stenosis. Am J Cardiol 1958;1:553.
14. Leatham A, Gray I. Auscultatory and phonocardiographic signs of pulmonary stenosis. Br Heart J 1956;18:193.
15. Shaver JA, Salerni R. Auscultation of the heart. In: Hurst JW, ed. The heart, ed 7. New York: McGraw Hill, 1990: 188–189.
16. Barlow JB, et al. The significance of late systolic murmurs. Am Heart J 1963;66:443.
17. Barlow JB, Bosman CK. Aneurysmal protrusion of the posterior leaflet of the mitral valve: an auscultatory-electrocardiographic syndrome. Am Heart J 1966;71:166.
18. Reid JVO. Mid-systolic clicks. S Afr Med J 1961;35:353.
19. Mathey DG, et al. The determinants of onset of mitral valve prolapse in the systolic click-late systolic murmur syndrome. Circulation 1976;53:872.
20. Fontana ME, et al. Postural changes in left ventricular and mitral valve dynamics in the systolic click-late systolic murmur syndrome. Circulation 1975;51:165.
21. Winkle RA, et al. Simultaneous echocardiographic-phonocardiographic recordings at rest and during amyl nitrite administration in patients with mitral valve prolapse. Circulation 1975;51:522.

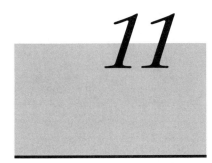

11

The Second Sound

The second sound (S2) plays an important role in diagnosis more often than any other transient. That is why Leatham called it the "key to auscultation of the heart."[1]

S2 approximately coincides with closure of the two semilunar valves, and it was long believed that it was closure of these valves that produced the sound. But meticulous scrutiny, with benefit of echocardiography and other modern techniques, has revealed that the sound does not begin until *after* the valves have closed.[2] Though audible closure has now proved to be a convenient fiction, there is no doubt that the sound is related to valvular closure—in the absence of closure the sound would not occur. And so it is reasonable to think of the two components of S2 as closure-related, and they are still often called "closure" sounds, and conveniently referred to as A2 and P2.

GENESIS

Three events occur in succession: ending of ventricular systole, closure of semilunar valves, and vibration of the closed valve leaflets, infundibu-

lum, and great vessel walls.[3] Some investigators believe that the sound is due mainly, if not entirely, to vibrations of the taut diaphragm created by the closed, compliant valve.[4,5] This is consistent with the fact that in congenital aortic stenosis the aortic component of S2 is preserved, whereas in acquired calcific valve stenosis it is diminished or absent.[6]

CLINICAL FEATURES

You can sometimes "see" S2 as a positive impact halting the recoil of the apex beat. You can often feel it when it is accentuated, as in hypertension of either circuit, or in normal subjects with thin chest walls. Its palpability at the left sternal border often gives the first clue to pulmonary hypertension—but one must always evaluate this palpability in its context: You can usually feel the second sound easily in normal children, and its absence, especially if associated with a systolic thrill, may indicate a semilunar valve stenosis; on the other hand, being unable to feel it in a patient with thick chest wall or emphysema does not rule out pulmonary hypertension. In occasional normal subjects, the sensitive hand can appreciate normal splitting, and sometimes the fixed or persistent splitting of atrial septal defect or of other lesions can be felt.

The best site for listening to and recording both aortic and pulmonic sounds is the 3rd left interspace, where "aortic" and "pulmonic" areas overlap. But one should listen to the second sound at all areas and specifically note:

1. The intensity, normal, increased, or diminished, of each component,
2. The quality of each component, and
3. The presence, absence, degree, and direction of splitting.

Intensity

The loudness of both components of S2 is obviously influenced by extracardiac factors such as thickness of the chest wall and the phase of respiration. Emphysema dampens all heart sounds, including both components of the second sound. Both may be diminished in heart failure, myocardial infarction, pericardial effusion, pulmonary embolism, and other causes of shock. Stenosis of the aortic or pulmonic valves may markedly diminish the respective component.

On the other hand, the early stages of semilunar valve stenosis not uncommonly produce accentuation of A2 or P2, presumably related to change in texture of the still pliant cusps. A2 is often accentuated in aortic regurgitation and in aneurysm of

the ascending aorta. Systemic and pulmonary hypertension, from whatever causes, produce accentuation of A2 and P2, respectively. And don't forget that quite marked accentuation of P2 is a fairly common finding in normal children and young adults.

Splitting

The second sound has undoubtedly been splitting as long as peas and personalities, though it was first recognized by Potain as recently as 1866. Because of higher aortic pressure, the aortic valve normally closes before the pulmonic. In expiration the interval between the two closures is so short that the ear usually cannot separate the two components; with inspiration, the gap widens, and in the majority of hearts the ear can detect this separation.

The interval between the aortic (A2) and pulmonic (P2) components of S2—the A2–P2 interval—normally averages 0.02 second in expiration and 0.04 second in inspiration,[7] and this is regarded as "physiologic" splitting (Fig. 11-1). The human ear finds it easier to recognize the change in the A2–P2 interval from 0.02 to 0.04 second than an equal change from 0.04 to 0.06 second.[8] In some normal subjects, the gap in inspiration may widen up to 0.08 or 0.09 second,[9] and the two components tend to drift apart in held inspiration at any phase.[10] Normal splitting should be evaluated during quiet, or only slightly exaggerated breathing, and is often better heard with the subject sitting.[11]

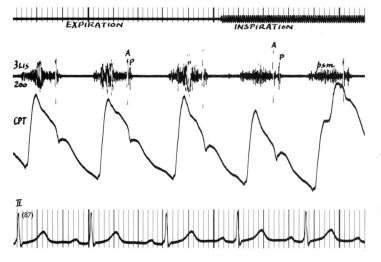

Figure 11–1. Physiologic splitting of S2. During expiration, the components (A,P) are barely separated; in inspiration they have clearly parted. The pansystolic murmur (psm) is of mitral regurgitation. CPT, carotid pulse tracing; 3LIS, recorded at 3rd left interspace; 200, at 200 cycles per second.

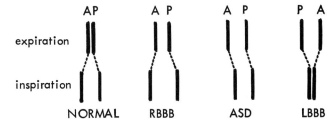

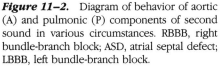

Figure 11–2. Diagram of behavior of aortic (A) and pulmonic (P) components of second sound in various circumstances. RBBB, right bundle-branch block; ASD, atrial septal defect; LBBB, left bundle-branch block.

Patterns of Splitting

Figure 11-2 diagrams the four main varieties of S2 splitting. In the normal heart, aortic (A) and pulmonic (P) sounds are close together in expiration but separate with inspiration: *physiologic splitting*. Their separation results from movements of both A and P relative to S1: A moves "to the left," nearer to S1, while P moves "to the right," away from S1.

In right bundle-branch block (RBBB) A and P are already widely apart in expiration (because of delayed right ventricular activation and consequent late P) and separate more widely with inspiration. They both move "physiologically" but are separated throughout: *persistent splitting*.

In atrial septal defect, A and P also are abnormally apart in expiration because of the increased output of the right ventricle, which delays P. With inspiration, both move about equally to the right, away from S1, retaining the same relationship to each other: *fixed splitting*.

In left bundle-branch block (LBBB), A is delayed so that in expiration it falls appreciably after P and produces perceptible splitting; in inspiration, P moves normally to the right and A to the left, bringing them closer together: *paradoxical* or *reversed splitting*.

Mechanisms of Splitting

The mechanisms responsible for the normal respiratory variation in the interval between the two components of S2 are thought to be as follows: Inspiration decreases intrathoracic and right atrial pressures, leading to increase in venous return to the right heart. The right ventricle, therefore, has more blood to handle and increases its stroke output; this increased output requires a longer ejection time, and this delays pulmonic closure and the subsequent sound-producing events. P2 therefore moves to the right, away from A2, and usually makes the major contribution to their separation; however, movement of A2 to the left, toward S1,

also makes a significant contribution, which various investigators have found to average 14%,[12] 35%,[7] and 44%.[8] According to Harris and Sutton,[13] earlier aortic valve closure contributes 21% to 36%, whereas delayed pulmonic closure contributes 64% to 79%.

The movement of A2 is explained as follows: During inspiration the capacity of the pulmonary vascular bed increases proportionately more than right ventricular output. Pooling in the lungs therefore occurs, with consequent reduction in return of blood to the left atrium, less output from the left ventricle with shortened left ventricular ejection time, and therefore earlier A2.[14,15] Others dispute that the pulmonary vascular capacity increases during inspiration, and even adduce evidence that it decreases.[16] An alternate postulate is that the increased right ventricular output of inspiration takes a few seconds to reach the left heart, by which time expiration is in progress and the left ventricular output rises; that is, the variation in left ventricular output is explained by the time it takes for the right ventricle to hand on its inspiratory load to the left ventricle.[17]

A peculiar form of splitting occurs in constrictive pericarditis, right at the onset of inspiration and lasting only one or two beats.[18] This splitting is apparently due exclusively to movement of A2, with P2 remaining motionless, and presumably results from an abrupt reduction in left ventricular stroke volume (pulsus paradoxus—see Chapter 4). It has also been described in tuberculous pericarditis,[19] and presumably might be seen in any form of restrictive disease.

Timing of Semilunar Valve Closure

The moment at which a semilunar valve closes depends on several factors:

1. Punctuality of ventricular activation—obviously, delay in activation, as in bundle-branch block, delays closure of the ipsilateral valve,

2. Duration of ventricular ejection,
   a. The following prolong ejection and delay closure:
      (1) Systolic overloading—as in aortic stenosis and systemic hypertension on the left side, pulmonic stenosis or hypertension on the right,
      (2) Diastolic overloading—as in mitral regurgitation or patent ductus on the left, atrial septal defect or anomalous pulmonary venous return on the right,
      (3) Ventricular failure,
   b. Double outlet—as in mitral regurgitation or ventricular septal defect (shortens left ventricular ejection and hastens aortic valve closure),
3. Gradient across valve—the higher the gradient, that is, the lower the relative pressure in the great artery concerned, the later the closure, and
4. Elastic recoil of great artery—in idiopathic dilation of the pulmonary artery, lack of elastic recoil postpones the moment of pulmonary valve closure[20]; a similar mechanism affects aortic valve closure.

The effects of such factors are sometimes complex; for example, in mitral regurgitation there may be a tug-of-war between two teams:

Double Outlet	—Shortens LVE	←A
Diastolic Overload	—Lengthens LVE	A→
2° Pulmonary Hypertension	—Lengthens RVE	P→
LV Failure	—Lengthens LVE	A→

The double outlet tends to shorten left ventricular ejection and increase splitting, whereas the diastolic overload tends to lengthen ejection and decrease splitting. Actual measurement of the duration of left ventricular ejection in six patients with severe mitral regurgitation found it to be in the upper range of normal or abnormally prolonged.[21] In the above example there are thus two factors tending to increase and two tending to decrease splitting, so that the net result depends on the relative influence of each.

In semilunar stenosis three factors combine to delay closure of the valve on the affected side. The stenosis itself imposes a systolic overload that lengthens ventricular ejection, whereas the gradient across the valve produces a relatively lower than normal arterial pressure to close the valve; in addition, if significant poststenotic dilation of the great vessel is present, slow recoil may further aggravate the delay.

The hemodynamic consequences of systolic overloading and its consequent effects on the behavior of S2 are summarized in Table 11-1.

Abnormal Forms of Splitting

Fixed Splitting

Fixed splitting may be defined as showing less than 0.01 second movement between the two components with respiration,[12] although for clinical purposes a cruder estimate must serve, and fixity is presumed when the ear can detect virtually no change in the degree of separation of the two components throughout the respiratory cycle. You

---

Table 11–1
Effects of Systolic Overloading on Second Sound

Lesion	Hemodynamic Consequence	Effect on S2
Systemic hypertension	Prolonged LVE	Loud, late A2 with narrow S2 or even reversed splitting
Pulmonic hypertension	Prolonged RVE	Loud, late P2 with normal respiratory variation
Aortic stenosis	Prolonged LVE Low closing pressure	Soft, late A2 with narrow S2 or even reversed splitting
Pulmonic stenosis	Prolonged RVE Low closing pressure	Soft, late P2 with normal or fixed splitting

LVE, left ventricular ejection; RVE, right ventricular ejection.

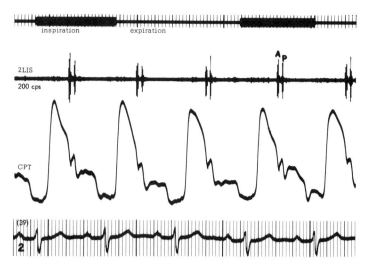

Figure 11–3. Fixed splitting of S2 in a patient with atrial septal defect. The separation of aortic (A) and pulmonic (P) components remains virtually unchanged during inspiration and expiration. CPT, carotid pulse tracing; 2LIS, recorded at 2nd left interspace; cps, cycles per second.

should always verify the presence of supposed fixed splitting with the patient sitting or standing, because some normal subjects manifest fixed splitting when supine, but when erect the movements of the second sound components become physiologic.[22] Splitting may seem to be fixed in the "straight back" syndrome.[23]

The prototypical mediator of fixed splitting is the atrial septal defect, in which the separation of A2 and P2 is little influenced by respiration (Fig. 11-3). Separation is already wide in expiration but does not widen appreciably in the majority with inspiration. There was no measurable alteration in the degree of splitting in 21 of 30 cases[24] or in 87 of 118.[12]

The explanation for this is that there is a reciprocal relationship between vena caval and transseptal inflow into the right atrium: In inspiration, when there is increased caval inflow, there is less room to accommodate the shunted flow, which is therefore reduced; but when caval flow decreases with expiration, more blood is shunted from left atrium to right, and less blood is handed on to the left ventricle. Left ventricular ejection is therefore shortened during expiration, and A2 occurs earlier. The net effect is that P2 and A2, instead of approaching and receding from each other like hands playing an accordion, move back and forth in the same direction like hands agitating a cocktail shaker. Evidence confirming the waxing and waning of the shunt is that the oxygen content of pulmonary artery blood during inspiration is higher than during expiration: The mean oxygen content in eight patients was 88.8% in expiration and 85.2% in inspiration.[12] When significant pulmonary hypertension complicates an atrial septal defect, it reduces the left-to-right shunt and narrows the splitting, which is no longer fixed.[25]

Although fixed splitting is characteristic of atrial septal defect, it is found elsewhere as well (Table 11-2). It is, of course, also found in the other left-to-right shunt at the atrial level, anomalous pulmonary venous return; and it is sometimes found in pulmonic stenosis, ventricular septal defect,[26] and in mitral stenosis with high pulmonary vascular resistance[27]; in mitral regurgitation with right ventricular failure, and in RBBB or LBBB with right ventricular failure[10]; in idiopathic dilation of the pulmonary artery,[28] and in African cardiomyopathy.[19]

Table 11–2
Causes of Fixed Splitting

Atrial septal defect

Anomalous pulmonary venous return

Pulmonic stenosis

Ventricular septal defect[24]

Mitral stenosis with high PVR[25]

Mitral regurgitation with RV failure

RBBB or LBBB with RV failure[8]

Idiopathic dilation of pulmonary artery[26]

Cardiomyopathy[17]

PVR, pulmonary vascular resistance.

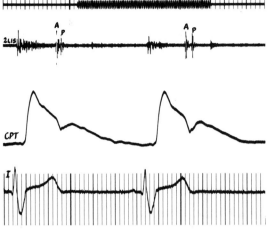

Figure 11–4. Persistent splitting of S2. Aortic (A) and pulmonic (P) components of S2 are already widely split at end of expiration, and open wider during inspiration. Note pattern of RBBB in ECG. 2LIS, recorded at 2nd left interspace; CPT, carotid pulse tracing.

Persistent Splitting

When the splitting is "persistent," the split is already evident in expiration and widens still further in inspiration. Far and away the most common cause of this form of splitting is RBBB (Fig. 11-4), but it can be found in many other situations (Table 11-3), including any of the conditions that can produce fixed splitting (Table 11-2). It is a feature of ectopic rhythms arising from the left ventricle[29] (Fig. 11-5), and it may result from anything that prolongs right ventricular ejection—outflow obstruction, pulmonary hypertension, increased right ventricular output, or impaired right ventricular efficiency—or that shortens left ventricular ejection.

Paradoxical Splitting

When splitting is "paradoxical" or "reversed," the exemplar is LBBB (Fig. 11-6), but other conditions that produce asynchrony of ventricular activation, with activation of the right before the left ventricle—ectopic rhythms arising from the right ventricle,[28] or preexcitation of the right ventricle in the Wolff-Parkinson-White syndrome[30]—may also cause reversed splitting (Table 11-3). So may numerous conditions that prolong left ventricular ejection enough to result in A2 falling perceptibly after P2, such as severe aortic stenosis and/or regurgitation, and systemic hypertension. Paradoxical splitting was present in 10 of 23 patients with aortic stenosis and in 10 of 29 patients with patent ductus.[31] It may also be heard in ischemic heart disease (in the absence of LBBB), especially after exercise or during acute episodes of angina or infarction.[32,33] Indeed, any lesion that materially impairs left ventricular function, such as rheumatic or viral myocarditis,[34] or primary cardiomyopathy, may produce paradoxical splitting. Dickerson and

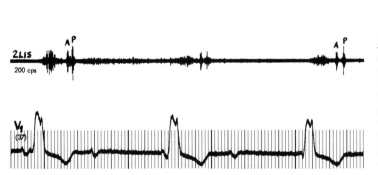

Figure 11–5. Persistent splitting in a patient with complete AV block during idioventricular rhythm arising in left ventricle. In ECG note typical pattern of left ventricular ectopy. At end of expiration, A and P are already widely split; during inspiration they become even more widely separated. 2LIS, recorded at 2nd left interspace; cps, cycles per second.

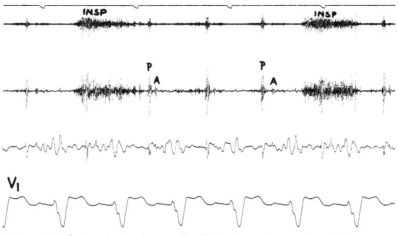

Figure 11–6. Paradoxical (reversed) splitting in a patient with LBBB. Upper two channels are high-frequency phonocardiograms—inspiratory artifact is fortuitously recorded in both channels. The pulmonic component (P) of S2 precedes aortic (A), and as expiration proceeds their separation increases.

Nelson drew particular attention to its value as an early and sometimes solitary sign of left ventricular embarrassment of any sort: "Unexplained paradoxical splitting may be a valuable bedside indicator of left ventricular dysfunction."[34]

Caution: As the lungs fill with air in inspiration, the heart sounds tend to become softer; an already soft P2, therefore, may disappear with inspiration and simulate reversed splitting—both sounds being heard in expiration but only a single sound in inspiration.

Paradoxical Persistent Splitting

Paradoxical splitting usually implies that S2 is audibly split in expiration but becomes single in inspiration—the converse of normal. In some situations, however, the second sound may remain split throughout the cardiac cycle—as in persistent splitting—but be more widely split in expiration than in inspiration; in such cases the split is both paradoxical and persistent. This form of splitting has been described in undeveloped right ventricle

---

Table 11–3
Causes and Mechanisms of Persistent and Paradoxical Splitting

	Persistent	Paradoxical
Asynchronous Ventricular Activation		
Block	RBBB	LBBB
Pre-excitation		WPW, type B
Ectopy	LV rhythms	RV rhythms
Prolonged Ventricular Ejection on One Side		
Systolic overloading	Pulmonic stenosis, pulmonary hypertension	Aortic stenosis, systemic hypertension
Diastolic overloading	Atrial septal defect, anomalous pulmonary venous drainage, ventricular septal defect, pulmonic insufficiency	Patent ductus, aortic insufficiency
Myocardial malfunction	RV failure	LV failure, angina, myocardial infarction, myocarditis, cardiomyopathy
Shortened Ventricular Ejection on Other Side		
Double outlet	Mitral insufficiency, ventricular septal defect	Tricuspid insufficiency

with pulmonic stenosis,[35] and in patients with giant left atria.[36]

Absence of Splitting

The unsplit or "single" S2 can provide useful information. It is observed when:

1. One component is unduly diminished, as in severe aortic or pulmonic stenosis, and severe tetralogy of Fallot,
2. The aortic component is enveloped by a long systolic murmur, as in ventricular septal defect, patent ductus, severe pulmonic stenosis, and ruptured sinus of Valsalva,
3. There is only one functioning semilunar valve, as in persistent truncus, pulmonary atresia, and in some cases of tricuspid atresia,
4. Pressures in the two ventricles are equal, as in single ventricle and the Eisenmenger syndrome, and
5. Abnormal posture of the heart and great vessels removes the pulmonic valve from its usual proximity to the chest wall and places the aortic valve anteriorly, as in transposition of the great vessels and tetralogy of Fallot with marked overriding.

Final Thoughts About the Detection of Splitting

Splitting of S2, like gold, is where you find it![34]

Although the aortic component of S2 is often reputed to be best heard at the "aortic" area, it is often far better heard to the left of the sternum than to the right. The pulmonic component, unless unusually loud, is not well heard at either the aortic or apical areas, but is quite often better heard at the 3rd or even 4th interspace than at the 2nd. Emphatically, then, the quest for splitting should not be abandoned if you cannot detect it at the "pulmonic" area: You must go prospecting in the neighborhood. In pulmonic stenosis, for example, you may not hear P2 where the murmur is loudest, but if you get out of range of the deafening murmur, P2 may come into earshot.

Because the second sound is mainly a high-frequency phenomenon, the diaphragm of the stethoscope is recommended. But the diaphragm can be a handicap at times: As a larger chestpiece, it gathers more sound and makes the already loud murmur even louder. If, therefore, there is a deafening murmur at the left upper sternal border, the components of S2 may be easier to hear if the murmur is attenuated by a smaller diaphragm—the firmly pressed bell.

REFERENCES

1. Leatham A. The second heart sound, key to auscultation of the heart. Acta Cardiol 1964;19:395.
2. MacCanon DM, et al. Direct detection and timing of aortic valve closure. Circ Res 1964;14:387.
3. Luisada AA. The second heart sound in normal and abnormal conditions. Am J Cardiol 1971;28:150.
4. Stein PD, Sabbah HN. Origin of the second heart sound: clinical relevance of new observations. Am J Cardiol 1978; 41:108.
5. Stein PD, Sabbah H. Second heart sound: mechanism and clinical utility of auscultatory changes. American Journal of Noninvasive Cardiology 1987;1:68.
6. Sabbah HN, et al. Determinants of the amplitude of the aortic component of the second heart sound in aortic stenosis. Am J Cardiol 1978;41:830.
7. Castle RF, Jones KL. The mechanism of respiratory variation in splitting of the second sound. Circulation 1961; 24:180.
8. Shafter HA. Splitting of the second heart sound. Am J Cardiol 1960;6:1013.
9. Ehlers KH, et al. Wide splitting of the second heart sound without demonstrable heart disease. Am J Cardiol 1969; 23:690.
10. Perloff JK, Harvey WP. Mechanisms of fixed splitting of the second heart sound. Circulation 1958;18:998.
11. Hall RJ. Auscultation: clinical evaluation and decision making. Houston: Texas Heart Institute, 1988:4–8.
12. Aygen MM, Braunwald E. The splitting of the second heart sound in normal subjects and in patients with congenital heart disease. Circulation 1962;25:328.
13. Harris A, Sutton C. Second heart sound in normal subjects. Br Heart J 1968;30:739.
14. Lauson HD, et al. The influence of the respiration on the circulation in man. Am J Med 1946;1:315.
15. Wiggers CJ. Physiology in health and disease, ed 5. Philadelphia: Lea & Febiger, 1950:659.
16. Visscher MB. The capacity changes in the pulmonary vascular bed with the respiratory cycle. Fed Proc 1948; 7:128.
17. Dornhorst AC, et al. Respiratory variation in blood pressure. Circulation 1952;6:553.
18. Beck W, et al. Splitting of the second heart sound in constrictive pericarditis, with observations on the mechanism of pulsus paradoxus. Am Heart J 1962;64:765.
19. Reid JVO: The second heart sound in biventricular failure due to African cardiomyopathy. Am Heart J 1964; 68:38.
20. Schrire V, Vogelpoel L. The role of the dilated pulmonary artery in abnormal splitting of the second heart sound. Am Heart J 1962;63:501.
21. Nixon PGF, Wagner GR. The duration of left ventricular systole in mitral incompetence. Br Heart J 1962;24:464.
22. Breen WJ, Rekate AC. Effect of posture on splitting of the second heart sound. JAMA 1960;173:106.
23. deLeon AC, et al. The straight back syndrome: clinical cardiovascular manifestations. Circulation 1965; 32:193.
24. Leatham A, Gray I. Auscultatory and phonocardiographic signs of atrial septal defect. Br Heart J 1956;18:193.
25. Leonard JJ, Kroetz FW. Examination of the heart: Part 4. auscultation. New York: American Heart Association, 1966:14.
26. Harris C, et al. "Fixed" splitting of the second heart sound in ventricular septal defect. Br Heart J 1971; 33:428.

27. Kardilinos A. The second heart sound. Am Heart J 1962; 64:610.
28. Karnegis JN, Wang Y. Phonocardiogram of idiopathic dilatation of the pulmonary artery. Circulation 1963; 28:747.
29. Haber E, Leatham A. Splitting of heart sounds from ventricular asynchrony in bundle branch block, ventricular ectopic beats and artificial pacing. Br Heart J 1965; 27:691.
30. Zuberbuhler JR, Bauersfeld SR. Paradoxical splitting of the second heart sound in the Wolff-Parkinson-White syndrome. Am Heart J 1965;70:595.
31. Gray I. Paradoxical splitting of the second sound. Br Heart J 1956;18:21.
32. Wood P. Acute and subacute coronary insufficiency. Br Med J 1961;1:1780.
33. Yurchak PM, Gorlin R. Paradoxical splitting of the second heart sound in coronary heart disease. N Engl J Med 1963;269:741.
34. Dickerson RB, Nelson WP. Paradoxical splitting of the second heart sound: an informative clinical notation. Am Heart J 1964;67:410.
35. Williams JCP, et al. Underdeveloped right ventricle and pulmonic stenosis. Am J Cardiol 1963;11:458.
36. Leachman RD, et al. Narrowed splitting of the second heart sound upon inspiration in patients with giant left atrium. Chest 1971;60:151.

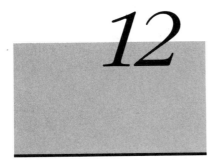

Opening Snaps and Tumor Plops

THE OPENING SNAP

As our attention moves into diastole, the earliest transient likely to interrupt the normal diastolic hush is the opening snap (OS), so named by Thayer in 1908. First recognized by Bouillaud in 1835, Potain called it "claquement d'ouverture de la mitrale" in 1844. An even earlier diastolic sound of uncertain origin and rare occurrence has been recorded in mitral valve prolapse.[1]

Genesis

Just as the first heart sound is not strictly due to valve closure, so the OS is not strictly due to opening. As diastole begins, the ventricle relaxes and the pressure within abruptly falls. When it has fallen below atrial pressure, the A-V ring and valve are drawn toward the ventricle. The snap occurs at the moment this descent is checked,[2] and the sound is thought to be due to the sudden deceleration of the mass of left atrial blood[3,4] and its loudness correlates with the volume of the left

atrium[5] and with the mobility of the mitral apparatus. In patients with mobile leaflets, echocardiography demonstrates that the snap occurs at the moment of maximal opening of the anterior mitral leaflet.[6,7]

Timing

The snap follows the aortic component of the S2 by a variable interval (the A2–OS, or simply the 2–OS interval), depending, among other things, on the severity of the valvular stenosis. If this is severe, the atrial pressure is high, atrial and ventricular pressures equalize more rapidly in early diastole, the valve apparatus begins and ends its downward descent sooner, and the 2–OS interval is comparatively short (0.04–0.06 second). If the stenosis is mild, or after successful valvotomy, the 2–OS interval is longer (0.09–0.12 second).[8,9] Unfortunately, the timing of the OS is also influenced by other factors besides the degree of stenosis, and so the 2–OS interval is not a reliable guide to severity.[10,11] When cycle length varies,

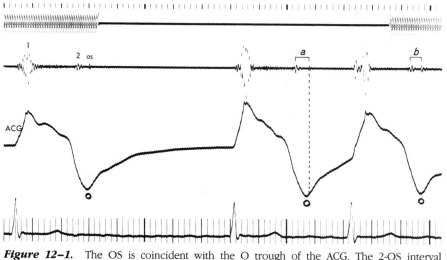

Figure 12–1.   The OS is coincident with the O trough of the ACG. The 2-OS interval **(A)** after a long cycle is longer than that **(B)** after a short cycle.

as in atrial fibrillation, the 2–OS varies with it: after a long cycle the 2–OS interval widens with it, and vice versa.[12] A short cycle gives the atrium less chance to decompress itself through the stenosed valve, so that at the end of a short cycle the A-V pressure difference ("gradient") is higher and atrial pressure remains high during the ensuing systole. At the beginning of diastole, therefore, the mitral valve opens earlier and produces a shorter 2–OS interval (Fig. 12-1).

Clinical Features

The OS is present in 75% to 90%[13,14] of patients with mitral stenosis, and is best heard in the "su-

pramammary area"—a point above and a little medial to the left male nipple[13]—or between the apex and the left sternal border. It radiates widely and may be heard over the entire precordium. If you begin auscultation at the base, you will often pick it up first in the 2nd interspace, left or right. As it is often well heard in the pulmonic area, it was long mistaken for the second component of a widely split second sound. It can sometimes be felt, and meticulous palpation may identify it as the trough of apical retraction (0-point in Fig. 12-1), in contrast with the later lift of S3.

The OS seems relatively high-pitched and is best heard with the diaphragm, yet spectral analysis determines that its peak frequency is in the moderately low range (50–90 Hz).[5] The OS of

Table 12–1
Clues for Differentiating OS from P2 and S3

2nd Component of S2 (P2)	Whereas the OS	Third Sound	Whereas the OS
1. Is loudest at LUSB	1. Is loudest between apex and LLSB	1. Is lower pitched	1. Is higher pitched
2. Separates from A2 on inspiration	2. Tends to close with S2 on inspiration	2. Occurs later	2. Occurs earlier
	3. Opens on standing	3. Is best heard at apex	3. Is best heard nearer sternum
		4. Is often louder on inspiration	4. Is louder on expiration

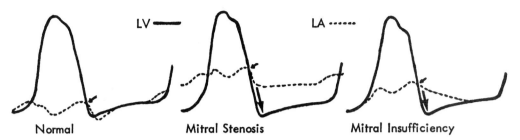

Figure 12–2. Simultaneous left atrial (LA) and left ventricular (LV) pressure curves. LA and LV pressures equalize when their curves cross on the downstroke of the LV curve (small arrow). In the normal, virtually no pressure difference develops. But in both mitral stenosis and mitral regurgitation, there is an abrupt descent of ventricular pressure to well below atrial (large arrow).

mitral stenosis must be distinguished from the second component of a widely split S2 and from S3; helpful pointers are summarized in Table 12-1.

Significance

Paul Wood[15] regarded the OS as a good sign of dominant stenosis and "an excellent talisman" against the presence of serious regurgitation. But the OS undoubtedly depends on other things besides stenosis of the valve, and is common in dominant mitral regurgitation, where it seems more related to mobility and pliancy of the aortic cusp of the mitral valve "moving abruptly under the influence of a high left atrial pressure."[16,17]

It is perhaps surprising that in mitral regurgitation, even in the complete absence of valvular obstruction, the pressure in the overfilled left atrium is often significantly elevated in early diastole. This means that early diastolic ventricular pressure drops markedly below atrial pressure with a sizeable A-V pressure difference (Fig. 12-2). This pressure difference drives the mitral ring vigorously toward the ventricular cavity, and when this vigorous descent is abruptly checked, a snap may be generated.

Presumably the changed texture of the diseased valve leaflets also favors the production of a snap. But opening snaps are not the monopoly of sick valves: The normal mitral valve may snap when flow across it is excessive, as in thyrotoxicosis, complete A-V block, patent ductus, ventricular septal defect, after a successful Blalock-Taussig shunt, or in tricuspid atresia with large atrial septal defect.[16,18,19]

Snaps of the tricuspid valve may appear in tricuspid stenosis,[20–22] but are neither so constant, so loud, or so diagnostically important as mitral snaps. Unlike the mitral OS, the tricuspid snap

becomes louder with inspiration. With excessive flow through the tricuspid valve, as with an atrial septal defect, an OS may occur,[23–25] but careful timing suggests to some that this is a ventricular filling sound rather than an OS.[26]

Two snaps, mitral first and then tricuspid, are sometimes audible in the same patient,[27] but their separation is virtually impossible at the bedside, and depends on careful measurement in simultaneous sound recordings.

THE TUMOR PLOP

This phenomenon is considered here because it has the same timing as the opening snap, occurring 0.08 to 0.12 second after the beginning of S2.[28] It was named by Abbott[29] in 1962, and a number of cases have been described.[30–32] The plop is coincident with the deepest excursion of the atrial myxoma through the A-V valve into the ventricle, and is therefore thought to be caused by tensing of the tumor's retaining stalk. The plop may be produced by a mobile myxoma in either atrium. Its importance lies in the likely confusion with an opening snap and in the consequent contentment with the diagnosis of mitral stenosis. You can quickly resolve any doubt by visualizing the agile tumor by echocardiography.

REFERENCES

1. Bonner AJ, et al. Early diastolic sound associated with mitral valve prolapse. Arch Intern Med 1976;136:347.
2. Ross RS, Criley JM. Cineangiocardiographic studies of the origin of cardiovascular physical signs. Circulation 1964;30:255.
3. McCall BW, Price JL. Movement of the mitral cusps in relation to the first heart sound and opening snap in patients with mitral stenosis. Br Heart J 1967;29:417.

4. Thompson ME, et al. Sound, pressure and motion correlates in mitral stenosis. Am J Med 1970;49:436.

5. Longhini C, et al. The genesis of the opening snap in mitral stenosis: correlations between spectral analysis and echocardiographic data. American Journal of Noninvasive Cardiology 1987;1:373.

6. Friedman NJ. Echocardiographic studies of mitral valve motion: genesis of the opening snap in mitral stenosis. Am Heart J 1970;80:177.

7. Salerni R, et al. Pressure and sound correlates of the mitral valve echocardiogram in mitral stenosis. Circulation 1978;56:119.

8. Mounsey P. The opening snap of mitral stenosis. Br Heart J 1953;15:135.

9. Tavel ME. Opening snaps: mitral and tricuspid. American Heart Association Monograph #46. New York: American Heart Association, 1975:85.

10. Haring OM, et al. The mitral patient before and after surgery. Am Heart J 1956;52:18.

11. Proctor MH, et al. The phonocardiogram in mitral valvular disease: a correlation of Q-1 and 2-OS intervals. Am J Med 1958;24:861.

12. Julian D, Davies LG. Heart sounds and intracardiac pressures in mitral stenosis. Br Heart J 1957;19:486.

13. Reddy PS, et al. Normal and abnormal heart sounds in cardiac diagnosis: II. diastolic sounds. Curr Prob Cardiol 1985;10:36.

14. Messer AL. The effect of cycle length on the time of occurrence of the first heart sound and the opening snap in mitral stenosis. Circulation 1951;4:576.

15. Wood P. An appreciation of mitral stenosis. Br Med J 1954;1:1051 and 1113.

16. Nixon PGF, et al. The opening snap in mitral incompetence. Br Heart J 1960;22:395.

17. Perloff JK, Harvey WP. Auscultatory and phonocardiographic manifestations of pure mitral regurgitation. Prog Cardiovasc Dis 1962;5:172.

18. Neill C, Mounsey P. Auscultation in patent ductus arteriosus. Br Heart J 1958;20:61.

19. Millward DK, et al. Echocardiographic studies to explain opening snaps in presence of nonstenotic mitral valves. Am J Cardiol 1973;31:64.

20. Kossmann CE. The opening snap of the tricuspid valve: a physical sign of tricuspid stenosis. Circulation 1955;11:378.

21. Perloff JK, Harvey WP. Clinical recognition of tricuspid stenosis. Circulation 1960;22:346.

22. Bousvaros GA, Stubbington D. Some auscultatory and phonocardiographic features of tricuspid stenosis. Circulation 1964;29:26.

23. Leatham A, Gray I. Auscultatory and phonocardiographic signs of atrial septal defect. Br Heart J 1956;18:193.

24. Aravanis C. Opening snap in relative tricuspid stenosis: report of two cases of atrial septal defect. Am J Cardiol 1963;12:408.

25. Tavel ME, et al. Opening snap of the tricuspid valve in atrial septal defect. Am Heart J 1970;80:550.

26. Baritt DW, et al. Heart sounds and pressures in atrial septal defect. Br Heart J 1965;27:90.

27. Luisada AA, et al. Double (mitral and tricuspid) opening snap in patients with valvular lesions. Am J Cardiol 1965;16:800.

28. Martinez-Lopez JI. Sounds of the heart in diastole. Am J Cardiol 1974;34:594.

29. Abbott OA, et al. Primary tumors and pseudotumors of the heart. Ann Surg 1962;155:855.

30. Pitt A, et al. Myxoma of the left atrium: hemodynamic and phonocardiographic consequences of sudden tumor movement. Circulation 1967;36:408.

31. Zitnik RS, et al. Left atrial myxoma: phonocardiographic clues to diagnosis. Am J Cardiol 1969;23:588.

32. Nasser WK, et al. Atrial myxoma: II. phonocardiographic, echocardiographic, hemodynamic and angiographic features in nine cases. Am Heart J 1972;83:810.

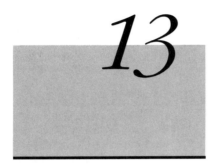

The Third Sound

The next event in diastole that may catch the ear is the third heart sound (S3). Contrasts between the opening snap and S3 were presented in Table 12-1 and are expanded in Table 13-1.

GENESIS

Everyone agrees that S3 coincides with the climax of early diastolic filling of the ventricles, and it occurs during the rapid filling wave between "O" and "F" points in the apexcardiogram (ACG). Its exact mechanism of production, however, is still controversial[1,2]: Is it generated in the valve apparatus of the ventricular myocardium? Or is it caused by impact of the heart against the chest wall?

Those who favored a *valvular* genesis pointed to the fact that the valvular apparatus consists of "structures easily set into audible vibration,"[3] or that when the valvular apparatus was removed and a prosthetic valve substituted the S3 disappeared.[4,5] Subscribers to this theory thought that the sound was probably produced by sudden taut-

ening of cusps and chordae with ascent of the mitral annulus as the inrush of blood abruptly elongates the left ventricle in early diastole,[6,7] producing a palpable shock that can be felt as the F-point in the ACG (Fig. 13-1).

On the other hand, there is conflicting evidence that the chief resonator is the *ventricular muscle*.[8] Others have adduced evidence that the sound source is *impact* of the left ventricle against the chest wall.[1,2,9]

Regardless of which tissues are the major source of the sound, certain factors seem clearly related to its intensity: The volume and the velocity of the blood flow across the mitral valve, and the degree of ventricular relaxation[10]; the greater the volume, the greater the velocity of inflow, and the less complete the myocardial relaxation, the louder the sound; and the sound appears to coincide with the rapid deceleration of the inflowing torrent.[11]

Any explanation of the mechanism must account for both the normal S3 and the S3 gallop. They both occur at the moment when ventricular pressure dips sharply below atrial in early diastole. As ventricular filling approaches completion, there

Table 13–1
Comparisons and Contrasts Between Opening Snap and Third Sound

	Characteristics of S3	Characteristics of OS
Pitch	Low-pitched, dull	Higher pitched, sharp
Preferred chestpiece	Bell	Diaphragm
Timing	Later	Earlier
Optimal site	Apex	Supramammary area
Relationship to apex impulse	At peak of F-point	At trough of O-point
Respiration	Often louder on inspiration	Louder on expiration; may approach S2 on inspiration
Exercise, etc.	Louder	
Turning on left	Louder	
Phenylephrine	Louder	Little or no effect
Tourniquets, standing	Abolishes	
Carotid sinus stimulation	Abolishes	

is an abrupt deceleration of the filling flood, the kinetic energy of which is converted to vibratory energy, and the third sound is generated.[8] Thus, its appearance and intensity are influenced by the following interdependent factors: Atrial pressure, ventricular pressure, volume and rate of inflow, and compliance of the ventricle.

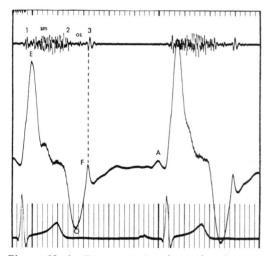

Figure 13–1. From a patient with mitral regurgitation showing the relationship of apical events (O-point and F-point) to opening snap (os) and third heart sound (3). sm, systolic murmur.

THE NORMAL THIRD SOUND

The normal S3 is heard in most if not all children, many teenagers, and in fewer—perhaps between 10% and 35%—young adults.[12] It is probably never audible after 40 years, though it was *recordable* in nearly 40% of adults between the ages of 40 and 62 years.[13] Its diminution or disappearance with advancing age has been attributed to decreased ventricular wall compliance, resulting in reduced early ventricular filling with consequent reduced deceleration of inflow.[13]

It occurs 0.14 to 0.22 second (average 0.15 second) after the beginning of S2 (Fig. 13-2). It is low-pitched and therefore best heard with the bell lightly applied. It is usually loudest at the apex, and turning the patient on to his left side approximately doubles its intensity.[3] Its response to respiration varies, but it often becomes louder with inspiration (Fig. 13-3). Exercise, raising arms and legs, inspiration and abdominal compression, all of which increase return of venous blood to the right heart, make the normal S3 louder.[14]

There are some unsettled points about the respiratory behavior of S3. The sound presumably can be produced in either or both ventricles, and, supposedly, that produced in the left ventricle is best heard at the apex, whereas that produced in the right ventricle is best heard at the left lower sternal border. But the normal S3 at the apex often

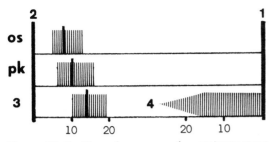

Figure 13–2. Time of occurrence (approximate range and average) of the diastolic transients. os, opening snap; pk, pericardial knock; 1,2,3,4, the four heart sounds; 10 and 20, 0.10 and 0.20 seconds after onset of S2 or before onset of S1. Limits to the left obviously cannot be set for S4 since its distance from S1 is dependent on the P–R interval.

waxes with inspiration and wanes with expiration (Fig. 13-3), and this suggests a right-sided origin. Furthermore, patients with severe mitral stenosis (which prevents rapid filling of the LV) and a loud S3 at the apex, often turn out to have tricuspid regurgitation as well[15]; one wonders if, in those patients in whom the sound is augmented by inspiration, perhaps the apex is formed by the RV and we are in fact hearing the right ventricular S3. This, however, leaves unexplained the inspiratory waxing of S3 when it is presumably a left ventricular event, as in pure mitral regurgitation.[16]

Fever, pregnancy, anemia, thyrotoxicosis, and mitral regurgitation all increase the volume and/or velocity of transmitral flow; left ventricular failure limits myocardial relaxation. Aortic regurgitation is often associated with a pathologic third sound, but probably only when it has produced left ventricular dysfunction; it may therefore be a useful sign in gauging prognosis and determining the time for surgery.[17]

GALLOP RHYTHM

It appears to be widely believed that normal and abnormal third sounds have identical mechanisms; auscultatorily they are certainly indistinguishable, and they are generally differentiated by the company they keep. When S3 is abnormal it becomes a protodiastolic or S3 "gallop."

Like many a medical term, "gallop" suffers from inadequate definition. Its meaning varies with the whim or logic of the user. It is variably applied to:

1. Any three sounds regardless of rate or cadence (this includes systolic "gallops" due to systolic clicks, triple cadences caused by normal third sounds or by opening snaps, etc.),
2. Any three-beat cadence that sounds like a gallop (this allows any added sound to complete the cadence, but obviously requires a tachycardia),
3. Any abnormal triple rhythm (this excludes the physiologic S3, but permits any abnormal sounds at any rate—"a gallop is a gallop regardless of the ventricular rate"),[18] and
4. An abnormal triple rhythm caused by the addition only of either S3 or S4, or both (this excludes systolic gallops and the triple cadences due to opening snaps, etc.).

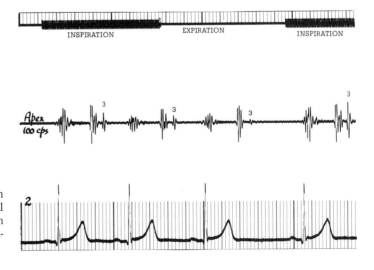

Figure 13–3. PCG recorded at apex in a normal boy. Notice how the normal third sound (3) progressively wanes with expiration and gets louder with inspiration.

Whichever use is espoused, "gallop" has become firmly attached to triple cardiac cadences, despite the fact that the equine gallop is a quadruple rhythm and it is the canter that provides the three-beat cadence![19] In view of prevalent ambiguity, but in deference to common custom, it is expedient to stick to "triple rhythm" as the generic term[20] for all three-beat cadences, and to reserve "gallop" for obviously pathologic triple rhythms that genuinely resemble the hoofbeats of the hurrying ungulate. Certainly few can take exception to this application of the term; it is here applied only to S3, S4, and summation gallops.

THIRD SOUND GALLOP
(SYNONYMS: S3, PROTODIASTOLIC, AND VENTRICULAR GALLOP)

It is almost universally agreed that the early diastolic gallop is a pathologic exaggeration of the normal S3. Clinical distinction from the normal sound is not always easy, and so the significance of an S3 is often arrived at by appraising its bedfellow: A third sound in a child with an otherwise normal heart is a normal S3, whereas a third sound in a 60-year-old with known heart disease is obviously an S3 gallop, although timing, tone, and intensity may be similar. Having the patient stand may be helpful, since it rapidly and regularly abolishes the normal third sound, whereas the abnormal one persists.[21]

The same things that augment the normal third sound—maneuvers that increase venous return, turning on the left side—also accentuate the gallop sound. Vasoconstrictors, such as phenylephrine, which increase the central blood volume, likewise intensify the sound.[22] The ventricular gallop may be accentuated and become audible for a few beats only after a ventricular extrasystole.[18] In differentiating a ventricular gallop from an opening snap or the second component of a widely split S2, carotid sinus stimulation[23] or venous pooling[24] may be helpful: These maneuvers abolish a ventricular gallop but leave the other two transients unaffected.

Although gallop rhythm has been characterized as "one of the two death rattles of the left ventricle" (the other being pulsus alternans), this is true only when it is associated with a failing myocardium owing to chronic irreversible disease; in this

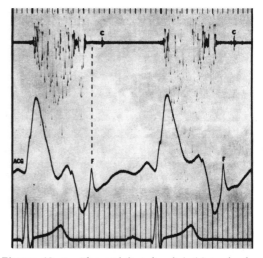

Figure 13–4. The mid-diastolic click (c) is clearly a high-frequency transient and occurs well after the F-point in the ACG—too late to be a third sound.

context a gallop usually presages death within a year or two. But gallops associated with exuberant flow, as with regurgitant valvular disease, and reversible states such as anemia and thyrotoxicosis, are attended by a much less dismal prognosis. The several clinical causes of both ventricular (S3) and atrial (S4) gallops are together tabulated in Chapter 14.

PERICARDIAL KNOCK

This variant of S3 is heard in constrictive pericarditis, and is presumably due to the sudden arrest of ventricular filling when the unyielding pericardium halts ventricular relaxation.[25] It may produce the loudest of all third sounds.[26] It tends to occur somewhat earlier (0.09–0.12 second after aortic closure)[25] and to be higher pitched than the usual S3 or ventricular gallop, and therefore may be readily mistaken for an opening snap. It was audible in 18 of 22 patients with constrictive pericarditis,[26] in whom the sound persisted after surgical decompression but occurred later, at the time of the usual S3. As with other third sounds, the pericardial knock may increase in intensity with inspiration, as Potain noted as long ago as 1846. It may also be brought to light or accentuated by squatting or the infusion of phenylephrine.[27]

MID-DIASTOLIC CLICKS

Clicks and sounds in mid-diastole have been described, but they are rare and their significance is uncertain. They are high-pitched and occur later than S3 (Fig. 13-4).

REFERENCES

1. Shaver JA, et al. Genesis of the physiologic third heart sound. American Journal of Noninvasive Cardiology 1987;1:39.
2. Shaver JA, Salerni R. Auscultation of the heart. In: Hurst JW, ed. The heart. 7th ed. New York: McGraw Hill, 1990:200.
3. Dock W, Grandell F, Taubman F. The physiologic third heart sound: its mechanism and relation to protodiastolic gallop. Am Heart J 1955;50:449.
4. Ikram H, et al. Genesis of diastolic sounds in mitral incompetence. Br Heart J 1969;31:762.
5. Fleming JS. Evidence for a mitral valve origin of the left ventricular third heart sound. Br Heart J 1969;31:192.
6. Nixon PGF. The third heart sound in mitral regurgitation. Br Heart J 1961;23:677.
7. Nixon PGF. The genesis of the third heart sound. Am Heart J 1963;65:712.
8. Timmis AJ. The third heart sound. Br Med J 1987; 294:326.
9. Reddy PS, et al. The genesis of gallop sounds: investigation by quantitative phono- and apexcardiography. Circulation 1981;63:922.
10. Van de Werf F, et al. Diastolic properties of the left ventricle in normal adults and in patients with third heart sound. Circulation 1984;69:1070.
11. Ozawa Y, et al. Origin of the third heard sound: II. studies in human subjects. Circulation 1983;67:399.
12. Sloan AW, et al. Incidence of the physiological third heart sound. Br Med J 1952;2:853.
13. Van de Werf F, et al. The mechanism of disappearance of the physiologic third heart sound with age. Circulation 1986;73:877.
14. Sloan AW, Wishart M. The effect on the human third heart sound of variations in the rate of filling of the heart. Br Heart J 1953;15:25.
15. Contro S. Ventricular gallop in mitral stenosis: its mechanism and significance. Am Heart J 1957;54:246.
16. Wood P. An appreciation of mitral stenosis. Br Med J 1954;1:1051 and 1113.
17. Abdulla AM, et al. Clinical significance and hemodynamic correlates of the third heart sound gallop in aortic regurgitation. Circulation 1981;64:464.
18. Harvey WP, Stapleton J. Clinical aspects of gallop rhythm with particular reference to diastolic gallops. Circulation 1958;18:1017.
19. Herder SL. More cardiac dressage: galop, gallop, gal(l)oppity glop. Letter to editor. JAMA 1989;262:352.
20. Evans W. Triple heart rhythm. Br Heart J 1943;5:203.
21. Rodin P, Tabatznik B. The effect of posture on added heart sounds. Br Heart J 1963;25:69.
22. Ruskin A, Garner B. Factors influencing gallop rhythm. Circulation 1959;20:761.
23. Read JL, Porter WB. The efficacy of carotid sinus pressure in the differential diagnosis of triple rhythm. Am J Med 1955;19:177.
24. Leonard JJ, et al. Modification of ventricular gallop rhythm induced by pooling of blood in the extremities. Br Heart J 1958;20:502.
25. Tyberg TI, et al. Genesis of pericardial knock in constrictive pericarditis. Am J Cardiol 1980;46:570.
26. Mounsey P. The early diastolic sound of constrictive pericarditis. Br Heart J 1955;17:143.
27. Nicholson WJ, et al. Early diastolic sound of constrictive pericarditis. Am J Cardiol 1980;45:378.

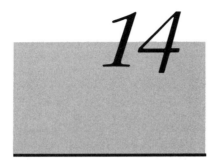

14

The Fourth Sound

The fourth sound is related to atrial contraction, and, like S3, is a low-pitched sound best heard with the bell lightly applied to the recumbent patient. Authorities differ in their expressed opinions regarding its normal audibility: It is probably a normal finding in some circumstances and age groups; but when it becomes accentuated, and especially if associated with a palpable "A" wave in the apical impulse, it is clearly abnormal and is then known as an S4, atrial, or presystolic gallop sound. Thus, like the S3 gallop, the atrial gallop is considered to be the abnormal accentuation of a normal event. Both S3 and S4 gallops may be seen or felt more readily than heard; the directly applied ear, as recommended by Potain in the 19th century, makes an excellent—though now abandoned!—"feeling-scope."

GENESIS

There is uncertainty about the genesis of the atrial sound. It is undoubtedly related to the ventricular filling[1] that is augmented by atrial contraction, but the exact mechanism of sound production is controversial. It is absent in atrial fibrillation,[2] where there is no effective atrial contraction: No contraction, no sound. In complete A-V block, where independent atrial sounds are otherwise audible, according to some observers, no sound may be heard when the atria contract against already closed A-V valves during ventricular systole[3]: No ventricular filling, no sound. Others, on the other hand, can hear and record atrial sounds even during ventricular systole,[4,5] and even the infirm contractions of atrial flutter and the disorganized twitches of coarse atrial fibrillation may at times produce audible sounds.[6] A third explanation, the "impact theory," is that the sound results from the thud of the left ventricle against the chest wall, impelled by the vigor of atrial contraction.[7]

Atrial sound vibrations, as recorded in the phonocardiogram (PCG), consist of two sets: The first, usually inaudible and presumably due to atrial contraction, and the second audible and associated with ventricular filling. It is possible that the first set may become audible in pathologic states, and may account for atrial sounds being

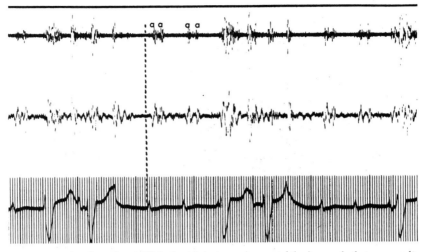

Figure 14–1. Complete A-V block with independent atrial (a,a) sounds that were split clearly on auscultation.

heard even when ventricular filling is prevented by closed A-V valves, and for the first component of reduplicated atrial sounds sometimes heard in complete A-V block (Fig. 14-1).[8] In complete A-V block the independent atrial sounds may sound single, double (as in Fig. 14-1), or like a short rumble.

TIMING

The abnormal S4 occurs 0.07 to 0.20 second after the beginning of the P wave of a simultaneous electrocardiogram (ECG), and the longer P–S4 intervals may bury it within the first sound—to which it presumably contributes.[3] Either disease or delayed A-V conduction separates it from S1 so that it becomes audible. The worse the disease or the longer the P–R interval, the greater is the S4–S1 separation, the more distinct the atrial sound, and the more frank the triple cadence. Without any change in the P–R interval, moderate disease may advance the audible atrial sound to within 0.15–0.18 second of the P wave, and severe disease to within 0.07–0.08 second.[3,9] Figure 14-2 illustrates a fourth sound[4] beginning 0.14 second after the onset of the P wave in the ECG.

With a borderline P–R of 0.20–0.22 second, the atrial sound may occur just before S1, perhaps giving the impression of a split S1, and a longer P–R (0.28–0.30 second) may produce a classical presystolic gallop cadence.

The auditory impression of an S4 that is barely diverging from S1 is hard to describe; it is not discrete enough to give the impression of a split S1 but rather sounds like a false start—a stuttering indecision on the part of S1 to get going. At this stage its presence may be confirmed by one of the maneuvers listed below as a means of accentuating S4.

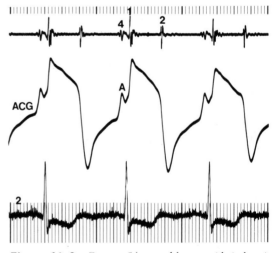

Figure 14–2. From a 54-year-old man with ischemic heart disease and classical angina. The low-frequency PCG recorded at the apex documents the loud fourth sound (4) coinciding with an abnormal and palpable "A" wave in the ACG.

CLINICAL FEATURES

The atrial gallop is a cry for help, the ventricular gallop a more desperate appeal.

An S4, when heard, is usually a left-sided event and is loudest at the apex with the patient in the left lateral position; its intensity varies with respiration, but it is usually best heard in full expiration and associated with a palpable "A" wave in the apex impulse. At times it is maximal at the base, even at the aortic area.[10] The right-sided atrial gallop is best heard at the lower left sternal border, is better heard in inspiration, and is often accompanied by a prominent "a" wave in the jugular pulse. On either side, its loudness and timing are related to the end-diastolic volume of the respective ventricle.

Most authorities agree that an audible S4 is seldom if ever a normal finding, and should always be viewed with suspicion of underlying pathology,[11-13] especially if associated with a palpable "A" wave; several other authorities, however, claim that it can be a normal auscultatory finding.[14-16] Some state that it is often heard in infancy and the early years. The fact that it is sometimes heard in the presumably healthy elderly person may be attributed to the fact that, with advancing age, the first sound loses intensity and the fourth sound, therefore, becomes *relatively*—though not absolutely—louder, reaching the threshold of audibility.[17]

There is a difference between audibility and recordability. Undoubtedly the fourth sound can be recorded by the sensitive PCG in many normal subjects: Spodick and coworkers[18] recorded an S4 in no less than 70% of normal middle-aged and elderly subjects, and found no higher prevalence in hypertensive patients. They also found that when the S4 was recordable in normal subjects, it also usually was audible.

The clinical contexts of the gallops are presented in Table 14-1. The atrial gallop does not have the same sinister ring as the ventricular gallop. It is often present in the absence of ventricular failure and it may persist, close to S1, for several years in asymptomatic patients with hypertension. When it is widely separated from S1 (unless due to A-V block), it is more ominous. A discrete S4 in aortic stenosis, usually associated with a palpable presystolic impulse, signifies a left ventricular pressure in excess of 160 mm Hg, a pressure dif-

Table 14–1
Causes of Gallops

S3 Gallops Are Found in	S4 Gallops Are Found in
LV diastolic overloading	LV systolic overloading
Mitral regurgitation	Hypertension
Aortic regurgitation	Aortic stenosis*
Left-to-right shunts	Coarctation of aorta
RV diastolic overloading	RV systolic overloading
Tricuspid regurgitation	Pulmonary hypertension
Pulmonic regurgitation	Pulmonic stenosis*
Atrial septal defects	Pulmonary artery stenosis
High output states	RA systolic overloading
Diminished ventricular compliance and/or raised ventricular diastolic pressure	Tricuspid stenosis or atresia
Cardiomyopathies	Diminished ventricular compliance and/or raised ventricular diastolic pressure
Ventricular failure	Mitral regurgitation†
Constrictive pericarditis	Cardiomyopathies
Ischemic heart disease‡	Ventricular failure
Ebstein's anomaly	Ischemic heart disease‡
	Ebstein's anomaly
	Systemic diseases
	Severe anemia
	Severe infections
	1° A-V block

*Including all forms of outflow tract obstruction.
†Secondary to rupture of chordae tendineae.
‡With or without myocardial infarction.

ference across the valve of over 75, and a left ventricular end-diastolic pressure of at least 12.[9] Subsequent observations suggest that these strictures may apply only to subjects under the age of 40 years.[19] When the atrium thus "cries for help," one ignores it at the patient's peril. Perhaps the cause of sudden death in patients with aortic stenosis is the abrupt failure of the left atrium to supply the supportive "atrial kick" required by the overtaxed left ventricle.

In the sick hypertensive heart with a classical atrial gallop, as clinical improvement takes place, S4 moves nearer to S1. As S4 nears S1, S1 may become louder.[20] Simply resting for several minutes to an hour or two may shorten the S4–S1 interval or may eliminate the atrial gallop entirely; so may peripheral venous pooling, as with tourniquets or standing,[21] drop in blood pressure induced by hypotensive agents, and amyl nitrite.

An atrial gallop may be brought to light or intensified by a cold pressor test,[22] and in hypertensive patients with left ventricular hypertrophy but without an audible S4, infusion of saline may evoke one.[23]

A fourth sound has to be differentiated from the first component of a split first sound, and this may be impossible without the aid of a PCG with simultaneous ECG. The first component of a split S1 is higher pitched and only narrowly separated (average 0.03 second) from the second component. The following characteristics of S4 may aid in its recognition:

1. It is lower pitched than S1,
2. It is usually more widely separated from S1 than the components of S1 are from each other,
3. With quiet breathing, it is loudest at the start of expiration, softest at mid-inspiration,
4. It is usually best heard at the left sternal border or at the base, sometimes maximal at the aortic area,
5. Carotid sinus stimulation may diminish it,[22,24]
6. Held exhalation may abolish it completely after several beats,[25]
7. Sitting, standing, or venous pooling (tourniquets) may abolish it,[25]
8. It disappears during a Valsalva strain, only to reappear after the strain much louder than before,[22] and
9. Lying down, exercise, or forcible inspiration with closed glottis makes it louder.[5]

The sequence S4–S1 at times requires differentiating from S1 followed by an ejection click. This often can be achieved by simply having the patient stand: Standing regularly makes S4 move closer to S1 or disappear, whereas the ejection click is unaffected.[20]

QUADRUPLE RHYTHM

Classical quadruple rhythm ("train-wheel rhythm") occurs when both third and fourth sounds are added to the cardiac cadence, as in Figure 14-3. However, any four sounds may produce a quadruple rhythm, and other foursomes include the wide splitting of both S1 and S2 in bundle branch block and in ectopic ventricular rhythms; and the combination of an opening snap and an S4. These have no special significance be-

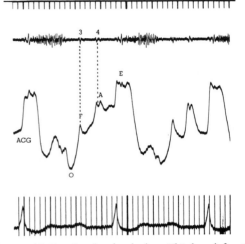

Figure 14–3. Quadruple rhythm. Third and fourth sound gallops correspond with "F" and "A" waves, respectively, in the ACG. The four step-like peaks in this quadrifid apex impulse were felt easily.

yond that of the individual components of the quadruplet. Quadruple rhythm may be palpable, as indeed it was in the patient of Figure 14-3.

The gallop sounds at times exhibit an interesting reciprocal relationship.[24] In patients with hypertensive or ischemic heart disease and a ventricular gallop, rest alone, or, if necessary, reinforced by sitting or venous pooling, induced the following salutary sequence: The S3 gallop was joined by an S4 gallop, making the rhythm quadruple; then the ventricular gallop disappeared while the S4 persisted; S4 then gradually drew nearer to S1 and disappeared within it. At this stage, the sequence could be reversed by any maneuver that increased venous return. At the quadruple stage (S3 + S4), inspiration increased the intensity of S3 while softening S4.

SUMMATION GALLOP

When third and fourth sounds coincide and augment each other, either because of critical lengthening of the P–R interval or critical increase in the cardiac rate, the triple cadence is called a summation gallop. Tachycardia shortens diastole and superimposes S4 on S3, or the P–R may lengthen to the point where atrial contraction reinforces early diastolic ventricular filling. Grayzel[4] developed a formula, taking rate and P–R into account, for determining when summation would occur. At normal P–R intervals (0.14–0.20 second), summation develops at rates between 104 and 120/minute. As the P–R lengthens, the rate at which summation develops progressively decreases, so that at a P–R of 0.30 second, summation would take place at a rate of about 85/minute.

The audible summation may result from a combination of (1) two silent filling phases that, when they are superimposed, become audible—this happens in normal children with tachycardia (Fig. 14-4); (2) one already audible sound (S3 or S4) and the other silent filling phase—called an "augmented" gallop; or (3) already audible third and fourth sounds. These three summations cannot be distinguished by simple auscultation, but they can be separated by observing the effect of slowing, as by carotid sinus stimulation: As the rate slows, type 1 loses the gallop sound; type 2 remains a triple rhythm but the gallop sound is much softer; and type 3 expands into a quadruple rhythm.

A concluding caveat: Don't be dogmatic about the presence, absence, intensity, or timing of a gallop in a patient you examined yesterday. THEY CHANGE.

THE JUGULAR FOURTH SOUND

The neglected neck veins may repay auscultation as well as inspection. A special variant of the atrial sound may be heard over the jugular vein in pa-

tients with right atrial hypertension—tricuspid stenosis, pulmonic stenosis, pulmonary hypertension, or right ventricular failure from any cause.[26] It may be loud over the jugular bulb just above the clavicle, yet inaudible just below the clavicle. You may hear it alone, or the other heart sounds may also be transmitted to this area, giving rise to a presystolic triple rhythm.

REFERENCES

1. Crevasse L, et al. The mechanism of generation of the third and fourth heart sounds. Circulation 1962;25:635.
2. Shaver JA, Salerni R. Auscultation of the heart. In: Hurst JW, ed. The heart, ed 7. New York: McGraw Hill, 1990: 175–242.
3. Kincaid-Smith P, Barlow J. The atrial sound and the atrial component of the first heart sound. Br Heart J 1959; 21:470.
4. Grayzel J. Gallop rhythm of the heart: II. quadruple rhythm and its relation to summation and augmented gallops. Circulation 1959;20:1053.
5. Sloan AW. Cardiac gallop rhythm. Medicine 1958; 37:197.
6. Neporent LM. Atrial heart sounds in atrial fibrillation and flutter. Circulation 1964;30:893.
7. Reddy PS, et al. Normal and abnormal heart sounds in cardiac diagnosis: Part II. diastolic sounds. Curr Probl Cardiol 1985;10:36–50.
8. Merrill JM, France R. Double atrial sounds and peripheral atrial impulses in a patient with complete heart block. Ann Intern Med 1963;58:867.
9. Goldblatt A, et al. Hemodynamic-phonocardiographic correlations of the fourth heart sound in aortic stenosis. Circulation 1962;26:92.
10. Castle RF, Craige E. Auscultation of the heart in infants and children. Pediatrics 1960;26:511.
11. Fowler NO, Adolph RJ. Fourth sound gallop or split first sound? Am J Cardiol 1972;30:441.
12. Tavel ME. The fourth heart sound: a premature requiem? Circulation 1974;49:4.
13. Abrams J. The fourth heart sound: a normal finding? Am J Cardiol 1975;36:534.
14. Spodick DH, Quary-Pigotti VM. Fourth heart sound as a normal finding in older persons. N Engl J Med 1973; 288:140.
15. Benchimol A, Desser KB. The fourth heart sound in patients without demonstrable heart disease. Am Heart J 1977;93:298.
16. Bethell HJN, Nixon PGF. Understanding the atrial sound. Br Heart J 1973;35:229.
17. Reddy PS, et al. The genesis of gallop sounds: investigation by quantitative phono and apexcardiography. Circulation 1981;63:922.
18. Swistak M, et al. Comparative prevalence of the fourth heart sound in hypertensive and matched normal persons. Am J Cardiol 1974;33:614.
19. Caulfield WH, et al. The clinical significance of the fourth heart sound in aortic stenosis. Am J Cardiol 1971;28:179.
20. Kincaid-Smith P, Barlow J. The atrial sound in hyper-

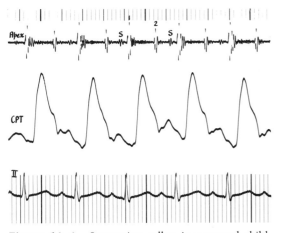

Figure 14–4. Summation gallop in a normal child. Because of the tachycardia at a rate of about 125/minute, S3 and S4 are superimposed and become audible, producing a transient (S) about 0.14 second after S2 and 0.08 second before S1.

tension and ischemic heart disease. Br Heart J 1959; 21:479.

21. Rodin P, Tabatznik B. The effect of posture on added heart sounds. Br Heart J 1963;25:69.

22. Harris WS, et al. Modification of the atrial sound by the cold pressor test, carotid sinus massage, and the Valsalva maneuver. Circulation 1963;28:1128.

23. Kontos HA, et al. Observations on the atrial sound in hypertension. Circulation 1963;28:877.

24. Read JL, Porter WB. The efficacy of carotid sinus pressure in the differential diagnosis of triple rhythms. Am J Med 1955;19:177.

25. Parry E, Mounsey P. Gallop sound in hypertension and myocardial ischemia modified by respiration and other manoeuvres. Br Heart J 1961;23:393.

26. Dock W. Loud presystolic sounds over the jugular veins associated with high venous pressure. Am J Med 1956; 20:853.

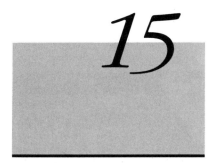

Systolic Murmurs

MURMURS IN GENERAL

Murmurs catch the ear and capture the imagination often out of proportion to their significance. The transients frequently have a more important, though more subtle, message for us, and we should not focus on murmurs to the neglect of sounds. Unfortunately, the murmur is established in the lay mind as the badge of heart disease, and even the medical mind is disproportionately murmur-conscious. Until experience has put murmurs in their proper perspective, a good rule is: Ignore All Murmurs Until You Have Evaluated All Sounds.

It is convenient to think of murmurs as organic, functional, or innocent:

Organic murmurs are due to intrinsic cardiovascular disease,
Functional murmurs are cardiovascular but are produced by disturbances of the circulation other than cardiovascular (eg, anemia, thyrotoxicosis, pregnancy), and
Innocent murmurs may be cardiovascular or extra-cardiac, and their precise origin may or may not

be known, but at least no disease, cardiac or otherwise, is recognized as a cause.

You should study the following attributes of all murmurs:

Timing: (1) systolic or diastolic; (2) position in systole or diastole (early, mid-, late, pan-),
Site: (1) of maximal intensity; (2) of propagation,
Loudness: grades 1 to 6,
Quality: blowing, harsh, musical, etc., and
Shape: plateau, diamond, crescendo, decrescendo, etc.

All murmurs should be graded from 1 (softest) to 6 (loudest) according to the following criteria:

Grade 1: so soft that it is not heard for the first beat or two after applying the stethoscope,
Grade 2: faint, but distinctly heard immediately,
Grade 3: moderately loud, but no associated thrill,
Grade 4: loud and accompanied by a thrill,
Grade 5: very loud and audible even if one edge of the bell is raised off the chest wall; associated thrill, and

Grade 6: so loud that it is audible with the entire bell's rim raised off the chest wall; associated thrill.

SYSTOLIC MURMURS

It was a real step forward when Leatham[1] proposed dividing systolic murmurs into Pansystolic Regurgitant and Midsystolic Ejection; it sensibly substituted physiology for geography. This laid the groundwork for excellent later studies, and it certainly embraces the most important murmurs. But, good as it is, it is not inclusive enough to be entirely satisfactory as a classification. It is like classifying widows into (1) old and (2) pretty: There are some that are not old and not pretty either. So there are systolic murmurs that are not pansystolic but are not ejection either. Several classifications are available, and none is wholly satisfactory. A practical one groups them into:

1. *Pansystolic (or holosystolic) or regurgitant*: begins with S1 and goes right up to and perhaps slightly beyond S2 (Fig. 15-1A),
2. *Midsystolic or ejection*: begins a little after S1 and proceeds for a variable time through systole, but never reaches the ipsilateral closure sound, A2 or P2 (Fig. 15-1B),
3. *Early systolic*: begins with S1 and finishes in midsystole, and
4. *Late systolic*: begins in midsystole or later and usually reaches S2.

Pansystolic murmurs result when blood is regurgitated from a high-pressure chamber into a relatively low-pressure system—ventricle to atrium, or systemic circulation to pulmonary. All the way to the end of systole, the pressure in the expelling chamber is higher than that in the receiving chamber, and so there is no reason for the regurgitant flow—or consequent murmur—to cease before systole ends; examples are mitral and tricuspid regurgitation and ventricular septal defect.

Ejection murmurs are produced when blood is ejected from a high-pressure chamber (ventricle) into a comparably high-pressure system (great artery). Pressures equalize before the end of systole, and the diamond-shaped murmur is consequently cut short before the second sound. Many normal (innocent) murmurs are of this type.

The turbulence responsible for abnormal ejection murmurs is produced in several ways, for example:

Narrow orifice, jet effect: aortic and pulmonary valvular, subvalvular, and supravalvular stenosis,
Deformity of valve without stenosis: bicuspid aortic valve; thickening of aortic cusps with aging[2]; infective endocarditis,
Dilation beyond orifice: dilated aorta from aortic regurgitation, coarctation, aneurysm, hypertension, atherosclerosis; idiopathic dilation of pulmonary artery, pulmonary hypertension; poststenotic dilation,
Increased flow (rate or volume): aortic or pulmonic regurgitation; atrial septal defect; anemia, thyrotoxicosis; fever, pregnancy, exercise, bradycardia,
Decreased viscosity: anemia; pregnancy, and Combinations of the above.

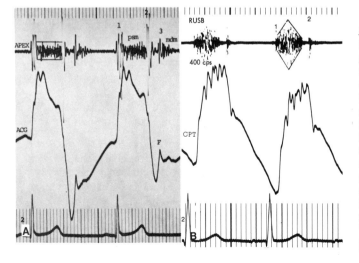

Figure 15–1. (A) Illustrates the characteristics of a pansystolic murmur (psm): Begins with the first heart sound (1) and continues right up to the second sound (2) with relatively little change in intensity ("plateau" shape). From a 10-year-old boy with mitral regurgitation; note also the loud third sound (3), coinciding with the F-point in the apexcardiogram (ACG), followed by a short mid-diastolic flow murmur (mdm). (B) Illustrates the features of an ejection murmur: Ends definitely before the second sound (2), and is crescendo–decrescendo ("diamond-shaped"); note the jagged summit of the carotid pulse tracing—carotid "shudder" (pictorial equivalent of the palpable thrill).

The great importance of FLOW in the production of murmurs is perhaps underappreciated; it is nicely illustrated by aortic valve lesions. When patients with aortic stenosis go into heart failure, the reduced cardiac output may eliminate a previously loud ejection murmur. On the other hand, a patient with severe aortic regurgitation (and no stenosis) may have a loud systolic murmur *and thrill* as a result of the greatly augmented stroke output.

Early systolic murmurs are sometimes innocent. They are also found at times as atypical expressions of mitral or tricuspid regurgitation; and in small ventricular septal defects of the muscular septum (which close before the end of systole) or in defects with curtailed left-to-right shunt because of increased pulmonary vascular resistance.

Late systolic murmurs were formerly regarded as innocent—and no doubt some are; certainly the prognosis of a patient with an isolated late systolic murmur is generally good.[3] But most such murmurs are recognized to be due to mild mitral regurgitation, usually due to a prolapsing posterior leaflet,[4–7] less often to rheumatic mitral regurgitation,[8,9] and they are frequently ushered in or punctuated by a mid–late systolic click. Late systolic murmurs may also characterize other syndromes, including hypertrophic cardiomyopathy,[8] papillary muscle dysfunction, and coarctation of the aorta[10]; and they may result from pericardial roughening following pericarditis. The mammary souffle may be audible only in late systole, and uncommon causes include perforate aneurysm of the membranous ventricular septum with minor left-to-right shunt.[11]

Sites

Of Maximal Intensity

When a murmur is heard well or best at the right upper sternal border, the most likely cause is an aortic ejection murmur. But the first thing you say to yourself when you hear a murmur there is, "This is probably not aortic stenosis." This caveat is useful to remind ourselves that there are many other causes of aortic ejection murmurs besides stenosis (Table 15-1), and some of them, in certain age groups, are more common than stenosis. Aortic ejection murmurs were heard in 47% of 473 elderly people aged 62 to 100 years; of these, only 54% had evidence of valvar stenosis.[12]

Table 15–1
Aortic Ejection Murmurs

Outflow obstruction
  Aortic stenosis
  Subaortic stenosis
  Supravalvar stenosis
Aortic dilation
  Hypertension
  Atherosclerosis
  Aneurysm
  Coarctation of aorta
Valve deformity
  Bicuspid
  Thickening with age
  Endocarditis
Increased flow
  Aortic regurgitation
  Anemia
  Thyrotoxicosis
  Fever
  Bradycardia
  Pregnancy
  Exercise

Also remember that severe mitral regurgitation, with or without ruptured chordae, may masquerade as aortic stenosis with murmur and thrill prominent at the aortic area, as well as at the apex.[13–16] This misleading acoustic freak is thought to be due to the regurgitant jet impinging on the atrial wall adjacent to the aortic root.[17] In the presence of pulsus alternans complicating severe aortic stenosis, the murmur may parallel the mechanical alternation, waxing and waning with alternate beats.[18]

When a murmur is heard well or best at the left upper sternal border, the most likely cause is a pulmonic ejection murmur (Table 15-2). Two other murmurs that may be maximal at the "pulmonic" area are those of patent ductus arteriosus and ventricular septal defect. For years a patent ductus may present only a systolic murmur with no diastolic spill-over. Remember also that aortic murmurs are often well, and sometimes best, heard at the left upper sternal edge—especially in youth.

The left lower sternal border is the classic site of maximal intensity for certain innocent and four important organic systolic murmurs: Ventricular septal defect, tricuspid regurgitation, infundibular pulmonic stenosis, and the muscular subaortic stenosis of hypertrophic cardiomyopathy.

The main systolic murmurs "at home" at the

Table 15–2
Pulmonic Ejection Murmurs

Outflow obstruction
  Pulmonic stenosis
  Infundibular stenosis
  Supravalvar stenosis
Pulmonary artery dilation
  Idiopathic
  Pulmonary hypertension
  Segmental pulmonary artery stenosis
Increased flow
  Atrial septal defect
  Pulmonic regurgitation
  Anemia, thyrotoxicosis, etc.
Innocent

apex are those of mitral regurgitation (from any of its many causes) and the occasional innocent murmur. The murmur of aortic stenosis may be well, and, not infrequently, best heard at the apex, where it may assume musical tones in contrast with its harsh and unmelodious timbre at the aortic area (Gallavardin effect). In addition, the murmurs of tricuspid regurgitation and ventricular septal defect may be quite well heard at the apex. In hypertrophic cardiomyopathy, no less than three systolic murmurs may be audible: At the left lower sternal border, the murmur of obstruction to left ventricular outflow; at the apex, the murmur of associated mitral regurgitation; and, less commonly, the ejection murmur of right ventricular outflow obstruction.[19]

When a systolic murmur is loudest in the back, one thinks first of extracardiac, vascular murmurs: Coarctation of the aorta, aortic aneurysm or dissection, pulmonary arterial stenoses, or pulmonary arteriovenous fistula.

Of Propagation

The direction and extent of murmur radiation is sometimes diagnostically significant but is probably the least valuable of all a murmur's attributes.

Aortic ejection murmurs are well transmitted upward into the neck and along the course of the carotids—louder at the root of the neck than higher, in contrast with the bruits of intrinsic carotid artery disease, which get louder as your bell ascends the carotid stalk. They are at times also well transmitted to the pulmonic area and to the apex.

Pulmonic ejection murmurs do not radiate so widely. They too may invade the neck, but usually only to the suprasternal notch, and they may be well heard at the lung bases. The loud, widely transmitted murmurs of patent ductus, ventricular septal defect, and mitral regurgitation may also be well heard in the neck.

The *murmur of a ventricular septal defect* is often well transmitted across the sternum to the right side of the chest, in contrast to that of pulmonic stenosis.

The *murmur of mitral regurgitation* may be extraordinarily widely propagated: To the lower left sternal border, to the base of the heart and into the neck, into the left axilla and through to the back, up and down the spine from occiput to sacrum. When mitral regurgitation develops acutely—as from rupture of a papillary muscle or of chordae—the loud, harsh pansystolic murmur is accompanied by loud S3 and S4, fades in late systole, and may seem to end before S2[20,21]; with radiation towards the base, it frequently mimics aortic stenosis.

The *murmur of tricuspid regurgitation* is much less widely transmitted; maximal at the left lower sternal border, it may be audible as far to the left as the apex, but is poorly radiated into the axilla; it can be distinguished from the murmur of mitral regurgitation by the fact that it becomes louder with inspiration, whereas the mitral murmur is little affected, and if anything gets softer, with inspiration. Compared with acute mitral regurgitation, acute tricuspid regurgitation—as from the surgical removal of the valve to combat infective endocarditis—produces a systolic murmur of low intensity and short duration.[22] Sometimes there is no precordial regurgitant murmur, but the massive reflux funnelled into the venous system produces a systolic murmur and thrill at the root of the neck.[23]

The main determinant of a murmur's propagation is its loudness. Undoubtedly the direction of regurgitant jets and the downstream direction of ejection murmurs influence the degree and direction of propagation. But the observations that the murmur of ventricular septal defect may be well heard in the neck, that of aortic stenosis over the olecranon (with blood pressure cuff inflated above systolic pressure), and that of mitral regurgitation even over the sacrum, cogently argue that the direction of the involved bloodstream is not the sole, nor even necessarily the main, determinant of propagation.[13,24]

REFERENCES

1. Leatham A. Systolic murmurs. Circulation 1958;17:601.
2. Bruns DL, Van Der Hauwaert LG. The aortic systolic murmur developing with increasing age. Br Heart J 1958;20:370.
3. Allen H, et al. Significance and prognosis of an isolated late systolic murmur: a 9- to 22-year follow-up. Br Heart J 1974;36:525.
4. Barlow JB, et al. The significance of late systolic murmurs. Am Heart J 1963;66:443.
5. Segal BL, Likoff WB. Late systolic murmur of mitral regurgitation. Am Heart J 1964;67:757.
6. Ronan JA, et al. Systolic clicks and the late systolic murmur. Am Heart J 1965;70:319.
7. Tavel ME, et al. Late systolic murmurs and mitral regurgitation. Am J Cardiol 1965;15:719.
8. Barlow JB, et al. Late systolic murmurs and non-ejection ("mid-late") systolic clicks. An analysis of 90 patients. Br Heart J 1968;30:203.
9. Steinfeld L, et al. Late systolic murmur of rheumatic mitral insufficiency. Am J Cardiol 1975;35:397.
10. Segal BL, Kalman P. Bedside diagnosis of heart disease: analysis of murmurs. Prog Cardiovasc Dis 1964;6:581.
11. Linhart JW, Razi B. Late systolic murmur: a clue to the diagnosis of aneurysm of the membranous ventricular septum. Chest 1971;60:283.
12. Aranow WS, Kronzon I. Correlation of prevalence and severity of valvular aortic stenosis determined by continuous-wave Doppler echocardiography with physical signs of aortic stenosis in patients aged 62 to 100 years with aortic systolic ejection murmurs. Am J Cardiol 1987;60:399.
13. Movitt E, Gasul B. Pure mitral insufficiency of rheumatic origin in adults. Ann Intern Med 1953;38:981.
14. Perloff JK, Harvey WP. Auscultatory and phonocardiographic manifestations of pure mitral regurgitation. Prog Cardiovasc Dis 1962;5:172.
15. Sleeper JC, et al. Mitral insufficiency simulating aortic stenosis. Circulation 1962;26:428.
16. Thomas JR. Mitral insufficiency due to rupture of chordae tendineae simulating aortic stenosis. Am Heart J 1966;71:112.
17. Antman EM, et al. Demonstration of the mechanism by which mitral regurgitation mimics aortic stenosis. Am J Cardiol 1978;42:1044.
18. Tavel ME, Nasser WK. Murmur alternans in aortic stenosis. Chest 1970;57:176.
19. Shah PM. Controversies in hypertrophic cardiomyopathy. Curr Prob Cardiol 1986;11:580.
20. Ronan JA, et al. The clinical diagnosis of acute severe mitral insufficiency. Am J Cardiol 1971;27:284.
21. DePace NL, et al. Acute severe mitral regurgitation: pathophysiology, clinical recognition and management. Am J Med 1985;78:293.
22. Rios JC, et al. Auscultatory features of acute tricuspid regurgitation. Am J Cardiol 1969;23:4.
23. Amidi M, et al. Venous systolic thrill and murmur in the neck: a consequence of severe tricuspid insufficiency. J Am Coll Cardiol 1986;7:942.
24. Levine SA, Likoff WB. Some notes on the transmission of heart murmurs. Ann Intern Med 1944;21:298.

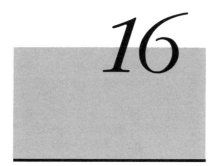

The Innocent Murmur

Recognizing the innocent murmur is one of the most important, and certainly sometimes one of the most difficult, responsibilities in cardiology. Muffing it can create a cardiac cripple or expose a minor lesion to the risks of serious aggravation. The innocent can usually be differentiated from the organic murmur by careful clinical examination alone, backed if necessary by noninvasive studies.[1] But there is no magic formula.

CLINICAL FEATURES

The innocent murmur is identified as much by the company it keeps as by its own characteristics (Table 16-1). It is accepted as innocent if it is soft, short, and systolic, and accompanied by no other clinical, electrocardiographic, x-ray or echocardiographic evidence of abnormality.

One should address especial attention to the second sound: It is always normal with innocent murmurs, whereas the common organic lesions confused with innocence—mild pulmonic steno-

sis, atrial septal defect—almost always have abnormal second sounds.

Although innocent murmurs are usually soft, there are exceptions—see below. Innocent murmurs are notoriously altered by simple maneuvers, like change of posture and deep respiration, and they may vary spontaneously from day to day. This is a useful differentiating rule of thumb, but some organic murmurs can be surprisingly influenced by respiration too. Exercise, often suggested as a means of differentiating innocent from guilty, is of no value: Most murmurs, both organic and innocent, become appreciably louder after exercise.

Innocent murmurs may be decrescendo, diamond-shaped, or crescendo; may be early, mid- or late systolic; may be heard in the midprecordium only, at the base only, apex only, base and apex, or over the entire precordium. Out of 80 innocent murmurs, Leatham[2] found 12 that were equally well heard at all areas. Soft ejection murmurs isolated at the aortic area are probably never innocent but indicate congenital bicuspid valves, minimal valve disease or a dilated aorta.[3]

Table 16–1
Salients of Innocent Murmurs

1. Always systolic
2. Usually not loud
3. Always short, *never* pansystolic
4. Modified by posture, respiration
5. In company with normal S2
6. Maximal at any area, most commonly at left sternal border
7. Often low-pitched, musical
8. Follow-up important

CLASSIFICATION

The classifications of innocent murmurs are unsatisfactory—quality, site and physiology are often intermingled as bases for classifying them. For example: basilar and apical;[4] vibratory, pulmonic ejection;[5] vibratory, pulmonic ejection and cardiorespiratory;[6] pulmonic, "fiddle-string," apical, and aortic;[7] precordial, coarse (vibratory) and fine, apical, pulmonic;[8] and parasternal-precordial, pulmonic, and cardiorespiratory.[9]

The two most commonly cited innocent murmurs are the "pulmonic ejection" (which may be aortic in origin—see below) and the "vibratory midprecordial." With minor variations in description, these comprise the great majority of most authors' series.

The Vibratory Midprecordial Murmur

This murmur is short, always ending before S2, and musical, variously described as groaning, twanging, fiddle-string, etc. (Fig. 16-1). It is commonest between the ages of two and seven years and is best heard in the 3rd and 4th left interspaces always inside the midclavicular line. Most observers believe that it is related to left ventricular ejection.[10] Some may be due to congenital bands strung across the outflow tract that vibrate during ejection,[11,12] or to increased ejection velocity into a narrow aortic diameter.[13]

The Pulmonic Ejection Murmur

This is short and blowing, is always associated with a normal S2, is loudest with the subject supine and is most often found in adolescents. It is hardly surprising if the normal current of blood coursing round the retrosternal crescent of the right ventricular outflow tract creates vibrations that sometimes reach the ear; and indeed, in one study all persons examined with intracardiac phonocardiography had systolic murmurs recorded in the root of the pulmonary artery.[14] In another series of patients with innocent murmurs, the murmurs were louder in the aortic root and therefore the so-called "pulmonic" murmur was ascribed to aortic flow.[15] All their patients, however, were aged between 38 and 69 years and had proven coronary

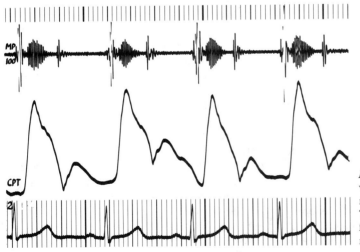

Figure 16–1. From a 12-year-old boy with an intensely musical systolic murmur but no evidence of heart disease. The PCG illustrates the typical "picket-fence" appearance of musical bruits. MP, midprecordium.

disease, and therefore their findings in no way exonerate the pulmonary artery in children.

INCIDENCE

Figures vary, but most authorities agree that innocent murmurs, whatever their origin, are audible in the majority of children; in Johannesburg, innocent murmurs were found in 84 percent of white children[3] and 72 percent of black children.[16] Opinions concerning the true innocence of these common murmurs also vary ranging all the way from the expressed possibility that such murmurs represent a restricted form of rheumatic or other valvulitis,[17] to the confirmed opinion that there is a potential innocent murmur in everyone. With special amplification and filtering, all of 71 adults, with no murmurs on ordinary clinical examination, had detectable systolic murmurs, most of them at the left sternal border.[18] This suggests that the necessary turbulence is universally present but the resulting murmur is often subaudible by our usual methods of examination. Although it still seems likely that those short systolic murmurs heard best at the left sternal border and localized there arise in the pulmonary outflow tract, it is probable that the short systolic murmur, heard well at both the apex and the aortic area and at points between, originates in the aortic outflow tract since its distribution is so similar to that of aortic murmurs.[2,19]

FOLLOW-UP

The follow-up is important. Out of 620 supposedly innocent murmurs, at the end of six years ten were diagnosed as ventricular septal defects and four as patent ductus; 386 were still audible and still regarded as innocent, while the remaining 220 had disappeared.[4] In another series of 96 innocent murmurs, 80 percent had disappeared at the end of a 20-year follow-up.[20]

Innocent murmurs are not the monopoly of children. Nor are they regularly "outgrown." Weaver[5] describes findings in 100 young adults known to have had innocent murmurs diagnosed 16 or more years previously. All still had murmurs of which 85 percent were "vibratory." Areas of maximal intensity were: left lower sternal border, 58 percent; left upper sternal border, 31 percent;

right upper sternal border and neck, 10 percent, and apex, 1 percent.

In summary, the most helpful features in establishing the innocence of a murmur are: its quality, its notable brevity, its normal companions, and the result of follow-up. These are often of greater importance than its loudness, site, response to exercise, respiration or posture, or its constancy or inconstancy.[21]

WHOOPS AND HONKS

The precordial "whoop," (like that of whooping cough), or "honk" (so called because it simulates the cry of a goose), usually maximal at the apex and extremely sensitive to respiratory and postural changes, may be an innocent finding in patients with no demonstrable heart disease; or at times may represent an exaggerated phase of an organic murmur.[22] Some honks have been identified with mild mitral regurgitation,[23,24] and a few with tricuspid regurgitation.[25,26] The tricuspid honk may be audible only on inspiration.[27]

A noisily fascinating phenomenon, the honk is a special exception to the general rule that innocent murmurs are of grade 3/6 intensity or less. Since some such honks are palpable by and even audible to dancing partners and lovers without benefit of stethoscope, they qualify by definition as grade 6 murmurs.

REFERENCES

1. Tavel ME. The systolic murmur—innocent or guilty? Am J Cardiol 1977;39:757.
2. Leatham A, et al. Auscultatory and phonocardiographic findings in healthy children with systolic murmurs. Br Heart J 1963;25:451.
3. Barlow JB, Pocock WA. The significance of aortic ejection systolic murmurs. Am Heart J 1962;64:149.
4. Lynxwiler CP, Donahoe JL. Evaluation of innocent heart murmurs. South Med J 1955;48:164.
5. Weaver WF, Walker CHM. Innocent cardiovascular murmurs in the adult. Circulation 1964;29:702.
6. Castle RF. Clinical recognition of innocent cardiac murmurs in children. JAMA 1961;177:1.
7. Wedum BG, Rhodes PH. Differential diagnosis of rheumatic fever in office practice. JAMA 1955;157:981.
8. Wells BG. The graphic configuration of innocent systolic murmurs. Br Heart J 1957;19:129.
9. Fogel DH. The innocent systolic murmur in children: a clinical study of its incidence and characteristics. Am Heart J 1960;59:844.
10. Shaver JA, Salerni R. Auscultation of the heart. In: Hurst

JW, ed. The heart, ed 7. New York: McGraw Hill, 1990:213

11. Durazs B, et al. The possible etiology of the vibratory systolic murmur. Clin Cardiol 1987;10:341.

12. Roberts WC. Anomalous left ventricular band: an unemphasized cause of a precordial musical murmur. Am J Cardiol 1969;23:735.

13. Schwartz ML, et al. Relation of Still's murmur, small aortic diameter and high aortic velocity. Am J Cardiol 1986;57:1344.

14. Lewis DH. Intracardiac phonocardiography. Prog Cardiovasc Dis 1959;2:85.

15. Stein PD, Sabbah HN. Aortic origin of innocent murmurs. Am J Cardiol 1977;39:665.

16. McLaren MJ, et al. Innocent murmurs and third heart sounds in black schoolchildren. Br Heart J 1980;43:67.

17. Luisada AA, et al. Murmurs in children: a clinical and graphic study in 500 children of school age. Ann Intern Med 1958;48:597.

18. Groom D, et al. The normal systolic murmur. Ann Intern Med 1960;52:134.

19. Stuckey D. Innocent systolic murmurs of aortic origin. Med J Aust 1957;1:38.

20. Marienfeld CJ, et al. A 20-year follow-up of "innocent" murmurs. Pediatrics 1962;30:42.

21. Mainzer W, et al. Systolic murmurs in children. Arch Dis Child 1959;34:131.

22. Rackley CE, et al. The precordial honk. Am J Cardiol 1966;17:509.

23. Leighton RF, et al. Mild mitral regurgitation: its characterization by intracardiac phonocardiography and pharmacologic responses. Am J Cardiol 1966;41:168.

24. Rizzon P, et al. The praecordial honk. Br Heart J 1971;33:707.

25. Keenan TJ, Schwartz MJ. Tricuspid whoop. Am J Cardiol 1973;31:642.

26. Upshaw CB. Precordial honk due to tricuspid regurgitation. Am J Cardiol 1975;35:85.

27. Kalyanasundaram V, et al. Musical murmurs: an echophonocardiographic study. Am J Cardiol 1978;41:952.

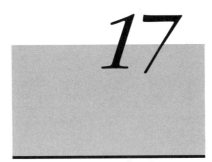

Continuous Murmurs

"Continuous" murmurs begin in systole and continue uninterrupted into diastole; they do not—as their name implies—necessarily occupy the whole of systole and diastole. They are not the same as "to-and-fro" murmurs, though many have used the two terms synonymously. The to-and-fro murmur is really two murmurs—a long systolic murmur immediately followed by an early diastolic murmur (Figs. 17-1**A**, 17-2**D**). Most to-and-fro murmurs are easily distinguished because the systolic murmur diminishes before S2 (arrow in Fig. 17-1**A**), just when most continuous murmurs are reaching their peak.[1] The rare combination of mitral regurgitation with end systolic crescendo immediately followed by a well heard murmur of aortic regurgitation is an exceptional mimic.

The recognition of continuous murmurs is important because they usually signal the presence of surgically correctable defects.[2]

Continuous murmurs develop when:

1. *Blood flows from a relatively high-pressure system or chamber into a relatively low-pressure system or chamber throughout the cardiac cycle:*

   a. From aorta to pulmonary artery (PA):
      Patent ductus arteriosus,
      Aortopulmonary window, and
      Ruptured aortic aneurysm into PA.
   b. From aorta to elsewhere:
      Ruptured sinus of Valsalva aneurysm,[3] and
      Ruptured aortic aneurysm into superior vena cava.
   c. From other systemic artery into venous circulation:
      Coronary A-V fistula,[4,5]
      Anomalous left coronary,[6]
      Intercostal or internal mammary A-V fistula, and
      Bronchial arteries to pulmonary arteries in pulmonic atresia, etc.
   d. From PA artery to pulmonary vein:
      Pulmonary A-V fistula.
   e. From left to right atrium:
      Mitral stenosis or atresia with atrial septal defect,[7,8] and
      Complication of transseptal catheterization for mitral stenosis.

2. *Blood flows across a severely constricted region in an artery:*

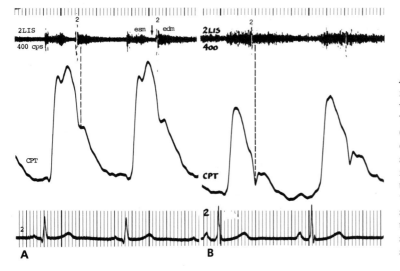

Figure 17–1. **(A)** "To-and-fro murmur" in a 37-year-old woman with traumatic aortic regurgitation. The ejection systolic murmur (esm) fades (arrow) before the second sound (2), and the early diastolic murmur (edm) begins immediately with S2, decreasing in the second half of diastole. **(B)** "Continuous" murmur of a Blalock anastomosis in a 14-year-old boy; the murmur reaches its maximum at about the time of the second sound (2).

Coarctation of aorta,
Segmental PA stenosis, and
Compression of PA by aortic aneurysm.

In these three situations the pressure proximal to the constriction is higher throughout the cardiac cycle than in the vessel distal to the constriction—so that, in effect, this is just a special form of mechanism 1 above.

3. *Blood flows through dilated, tortuous anastomotic channels*:
Dilated intercostals in coarctation of aorta,
Dilated bronchial arteries in pulmonic atresia, etc., and
Mammary souffle.[9]

In these cases the precise mechanism is uncertain, but it seems likely that tortuosity may be an important factor in producing audible turbulence. This mechanism is invoked by some but denied by others[10] to explain the continuous murmur of coarctation.

4. *Venous flow is turbulent*: This occurs as part of the exuberance of normal youth—all children have venous hums when erect; and in abnormal states when venous return is swift and turbulent:
Normal venous hum,
Venous hum from intracranial A-V fistula,
Total anomalous pulmonary venous return,[11] and
Possibly some mammary souffles.[12]

Most continuous murmurs reach their peak intensity at about the time of the second sound (Figs. 17-1**B**, 17-2**A**). Exceptions to this are the coronary A-V fistula, which tends to be crescendo-decrescendo in both systole and diastole and louder in diastole (Fig. 17-2**B**); and venous hum and ruptured sinus of Valsalva aneurysm into the right ventricle, both of which usually peak in diastole (Fig. 17-2**C**). Most are best heard on expiration and are diminished by inspiration; exceptions to this are the venous hum again, anomalous left coronary artery, pulmonary A-V fistula, and small atrial septal defect in the presence of mitral ste-

A | ~~~~~~~~~~~~~~~~~~ | PDA
B | ~~~~~~~~~~~~~~~~~~ | CAVF
C | ~~~~~~~~~~~~~~~~~~ | Venous hum
D | ~~~~~~~~~~~~~~~~~~ | "To-and-fro"

Figure 17–2. Diagrammatic representation of several systolic/diastolic murmurs. **(A)** The continuous, "machinery" murmur of patent ductus arteriosus (PDA); **(B)** coronary arteriovenous fistula; **(C)** venous hum; **(D)** "to-and-fro" murmur of aortic valve disease.

nosis or atresia—all of which tend to be accentuated by inspiration.

The quality and site of continuous murmurs are variable. The usual qualities attributed to the more common continuous murmurs are presented in Table 17-1, and the likely site of maximal intensity of those continuous murmurs that have a preferred precordial site is indicated in Figure 17-3.

Approximately 4% of all patients with cyanotic congenital heart disease have continuous murmurs, and such a murmur is three times more likely due to dilated bronchial arteries than to a patent ductus.[13] When the murmur is due to dilated bronchials, it may be maximal almost anywhere,[14] and is often widely disseminated over both sides, axillae and back.

When cyanosis and a continuous murmur are associated, you should think of the following syndromes:

1. Pulmonary atresia with dilated bronchials,
2. Persistent truncus with dilated bronchials,
3. Tetralogy of Fallot with dilated bronchials,
4. Pulmonary atresia with patent ductus, and
5. Mitral atresia or stenosis with atrial septal defect.

Table 17–1
Pathologic Continuous Murmurs

Lesion	Shunt	Murmur Mechanism	Murmur Description
Patent ductus			Harsh, rasping, uneven machinery (Gibson, 1900)
AP window			Similar (much less often continuous)
Blalock anastomosis	Aorta → PA	S/D flow from hi to lo	
Potts anastomosis			
Anomalous PA			
Ruptured aortic aneurysm	Aorta → PA, SVC	S/D flow from hi to lo	
Ruptured sinus of Valsalva aneurysm	Aorta → PA, RA, RV	S/D flow from hi to lo	Superficial, harsh, rasping
Coronary arteriocameral fistula	CA → RV, RA, LA	S/D flow from hi to lo	Superficial, harsh, rasping
Coronary A-V fistula	CA → CV or CS		
Anomalous left CA	RCA → LCA → PA	S/D flow from hi to lo	High-pitched, increasing on inspiration
Coarctation of aorta	Proximal aorta → distal aorta	1. S/D flow from hi to lo 2. collateral flow (?)	Soft, high-pitched
Segmental PA stenosis	Proximal PA → distal PA	S/D flow from hi to lo	
MS with LA hypertension and ASD	LA → RA	S/D flow from hi to lo	Increasing with inspiration
Intercostal or internal mammary A-V fistula	IC or IM artery → IC or IM vein	S/D flow from hi to lo	
Pulmonary A-V fistula	PA → PV	S/D flow from hi to lo	Soft, increasing with inspiration
PA atresia	1. bronchials → PA	1. S/D flow from hi to lo	Like PDA, or softer when due to collaterals; humming
Persistent truncus	2. PDA	2. Collateral flow	
Tetralogy of Fallot			
Total anomalous pulmonary venous return	Pulmonary veins → left innominate or SVC	Venous turbulence	Faint, high-pitched, *not* louder in diastole like venous hum

AP, aortopulmonary; PA, pulmonary artery; SVC, superior vena cava; RA, right atrium; RV, right ventricle; CA, coronary artery; LA, left atrium; CV, coronary vein; CS, coronary sinus; IC, intercostal; IM, internal mammary; PV, pulmonary vein; MS, mitral stenosis; ASD, atrial septal defect; PDA, patent ductus arteriosus; S/D, systolic/diastolic.

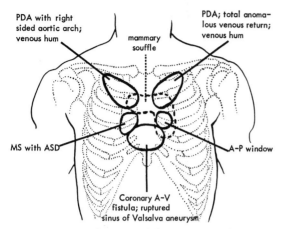

Figure 17–3. The precordial sites of several "continuous" murmurs. PDA, patent ductus arteriosus; MS, mitral stenosis; ASD, atrial septal defect; A–P, aortopulmonary; A–V, arteriovenous.

When a continuous murmur is loudest in the back, think of coarctation of aorta, segmental PA stenosis, or pulmonary A-V fistula, or one of the syndromes with dilated bronchials. The murmur of segmental PA stenosis is often best heard in the axillae.

MAMMARY SOUFFLE

This is an important murmur because of its innocence and because it can simulate a patent ductus with disastrous, or at least disturbing, results for its pregnant owner. It is high-pitched and usually systolic with spillover into diastole; less often it is confined to systole or continuous. It occurs in about 15% of pregnant women in the second and third trimesters and during lactation,[15] and is presumably due to increased blood flow through arteries—branches of internal mammary and intercostals—supplying the breasts. Some may be due to increased flow in the superficial veins.[12]

The souffle is best heard with the patient lying flat, and is loudest in the 2nd right, or 2nd, 3rd, and 4th left interspaces near the sternum. It is often associated with palpable arterial pulsation in the relevant interspace; often shows marked variation in intensity from day to day and even from beat to beat; is diminished but not obliterated by the Valsalva maneuver; and can be eliminated by pressure with the bell, or with the finger lateral to the listening bell.

Table 17–2
Differentiating Venous Hum from Ductus Murmur

	Venous Hum	Ductus Murmur
Diastole	↑	↓
Sitting up	↑	↓
Lying down	↓	↑
Inspiration	↑	—
Amyl nitrite	↑	↓
Vasopressor	?↓	↑

↑ murmur increases; ↓ murmur decreases; — little effect.

VENOUS HUM

This is present in all children, and in many adults if sought. Jones[16] found a venous hum in 27% of adults (average age, 32 years). Loudest in the neck, its importance lies in the fact that it may be well transmitted down over the precordium and be mistaken for the continuous murmur of a patent ductus or other A-V fistula. The several points that help to differentiate the venous hum from a patent ductus murmur are summarized in Table 17-2.

The hum is best heard at the root of the neck, usually better on the right, and is loudest when the subject sits or stands, often disappearing and always diminishing when he lies down. Inspiration, or turning the head away from the side of auscultation—so putting the veins on the stretch—usually increases its intensity; whereas turning the head toward the side of auscultation, or compressing the jugulars above the stethoscope, abolishes it.[16–18] Its quality is variable: Sometimes rough and groaning, sometimes higher-pitched, squeaking or blowing. It tends to be higher-pitched, louder, and more musical in diastole than in systole.

REFERENCES

1. Leatham A. Auscultation of the heart. Lancet 1958; 2:703 and 757.
2. Craige E, Millward DK. Diastolic and continuous murmurs. Prog Cardiovasc Dis 1971;14:38.
3. Holmes JC, et al. Coronary arteriovenous fistula and aortic sinus aneurysm rupture. Arch Intern Med 1966; 118:43.
4. Gasul BM, et al. Congenital coronary arteriovenous fis-

tula: clinical, phonocardiographic, angiocardiographic and hemodynamic studies in five patients. Pediatrics 1960;25:531.

5. Muir CS. Coronary arteriovenous fistula. Br Heart J 1960; 22:374.

6. Lampe CFJ, Verheugt APM. Anomalous left coronary artery: adult type. Am Heart J 1960;59:769.

7. Aykent Y, et al. Continuous murmur in mitral stenosis. Am J Cardiol 1965;15:715.

8. Ross J, et al. Interatrial communication and left atrial hypertension: a cause of continuous murmur. Circulation 1963;28:853.

9. Scott JT, Murphy EA. Mammary souffle of pregnancy: report of two cases simulating patent ductus arteriosus. Circulation 1958;18:1038.

10. Spencer MP, et al. The origin and interpretation of murmurs in coarctation of the aorta. Am Heart J 1958;56:722.

11. Keith JD, et al. Complete anomalous pulmonary venous return. Am J Med 1954;16:23.

12. Hurst JW, et al. Precordial murmurs during pregnancy and lactation. N Engl J Med 1958;259:515.

13. Campbell M, Deuchar DC. Continuous murmurs in cyanotic congenital heart disease. Br Heart J 1961;23:173.

14. Taussig HB. Congenital malformations of the heart, vol 2. Cambridge: Harvard University Press, 1960:295.

15. Tabatznik B, et al. The mammary souffle of pregnancy and lactation. Circulation 1960;22:1069.

16. Jones FL. Frequency, characteristics and importance of the cervical venous hum in adults. N Engl J Med 1962; 267:658.

17. Groom D, et al. Venous hum in cardiac auscultation. JAMA 1955;159:639.

18. Fowler NO, Geause R. The cervical venous hum. Am Heart J 1964;67:135.

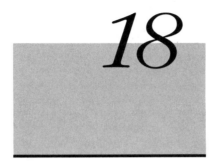

Diastolic Murmurs

Three main mechanisms produce diastolic murmurs: Semilunar valve regurgitation, A-V valve stenosis, and increased blood flow across A-V valves (Table 18-1). Most diastolic murmurs created at the semilunar valves begin the moment they are slammed supposedly shut, that is, immediately following S2 (Figs. 18-1**A**, 18-2**A**). On the other hand, murmurs at the A-V valves can begin only after they have "opened" (ie, an appreciable time after S2) (Figs. 18-1**D**, 18-2**B**); they are ventricular filling murmurs (just as S3 and S4 are "filling" sounds) and therefore occur at the two phases of most rapid ventricular filling:

Mid-diastolic: beginning with or at the time of an S3 (Fig. 18-2**B**), and
Late diastolic: beginning at the time of atrial contraction (Fig. 18-1**E**).

Since mid-diastolic murmurs begin an appreciable interval after S2, they produce a distinct triple cadence to the ear:

LUB–DUP—PRRRrr

This contrasts to the two-phase cadence of the early diastolic murmur:

LUB–DUFFFfff

The triple cadence of the mid-diastolic murmur is one of the most distinctive inflections in the voice of mitral stenosis. This cadence alone makes it quite impossible to mistake it for the loud, early murmur of aortic regurgitation when well transmitted to the apex—a confusion that may be experienced by the beginner.

Because the mid-diastolic murmur is not really "mid"—it begins well within the first third of diastole, and is therefore still relatively early—the term "delayed"[1] (as opposed to "immediate" for the murmur of semilunar regurgitation beginning with S2) has much to be said for it.

The two most common and important diastolic murmurs are sometimes missed by the beginner—and too often even by the more experienced—because they are not properly and thoroughly listened for. Before abandoning search for either of these

Table 18–1
Mechanisms of Diastolic Murmurs

Mechanism	Lesion	Timing
Semilunar valve incompetence	Aortic regurgitation	Early
	Pulmonic regurgitation	Early
	Austin Flint murmur	Mid/late
Inflow tract obstruction	Atrial tumors	
At atrial level	Mitral stenosis	
At valve	Tricuspid stenosis	Mid
	Obstructive cardiomyopathy	
At ventricular level		
High diastolic flow across A-V valve	Mitral regurgitation	
	Tricuspid regurgitation	
	VSD, PDA, A-V fistulas, ASD, APVR	Mid
	Anemia, thyrotoxicosis	
A-V valve deformity	Rheumatic valvulitis (Carey Coombs)	Mid
Enlarged ventricle ("relative" stenosis)	Ischemic heart disease	
	Hypertension	
	Cardiomyopathy	Mid
	Complete A-V block, etc.	
Interatrial flow	Ostium primum ASD + MR	Early
Diastolic gradient from PA to aorta	Reversed ductus	Pan
String across A-V valve	Ectopic chorda	Mid/late

VSD, ventricular septal defect; PDA, patent ductus arteriosus; ASD, atrial septal defect; APVR, anomalous pulmonary venous return; MR, mitral regurgitation.

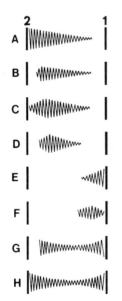

Figure 18–1. The various configurations of diastolic murmurs.

murmurs, you must always use five maneuvers as set out in the accompanying "five-step" table (Table 18-2).

These maneuvers look as though they added up to a complicated performance, but in fact they are all synthesized into about 1 minute's effort. If you are looking for the murmur of mitral stenosis, the patient sits up and touches her toes ten or 12 times, or climbs up and down steps, immediately lies down, turns partly on to her left side, blows out her breath, and the rest is up to you: Using the bell of your stethoscope with the *lightest possible touch*, you comb every square centimeter of the apical region as quickly as possible, with special attention at the site of maximal impulse (the apex beat).

To look for aortic regurgitation, after exercise the patient is instructed to sit on the edge of the examining table or bed, leaning forward, and blow his breath out, and then you listen carefully with the *firmly pressed* diaphragm up and down both

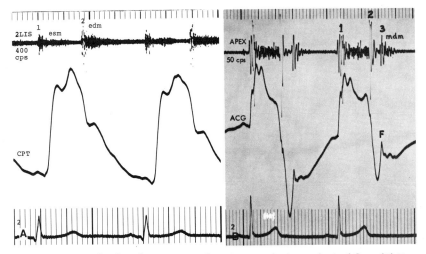

Figure 18–2. The diastolic murmurs of aortic regurgitation and mitral flow. **(A)** From a 37-year-old woman with traumatic aortic regurgitation; note that the early diastolic murmur (edm) begins immediately with S2 (2) and fades in the second half of diastole. **(B)** From a 10-year-old boy with mitral regurgitation; note the short, rapidly fading mid-diastolic murmur (mdm) beginning with S3 (3), well after S2 (2). 2LIS, 2nd left interspace; 1, first heart sound; esm, ejection systolic murmur; CPT, carotid pulse tracing; ACG, apexcardiogram; F, rapid filling wave.

sternal borders, giving particular attention at the left border.

Analogous murmurs on the right side—due to tricuspid stenosis and pulmonic regurgitation—are much less common. The Austin Flint (1862) murmur is a mitral flow murmur found in patients with aortic regurgitation, and a similar murmur of tricuspid flow may be found in patients with pulmonic regurgitation.[2] When the murmur of pulmonic regurgitation is secondary to pulmonary hypertension, it is known as the Graham Steell

(1888) murmur, which, although widely regarded as rare, is indeed a definite entity.[3]

Mid-diastolic flow murmurs at the A-V valves are fairly common in the presence of incompetent valves and in sizeable left-to-right shunts—as with atrial and ventricular septal defects and patent ductus arteriosus.

Some rare and bizarre causes of diastolic murmurs are listed in Table 18-3. Atrial tumors[7] can produce mid-diastolic murmurs, and so can diastolic flow through a moderately obstructed left anterior descending coronary artery.[8] Rarely, a floating atrial thrombus is responsible for marked variation in the timing and intensity of the diastolic murmur of mitral stenosis.[17]

Diastolic murmurs are generally regarded as conclusive evidence of abnormality, but short, early, diastolic murmurs at the left sternal border—possibly caused by normal coronary flow—have been heard and recorded within the cavity of the left ventricle (though not by external phonocardiography) in a few normal children.[18]

TIMING AND SHAPE

The timing, approximate duration, and shape of most diastolic murmurs are indicated in the dia-

Table 18–2
Five-Step Elicitation of Mitral and Aortic Diastolic Murmurs

Mitral Stenosis	Aortic Regurgitation
	Exercise
	Exhale
Turn half left	Sit, lean forward
Bell	Diaphragm
Quarter*	Right and left

*Key word in Osler's aphorism: "The murmur of mitral stenosis may be concealed under a *quarter* of a dollar."

Table 18–3
Unusual Causes of Diastolic Murmurs

Lesion	Tentative Mechanism
Immediate Diastolic Murmurs	
Pulmonary cusp prolapsed through VSD[4]	Pulmonic incompetence
Coronary artery–LV fistula	A-V gradient present only in diastole
Ostium primum ASD + MR[5]	Left atrial hypertension
Reversed flow through PDA[6]	Decompression of aneurysmal PDA only in diastole
Delayed Diastolic Murmurs	
Atrial tumors[7]	Obstruction to A-V valve
Coronary artery obstruction[8]	Diastolic coronary flow
Carcinoid syndrome	Tricuspid stenosis
Pulmonic regurgitation[9]	Right-sided Flint murmur
Rheumatic chorda[10]	Twanging string across mitral orifice
Obstructive cardiomyopathy[11]	Myocardial hypertrophy— inflow obstruction
Coarctation of aorta[12]	
Aortic stenosis[13]	Ventricular enlargement ("relative" stenosis)
Eisenmenger syndrome[14]	
Primary pulmonary hypertension[14]	
Complete A-V block[15,16]	Increased A-V flow
	Ventricular enlargement
	Atrial contraction augmenting flow

VSD, ventricular septal defect; LV, left ventricle; ASD, atrial septal defect; MR, mitral regurgitation; PDA, patent ductus arteriosus.

grams in Figure 18-1. Notice that the murmur of organic pulmonic regurgitation (Fig. 18-1**D**) differs from that secondary to pulmonary hypertension (Graham Steell murmur, Fig. 18-1**A**) in that it begins later, separated from the second sound by an appreciable gap. Rarely, the murmur of aortic regurgitation is similarly delayed (Fig. 18-1**B**)[19] or is crescendo-decrescendo (Fig. 18-1**C**).

In mitral valve stenosis, the best guide to severity is the duration of the diastolic murmur—the *longer the tighter*.[1] Tachycardia, including the rapid ventricular response in atrial fibrillation, may make a mid-diastolic murmur presystolic and defeat one's attempts to judge its duration. The long

diastolic pauses that follow extrasystoles, or the longer cycles during atrial fibrillation, should be patiently awaited, since they provide an ideal opportunity for estimating the murmur's length. Carotid sinus stimulation may be used to induce lengthened cycles in atrial fibrillation. In contrast to the organic murmur of A-V value stenosis, the mid-diastolic murmur of increased flow is always short—coinciding with the early rapid filling phase.

In mitral stenosis the murmur may be mid-diastolic only (Fig. 18-1**D**), presystolic only (Fig. 18-1**E**), or the two may combine to form a decrescendo-crescendo murmur occupying all but the first moments of diastole (Fig. 18-1**G**). In tricuspid stenosis the presystolic murmur begins earlier than that of mitral stenosis and often assumes a diamond shape (Fig. 18-1**F**); it used to be thought that this was because the right atrium begins to contract before the left, and that presystolic murmurs were atrial ejection murmurs.

Indeed, it was only natural to suppose that accelerated transvalvar blood flow was responsible for both the mid-diastolic and presystolic murmurs—the mid-diastolic occurring during the early rapid filling phase when atrial blood first gushes through the recently opened orifice, and the presystolic when the entering blood receives added impetus from atrial contraction.

Careful echocardiographic correlation, however, of the diastolic murmurs with mitral valve movement has demonstrated that the murmurs develop as the leaflets are *closing*; and, although the notion has not gained universal acceptance,[20] there is good reason to believe that mid-diastolic A-V valve murmurs result from the confrontation between entering blood and closing leaflets.[21–24] The closing leaflets progressively reduce the valve's orifice and so enhance the relative velocity of transvalvar flow. This could explain, not only the mid-diastolic murmur of mitral stenosis, but also the mid-diastolic "flow" murmurs of mitral and tricuspid regurgitation, of large left-to-right shunts, and of complete A-V block. In an unusual patient reported from Athens who had mitral stenosis, atrial fibrillation, and complete heart block, there were two distinct and separate murmurs in diastole, and precise echocardiographic correlation demonstrated that the mitral leaflets were closing at the time of both murmurs.[25]

The Austin Flint murmur, which was thought to be due to the anterior mitral leaflet fluttering between the two entering streams, may also be explicable by valve closure in the face of the entering stream[26]; but one need not entirely abandon the notion that it is caused by the shuddering leaflet as the regurgitant aortic jet impinges upon it.[27]

The crescendo presystolic murmur of mitral stenosis, often heard at the end of short cycles in atrial fibrillation—when atrial contraction is clearly not responsible—is also probably best explained by the noisy confrontation of entering blood and closing leaflets in the presence of a persisting A-V gradient.[21]

SITES

The usual sites of maximal intensity of the four important diastolic murmurs are shown in Figure 18-3. The murmur of aortic regurgitation is usually best heard at the left sternal border in the 3rd or 4th interspace. But it is often well heard at the right and left upper sternal borders, and the apex. Less often it is well transmitted down the right sternal border, and then suggests an etiology other than rheumatic. Good transmission to the apex sometimes prevents the ready recognition of a superadded Austin Flint murmur, if everything heard

at the apex is assumed to be transmitted. Closer attention to the duration and shape of the murmur as heard at the apex, contrasted with the murmur heard at the left lower sternal border, reveals that the apical (Flint) murmur at the end of diastole *gathers momentum* (Fig. 18-1**H**), whereas at the left lower sternal border the aortic regurgitant murmur is an unremitting diminuendo (Fig. 18-1**A**).

The murmur of pulmonic regurgitation is not transmitted down the right sternal border, so that a semilunar regurgitant murmur in this region is certainly aortic. Rarely, the murmur of mitral stenosis may radiate medially and upward to the 3rd and even 2nd left interspace, where it may sound higher-pitched and blowing, and so simulate semilunar regurgitation.[28]

The location of the rare murmur caused by mild obstruction of the left anterior descending coronary artery obstruction is precise: In the 3rd left interspace, 3 or 4 cm from the midline; it is better heard with the patient sitting.[8]

LOUDNESS

Like systolic murmurs, diastolic murmurs should also be graded from 1 to 6, but intensity does not parallel severity. Increased flow greatly increases the intensity of A-V valve murmurs; on the other hand, significant mitral stenosis, aortic regurgitation, and tricuspid stenosis can all be murmurless or "silent."[29] Silent aortic regurgitation can sometimes be made to talk by the administration of pressor agents—raising systemic pressure increases regurgitant flow; and the coy murmur of mitral stenosis may be evoked by amyl nitrite.

Inspiration diminishes the intensity of almost all diastolic murmurs; that of tricuspid stenosis is a notable exception, and its loudening with inspiration (Carvallo's sign) is an important diagnostic attribute. However, conduction of a murmur to the chest wall depends on other factors beside the hemodynamic effects of respiration; and, in fact, simultaneous intracardiac and precordial phonocardiograms show that the respiratory response of a precordial murmur is not necessarily a reflection of its intracardiac behavior.[30] When the external murmur becomes *louder* with inspiration, it is good evidence for a right-sided origin; when it does not become louder, it is poor evidence against such an origin.

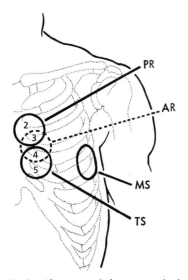

Figure 18–3. The precordial areas at which the main diastolic murmurs are usually best heard; 2nd, 3rd, 4th, and 5th interspaces are numbered 2, 3, 4, and 5. PR, pulmonic regurgitation; AR, aortic regurgitation; MS, mitral stenosis; TR, tricuspid stenosis.

QUALITY

The murmur of aortic regurgitation is typically high-pitched and blowing (Fig. 18-2**A**), but when transmitted to the apex it often assumes lower tones—which do not help to distinguish it from a mitral murmur. At times the aortic regurgitant murmur is quite harsh, at others it may be musical; and when a cusp is retroverted, perforated, or otherwise deformed it may produce the classical "seagull" tone.

The Graham Steell murmur of pulmonic regurgitation (secondary to pulmonary hypertension), is similar to that of aortic regurgitation. When pulmonic regurgitation is due to organic valvular disease, the murmur is lower-pitched, harsher, and more rumbling.[28] Functional pulmonic regurgitation is not uncommon in patients with renal failure and fluid overload, and its murmur disappears with successful dialysis.[31]

The murmur of mitral stenosis is low-pitched and "like an oxcart rumbling over a wooden bridge," whereas the mitral flow murmur is softer and less rumbling. Austin Flint described his similar murmur as "blubbering." The murmur of organic tricuspid stenosis is coarser, higher-pitched, and closer to the ear than the soft, low-pitched murmur of increased tricuspid flow.

The diastolic murmur of Ebstein's anomaly has a scratchy, "rub-like" quality.[32] An anomalous chorda strung across the mitral orifice can produce a musical mid-diastolic and/or presystolic murmur.[33]

Table 18–5
Pharmacodiagnosis of Diastolic Murmurs (DM)

DM	Amyl nitrite	Methoxamine	Serotonin
MS	+		
Austin Flint	−		
AR	−	+	0
PR	+	0	+

MS, mitral stenosis; AR, aortic regurgitation; PR, pulmonic regurgitation; +, increases; −, decreases; 0, no change.

The timing, quality, and site of the more common diastolic murmurs are summarized in Table 18-4.

PHARMACOLOGIC DIAGNOSIS

Pharmacologic aids in the diagnosis of diastolic murmurs are presented in Table 18-5. *Amyl nitrite* may bring to light the otherwise inaudible murmur of mitral stenosis, and may be used when the measures listed in Table 18-2 have not achieved their purpose.[34] Amyl nitrite—by increasing venous return to the right heart, and, in the presence of mitral stenosis, by increasing left atrial and pulmonary artery pressures—also may augment the intensity of the murmur of pulmonic regurgitation,

Table 18–4
Timing, Quality, and Site of Important Diastolic Murmurs

Murmur	Timing	Quality	Site
Mitral stenosis	Mid/late	Low-pitched, rumbling	Apex
Mitral valve flow	Mid	Low-pitched, softer, shorter	Apex
Austin Flint	Mid/late	Low-pitched, rumbling	Apex
Tricuspid stenosis	Mid/late	Higher-pitched	LLSB 4–5 LIS
Tricuspid valve flow	Mid	Soft, short, low-pitched	LLSB 4–5 LIS
Aortic regurgitation	Early	Blowing, high-pitched	3–4 LIS
Pulmonic regurgitation (Graham Steell)	Early	Blowing, high-pitched	2–3 LIS
Pulmonic regurgitation (organic)	Mid	Lower-pitched, harsher, rumbling	2–3 LIS

LLSB, left lower sternal border; LIS, left intercostal spaces.

but may decrease that of aortic regurgitation, and therefore help to differentiate between the two.

These may also be differentiated by comparing the effects of methoxamine and serotonin: *Methoxamine*, by increasing systemic pressure, increases the murmur of aortic regurgitation, leaving that of pulmonic regurgitation unchanged; whereas *serotonin*, by elevating pulmonary pressure, increases pulmonic regurgitation, leaving aortic regurgitation unchanged.[35]

REFERENCES

1. Leatham A. Auscultation of the heart. Lancet 1958;2: 757.
2. Green EW, et al. Right-sided Austin Flint murmur: documentation by intracardiac phonocardiography, echocardiography and postmortem findings. Am J Cardiol 1973; 32:370.
3. McArthur JD, et al. Reassessment of Graham Steell murmur using platinum electrode technique. Br Heart J 1974; 36:1023.
4. Gould L, Lyon AF. Prolapse of the pulmonic valve through a ventricular septal defect. Am J Cardiol 1966; 18:127.
5. Somerville J. Ostium primum defect: factors causing deterioration in the natural history. Br Heart J 1965;27:413.
6. Rosenthal R. Diastolic murmur in patent ductus arteriosus with flow reversal. Arch Intern Med 1964;114:760.
7. Peters MN, et al. The clinical syndrome of atrial myxoma. JAMA 1974;230:695.
8. Sangster JF, Oakley CM. Diastolic murmur of coronary artery stenosis. Br Heart J 1973;35:840.
9. Sloman G, Wee KP. Isolated congenital pulmonary valve incompetence. Am Heart J 1963;66:532.
10. Schrire V, Vogelpoel L. The loud musical diastolic murmur of an abnormal rheumatic chorda. Am Heart J 1961; 62:315.
11. Goodwin JF, et al. Obstructive cardiomyopathy simulating aortic stenosis. Br Heart J 1960;22:403.
12. Perloff JK. The clinical recognition of congenital heart disease, ed 3. Philadelphia: WB Saunders, 1987:141.
13. Nadas AS. Combined aortic and pulmonic stenosis. Circulation 1962;25:346.
14. Hurst JW, Cobbs BW. Diastolic rumbles. Bull Emory Univ Clin 1963;2:69.
15. Paul MH, et al. Congenital complete atrioventricular block: problems of clinical assessment. Circulation 1958; 18:183.
16. Rytand D. An auricular diastolic murmur with heart block in elderly patients. Am Heart J 1946;32:579.
17. Chen CC, et al. Variable diastolic rumbling murmur caused by floating left atrial thrombus. Br Heart J 1983; 50:190.
18. Liebman J, Sood S. Diastolic murmurs in apparently normal children. Circulation 1968;38:755.
19. Leatham A. Rheumatic aortic incompetence with delayed diastolic murmurs on auscultation. Proc R Soc Med 1950; 43:309.50.
20. Tavel ME, Bonner AJ. Presystolic murmur in atrial fibrillation: fact or fiction? Circulation 1976;54:167.
21. Criley JM, Hermer HA. Crescendo presystolic murmur of mitral stenosis with atrial fibrillation. N Engl J Med 1971;285:1284.
22. Criley JM, et al. Mitral valve closure and the crescendo presystolic murmur. Am J Med 1971;51:456.
23. Fortuin N, Craige E. Echocardiographic studies of genesis of mitral diastolic murmurs. Br Heart J 1973;35:75.
24. Toutouzas P, et al. Mechanism of diastolic rumble and presystolic murmur in mitral stenosis. Br Heart J 1974; 36:1096.
25. Toutouzas P, et al. Double diastolic murmur in mitral stenosis with atrial fibrillation and complete heart block. Br Heart J 1980;43:92.
26. Fortuin N, Craige E. On the mechanism of the Austin Flint murmur. Circulation 1972;45:558.
27. Rahko PS. Evaluation of mechanisms producing the Austin Flint murmur. Circulation 1987;76(Suppl 4):316.
28. Runco V, Booth RW. Basal diastolic murmurs. Am Heart J 1963;65:697.
29. Likoff W, et al. Silent rheumatic valvular heart disease. Dis Chest 1966;49:362.
30. Levin HS, et al. The effect of respiration on cardiac murmurs: an auscultatory illusion. Am J Med 1962;33:236.
31. Perez JE, et al. Pulmonic valve insufficiency: a common cause of transient diastolic murmurs in renal failure. Ann Intern Med 1985;103:497.
32. Perloff JK. The clinical recognition of congenital heart disease, ed 3. Philadelphia: WB Saunders, 1987:244.
33. Schrire V, Vogelpoel L. The loud musical diastolic murmur of an abnormal rheumatic chorda. Am Heart J 1961;62:315.
34. Bousvaros G. Response of phonocardiographic and hemodynamic features of mitral stenosis to inhalation of amyl nitrite. Am Heart J 1962;63:101.
35. Endrys J, Bartova A. Pharmacological methods in the phonocardiographic diagnosis of regurgitant murmurs. Br Heart J 1962;24:207.

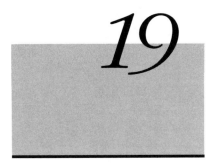

Aortic Stenosis

Left ventricular outflow obstruction may take place at the aortic valve, above the valve, or below it (Table 19-1).

VALVULAR STENOSIS

A simple and practical classification divides aortic stenosis (AS) into congenital, rheumatic, and degenerative-calcific.[1] Congenital and rheumatic disease—and rarely the exuberant vegetations of endocarditis—produce valvular stenosis without aid of calcium. Bicuspid valves may be congenital or acquired (fusion following rheumatic involvement), and both invite the deposition of stiffening and obstructing calcium.[2,3] Calcium is also apparently attracted to normal aging cusps as a result of the physiologic trauma of slapping shut 100,000 times a day. The frequency with which each valve is affected by rheumatic disease is also probably related to the trauma of closure, since the incidence of involvement runs closely parallel with the height of their closing pressures (Table 19-2).[4] Brucellosis as a cause of valvular stenosis has been

enthusiastically proposed,[5] and as enthusiastically rejected.[6]

Calcific stenosis is clearly the final common path for many different pathologic processes (Table 19-1). It afflicts men four times more often than women, and a history of rheumatic fever is found in only about one-third.[7,8] Thus the majority fit into the degenerative-calcific category, and these tend to progress and deteriorate more rapidly than the congenital or rheumatic varieties.[1]

SYMPTOMS

The area of the normally open aortic valve is 3 to 4 cm^2. Symptoms usually do not develop until the area is reduced to about a third of normal (1–1.5 cm^2), and patients with this degree of narrowing may remain asymptomatic for decades. Some are symptom-free with orifices of only 0.5 cm^2.[9]

Symptoms fall into two categories: Angina, dizziness, and syncope, which result from the hemodynamic effects of the narrowed valve; and dyspnea, which results later from failure of the left

Table 19–1
Causes of Aortic Stenosis

Valvular

Noncalcific ⟶ Congenital
⟶ Rheumatic
Secondary ⟶ Atherosclerotic
calcific ⟶ Bacterial endocarditis
⟶ ?Brucellosis
⟶ Bicuspid (congenital or rheumatic)

Primary calcific

Supravalvular

Constricting ring (coarctation)
Membrane or shelf
Hypoplastic ascending aorta

Subvalvular

Discrete membrane
Fibromuscular tunnel
Diffuse muscular
  Idiopathic hypertrophic
  Secondary hypertrophic

Table 19–3
Incidence (%) of Symptoms in Aortic Stenosis (AS)

Author	No. Cases	Dyspnea	Angina	Syncope
Bergeron[19]	100	76	32	12
Mitchell[7]	131	—	37	21
Wood[20]	250*	45	70	33
Uricchio[11]	350	89	49	31
Hancock[17]	41	61	59	37
Anderson[8]	100	94†	54	27
Braunwald[18]	100	54	29	23
Rotman[32]	158	31	50	48

*Percentages based on those with symptoms.
†Based on 51 patients operated on for AS.

ventricle.[9] Dyspnea, however, is the initial symptom in 38% of patients, angina in 34%, and syncope in 15%.

It is not easy to glean their true relative occurrence rate since reports vary greatly: Table 19-3 compares percentages from several representative series. Evidently dyspnea eventually occurs in the majority, angina in perhaps half, and syncope in about one-quarter of the patients. Tiredness and fatigability are also common complaints, but they are so frequently voiced by patients with any form of heart disease—and indeed by the average bored modern man or woman without disease!—that their significance is hard to evaluate.

If dizziness or syncope is brought on by exertion, one should be particularly suspicious of AS.[10] For some reason, angina and syncope appear to be twice as common in pure AS as in combined aortic and mitral stenosis.[11] Sudden death is a well recognized complication of AS, and it may close the eventful history in as many as 23% of cases[7]; most have not suffered from previous syncope. It is seldom sudden in the sense of instantaneous,[12] and is better called "unexpected."

The exact cause or causes of dizziness, syncope, angina, and unexpected death have not been determined. The *angina* may be due to hypertrophied myocardium outgrowing its blood supply; to associated coronary disease; to reduced cardiac output; to partial occlusion of a coronary ostium by an overhanging crag of calcium; to a calcific embolus into coronary artery; or to some combination of these. *Syncope* may result from cerebral ischemia secondary to a reduced cardiac output; from an arrhythmia; from calcific involvement of the A-V junction producing A-V block; from a hypersensitive carotid sinus; or possibly from sudden development of functional subaortic stenosis. *Unexpected death* may result from arrhythmia (ventricular fibrillation), heart block, a coincidental coronary occlusion, or possibly from sudden

Table 19–2
Valve Closing Pressure and Rheumatic Involvement

	Mitral	Aortic	Tricuspid	Pulmonic
Closing pressure in a 10-year-old (mm Hg)	100	60	15	6
Relative rheumatic involvement rate	85%	44%	10%–16%	1%–2%

Table 19–4
Average Survival After Development of Serious Symptoms

Symptom	Survival
Angina of effort	5 years
Syncope	3–4 years
Congestive heart failure	2 years

atrial failure. Among symptomatic patients, unexpected death retires 15% to 20%. Dyspnea and other manifestations of cardiac failure are dreaded complications, as is atrial fibrillation,[13] which develops in about 10%.[9] Average life expectancy after the development of the serious symptoms is summarized in Table 19-4. Once diagnosed, the prognosis of AS is significantly worse than that of aortic regurgitation, mitral stenosis, or mitral regurgitation.[14]

Calcific emboli can produce a variety of symptoms, including visual defects; in fact, the first indication of calcific AS may be sudden blindness in one eye from embolization to a retinal artery.[15]

An unexplained association of AS with massive gastrointestinal bleeding has been reported.[16] Infective endocarditis is a rare complication.

PHYSICAL SIGNS

As with the symptoms of AS, so with the signs it is extremely difficult to achieve meaningful estimates of their relative incidence. Most published series consist of heterogeneous groups of mild, moderate, and severe; congenital and acquired; subvalvular and supravalvular, with and without additional valvular involvement. Since most of these variables influence the clinical manifestations, a numerical analysis of clinical findings is inexact, to say the least.

The Pulse and Blood Pressure

The pulse is normal in mild stenosis; if severe enough, the slow-rising, "anacrotic" pulse (Fig. 19-1) may be perceptible to the trained finger. The pulse contour is better appreciated in the larger accessible arteries (carotid, femoral). The small, slowly rising and falling pulse (pulsus parvus et tardus) is classic but uncommon. A carotid thrill—commonly called carotid "shudder" (Fig. 19-2)—is often palpable.

Surprisingly, the cardiac output and pulse pressure are normal or even elevated in many patients with severe AS[17,18]; this presumably reflects the fact that AS is the only valvular stenosis that makes extra demands on the left ventricle, which in turn demands an increased coronary flow.

Mechanical alternans is often recorded within the left ventricle (Fig. 19-3) in significant AS, but its peripheral influence is damped by the stenosis, and pulsus alternans is much less often detected. If it is found in the peripheral pulse, it indicates that the aortic gradient is not great. In severe stenosis, alternans is sought at the bedside by listening for alternation in intensity of the ejection mur-

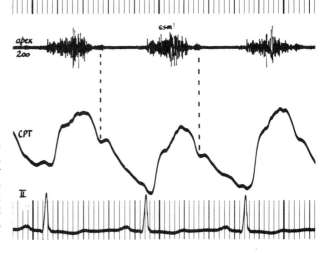

Figure 19–1. From a 57-year-old woman with severe AS (and regurgitation). Note the anacrotic, "stoop-shouldered" upstroke and the poorly formed incisura in the carotid tracing (CPT). In the PCG, the diamond-shaped murmur peaks in the second half of systole and the second sound is barely recorded (dashed line correlates incisura with S2).

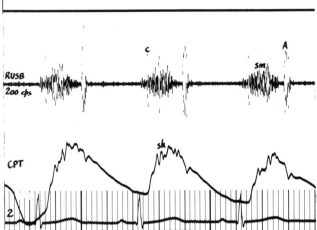

Figure 19–2. From an 8-year-old boy with left ventricular (LV) outflow tract obstruction at two levels: A pressure difference of 33 mm Hg between LV apex and outflow tract, and across the aortic valve a difference of 17 mm Hg. Note the loud ejection click (c), loud A2, and murmur peaking in first half of systole—all typical features of relatively mild stenosis. The carotid tracing shows the jagged contours of a "shudder" (sh)—visible expression of a palpable thrill.

mur, especially following a premature beat[17]; when detectable only in this way, it indicates that the stenosis is indeed severe.

The systolic peak in the left ventricle in severe stenosis may reach 400 to 500 mm Hg,[17] but a brachial systolic pressure over 200 mm Hg is rare in significant stenosis. High pressure can occur, however, and Bergeron[19] reported two cases with pressures of 280/140 and 260/130. Among 41 patients with moderate to severe pure stenosis, the pulse pressure averaged 35 mm Hg but ranged from 12 to 80,[17] and it was over 70 mm Hg in 29% of another series of patients with severe stenosis.[19] Clearly a high pulse pressure does not exclude severe stenosis; but if a low pulse pressure is found (under 20 mm Hg), it is good evidence that the stenosis is severe.

Precordial Findings

Inspection and Palpation

The left ventricular impulse is "quietly heaving,"[20] and not displaced to the left until failure with left ventricular dilation sets in. In severe stenosis a visible and palpable presystolic wave ("atrial kick") may appear (Fig. 19-4), and this is ominous—a plaintive ventricular cry for help. This is closely correlated with an audible S4, and

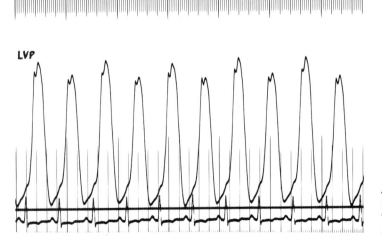

Figure 19–3. Mechanical alternans in pressure tracing recorded from left ventricular cavity (from a patient with ischemic myocardial disease).

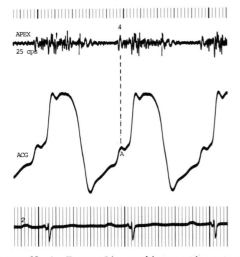

Figure 19–4. From a 54-year-old man with aortic stenosis and regurgitation. Note the loud S4 (4) in the low-frequency PCG coinciding with an abnormal "A" wave in the ACG.

when one or both appear the gradient across the valve is usually over 70 mm Hg, the peak left ventricular systolic pressure is over 160 mm Hg, the end diastolic pressure is 12 mm Hg or more, and there is an "a" wave in the left atrial pressure curve of 14 mm Hg or more.[21]

A systolic thrill is present in 50% to 90% of cases[20,22–24]; it may be well felt all over the precordium and in the neck—carotid "shudder" (see Fig. 19-2)—but is usually maximal either at the aortic area or at the apex. Occasionally it is maximal at the left sternal border, and at other times

it may be felt only in the next.[23] But all thrills in the neck are not due to AS (see Chapter 4).

Auscultation

In the 1950s, such giants of auscultation as Wood and Leatham found an ejection click (see Fig. 19-2; Fig. 19-5) to be much more common in mild than in severe AS, and Braunwald echoes agreement.[18] But other clinicians found the ejection click to be almost invariable in valvular AS, mild or severe, unless heavily calcified.[24,25] In contrast, it is usually absent in subaortic or supravalvular stenosis.[26] Although the association with a dilated aorta is unquestioned, and some authorities favor jet impingement on the dilated wall as the mechanism of production of ejection sounds,[18] there is good reason to believe that their presence depends on mobile valve cusps, since one less often hears an ejection click when the valve is heavily calcified (even though the aorta is dilated), and its intensity parallels that of aortic closure (A2). According to this view, the ejection click is best thought of as an "opening snap" of the aortic valve.

The second sound is variable. In mild stenosis A2 is often accentuated (Figs. 19-2, 19-5); in severe stenosis it is often subdued, sometimes absent (Fig. 19-1), but it is surprisingly often normal even in severe AS. Paradoxical splitting may occur either because of associated left bundle-branch block, or because severe stenosis has sufficiently prolonged left ventricular ejection time; in congenital AS it was found in four of 60 patients with gradients greater than 70 mm Hg,[18] and Wood re-

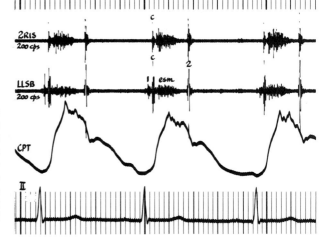

Figure 19–5. From an 11-year-old boy with mild aortic stenosis (pressure difference across valve, 32 mm Hg). Illustrates the value of two simultaneous PCGs in identifying an ejection click: At the aortic area (2RIS), the first identifiable transient is the click (c), whereas the simultaneous record at the LLSB demonstrates that this transient is preceded by another—the first sound (1). The systolic murmur (esm) peaks early and ends well before the loud second sound (2).

ported it in 25% of his cases.[20] An audible S4, in patients under the age of 40 years, usually indicates severe stenosis.[27]

The systolic, crescendo-decrescendo, diamond-shaped ejection murmur begins after S1 and ends before A2 (Figs. 19-1, 19-2, 19-5). It is usually maximal at the aortic area, but it may be loudest to the left of the sternum or at the apex. It was maximal at the apex in 16%,[7] and in 100 autopsy-proven instances of AS, the only murmur in 29 was an apical systolic[19]; such figures may reflect failure to listen attentively to the right of the sternum. At the apex, the murmur may assume a musical quality (Gallavardin effect). The early diastolic murmur of associated aortic regurgitation is obviously a common finding.

In differential diagnosis, remember also that the murmur of mitral regurgitation may be loudest at the ''aortic'' area, and both this murmur and those of pulmonic stenosis, patent ductus, and ventricular septal defect, as well as innocent murmurs, may be well heard in the neck. The pulmonic ejection murmur in the neck is louder on the left, and does not precisely follow the course of the carotids.[28] Behavior of the murmur in relationship to cycle length may help to differentiate the ejection murmur of AS from the regurgitant murmur of mitral regurgitation: The ejection murmur's intensity is proportional to the preceding cycle—louder after a long preceding cycle, softer after a short (Fig. 19-6)—whereas the loudness of the regurgitation murmur is relatively unaffected by changes in the cycle (cf. Fig. 23-4).

Profile: *Aortic Stenosis*

M:F = 4:1
Tiredness, dyspnea
Dizziness, syncope; angina; sudden death

Inconspicuous carotid pulsation
Pulse pressure variable; occasionally low, but
   don't depend on it; sometimes even high
Anacrotic pulse (feel carotids or femorals)—if
   severe
Thrill over carotids and in suprasternal notch
Thrill at RUSB, apex and/or LSB
Sustained LV impulse, with presystolic A wave
   if severe

S2 variable: loud, normal or absent (if severe)
Ejection click—almost invariable: maximal at
   RUSB, apex or LUSB, varying little with
   respiration
S4 at apex (and elsewhere) if severe stenosis
Systolic ejection murmur: maximal at RUSB,
   apex, or LUSB

THE INNOCENT SUPRACLAVICULAR BRUIT

Just above the clavicle in most children, in many young and in fewer older adults, a short vascular bruit is audible.[29-31] It is brief, lasting less than

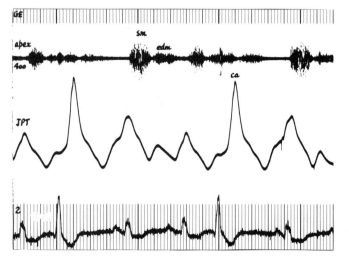

Figure 19-6. Illustrates the effect of cycle length on subsequent ejection murmur: After the long cycle, the murmur greatly intensifies. Compare with regurgitant murmurs which do not intensify (see Figs. 23-4 and 29-6).

half of systole, and is much more common on the right side. It may be well heard below the clavicle and so simulate the murmur of AS or of pulmonic stenosis; but it is louder in the neck, begins later, and is shorter than the ejection murmur of valvular stenosis. It is brought out or accentuated by exercise (like most murmurs), tachycardia, isoproterenol, or epinephrine; it is lengthened and intensified by partial occlusion of the subclavian artery against the first rib, and eliminated by complete occlusion.[31]

REFERENCES

1. Wagner S, Selzer A. Patterns of progression of aortic stenosis: a longitudinal hemodynamic study. Circulation 1982;65:709.
2. Bacon APC, Matthews MB. Congenital bicuspid aortic valves and the aetiology of isolated aortic valvular stenosis. Q J Med 1959;28:545.
3. Edwards JE. On the etiology of calcific aortic stenosis. Circulation 1962;26:817.
4. Wood P. An appreciation of mitral stenosis. Br Med J 1954;1:1051.
5. Peery TM. Brucellosis and heart disease. JAMA 1958;166:1123.
6. Griffith GC, Norris HT. Is brucellosis implicated in calcific aortic stenosis? Ann Intern Med 1961;54:254.
7. Mitchell AM, et al. The clinical features of aortic stenosis. Am Heart J 1954;48:684.
8. Anderson MW. The clinical course of patients with calcific aortic stenosis. Proc Mayo Clin 1961;36:439.
9. Selzer A. Changing aspects of the natural history of valvular aortic stenosis. N Engl J Med 1987;317:91.
10. Leak D. Effort syncope in aortic stenosis. Br Heart J 1959;21:289.
11. Uricchio JF, et al. A study of combined mitral and aortic stenosis. Ann Intern Med 1959;51:668.
12. Bean WB. Calcific aortic stenosis. Modern Concepts of Cardiovascular Disease 1956;25:343.
13. Myler RK, Sanders CA. Aortic valve disease and atrial fibrillation. Arch Intern Med 1968;121:530.
14. Rapaport E. Natural history of aortic and mitral valve disease. Am J Cardiol 1975;35:221.
15. Brochmeier LB, et al. Calcium emboli to the retinal artery in calcific aortic stenosis. Am Heart J 1981;101:32.
16. Williams RC. Aortic stenosis and unexplained gastrointestinal bleeding. Arch Intern Med 1961;108:859.
17. Hancock EW, Fleming PR. Aortic stenosis. Q J Med 1960;29:209.
18. Braunwald E, et al. Congenital aortic stenosis: I. clinical and hemodynamic findings in 100 patients. Circulation 1963;27:426.
19. Bergeron J, et al. Aortic stenosis: clinical manifestations and course of the disease: review of 100 proved cases. Arch Intern Med 1954;94:911.
20. Wood P. Aortic stenosis. Am J Cardiol 1958;1:553.
21. Goldblatt A, et al. Hemodynamic-phonocardiographic correlations of the fourth heart sound in aortic stenosis. Circulation 1962;26:92.
22. Smith JE, et al. Aortic stenosis: a study with particular reference to an indirect carotid pulse recording in diagnosis. Am Heart J 1959;58:527.
23. Cosby RS, et al. A critical review of aortic stenosis. Am J Cardiol 1962;9:203.
24. Gamboa R, et al. Accuracy of the phonocardiogram in assessing severity of aortic and pulmonic stenosis. Circulation 1964;30:35.
25. Vogel JHK, Blount SG. Clinical evaluation in localizing level of obstruction to outflow from left ventricle: importance of early systolic ejection click. Am J Cardiol 1965;15:782.
26. Hancock EW. The ejection sound in aortic stenosis. Am J Med 1966;40:569.
27. Nugent EW, et al. The pathology, abnormal physiology, clinical recognition and medical and surgical treatment of congenital heart disease. In: Hurst, JW, ed. The heart. 7th ed. New York: McGraw Hill, 1990:708.
28. Barlow JB, Pocock WA. The significance of aortic ejection systolic murmurs. Am Heart J 1962;64:149.
29. Stapleton JF, El-Hajj MM. Heart murmurs simulated by arterial bruits in the neck. Am Heart J 1961;61:178.
30. Hammond JH, Eisinger RP. Carotid bruits in 1,000 normal subjects. Arch Intern Med 1962;109:563.
31. Fowler NO, Marshall WJ. The supraclavicular arterial bruit. Am Heart J 1965;69:410.
32. Rotman M, et al. Aortic valve disease: comparison of types and their medical and surgical management. Am J Med 1971;51:241.

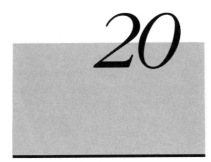

20

Supravalvar and Subvalvar Aortic Stenosis

In addition to aortic valve stenosis, obstruction to outflow from the left ventricle can occur both above and below the valve. The relative frequency of each lesion according to Wood[1] is presented in Table 20-1.

Since both medical and surgical management may radically differ, it is important to determine the level of left ventricular outflow obstruction. Both supravalvar and subvalvar obstruction may present quite distinctive features (Table 20-2) that enable them to be suspected, if not clinched, by physical examination alone, though definitive diagnosis will depend on echocardiography.

SUPRAVALVAR STENOSIS

The aortic obstruction may take the form of hypoplasia, a membrane, an hourglass constriction of the aorta, or diffuse narrowing of the ascending aorta; a number of distinguishing clinical features result (Table 20-2).

Some of these young patients, thanks to an unusual and distinctive "elfin" or "puckish" facies, can be diagnosed at first sight. They have a full head of hair, bright, staring eyes, full lips, flaring nostrils, and short philtrum—obviously they are better seen than described, and excellent photographs have been reproduced by several authors.[2-6] They have acquired a reputation as "charming characters."[3] When a measure of mental retardation is added, the patients are said to have Williams' syndrome, and this is often associated with idiopathic hypercalcemia of infancy.[7] They may have a history of cyanosis in infancy, blue irises, tortuous retinal vessels, strabismus, and hypoplasia of the mandible with a receding chin and teeth with malocclusion. Sometimes they have multiple peripheral pulmonary artery stenoses,[4] or abnormalities of the aorta or its branches distal to the stenosis (eg, a patent ductus arteriosus or stenosis of a subclavian artery). There is a familial tendency[8] among some, but these lack the facial and mental traits.[9]

Table 20–1
Levels of LV Outflow Obstruction[1]

Supravalvar	3%
Valvar	70%
Subvalvar	15%
Muscular	12%
	100%

Examination of the cardiovascular system uncovers an inequality in carotid pulses and arm pulse pressures, with marked pulsation of the right carotid, and with systolic or pulse pressure greater in the right arm.[9] The point of maximal thrill and murmur is higher than with valvar stenosis—in the 1st right interspace and suprasternal notch—and both are well transmitted to the carotids. Ejection click, aortic diastolic murmur, and dilated ascending aorta are *not* in evidence, and A2 is not diminished.

Infective endocarditis and sudden death are ever-present threats.

DISCRETE SUBVALVAR STENOSIS

Narrowing of the left ventricular outflow tract below the aortic valve can be caused by a membrane or by a fibromuscular tunnel; males are affected at least twice as frequently as females, and the membranous type is about five times more common than the tunnel. The obstruction is usually severe, and may worsen progressively.[10] Associated congenital cardiac defects are found in at least half the patients, making the diagnosis of the subvalvar stenosis more difficult; and a few—in one series as many as 10%[11]—have an associated valvar stenosis.

Symptoms are what one would expect with any form of outflow tract obstruction: Fatigue, dyspnea, angina, and dizziness or syncope. Congestive heart failure may eventuate.

The ejection systolic murmur is usually best heard at the mid left sternal border and may be mistaken for the murmur of a ventricular septal defect. There is no ejection click (unless valvar stenosis is associated), and half the patients develop the murmur of aortic regurgitation.

HYPERTROPHIC CARDIOMYOPATHY

In the past, hypertrophic cardiomyopathy has been a terminological battleground, so that McKenna and Goodwin[12] in 1981 were able to list over 40 terms introduced for it in the 15 years between 1957 and 1972. "Cardiomyopathy" was coined by Brigden in 1956 to signify disease of the heart's muscle that was not secondary to coronary, hy-

Table 20–2
Differential Points in LV Outflow Obstruction

	Valvar	Supravalvar	Discrete Subvalvar	HCM
Valve calcification	Common after 40	0	0	0
Dilated asc. aorta	*Common*	Rare	Rare	Rare
PP after VPB	Increased	Increased	Increased	*Decreased*
Valsalva effect on SM	Decreased	Decreased	Decreased	*Increased*
Mitral involvement	Common	0	0	Sometimes MR
Murmur of AR	Common	Rare	Sometimes	0
S4	If severe	Uncommon	Uncommon	*Common*
Intensity of A2	Variable	Variable	Diminished	Normal or diminished
Paradoxic splitting	Sometimes	0	0	Rather common
Ejection click	*Most* (unless valve calcified)	0	0	Uncommon or 0
Max. thrill & murmur	2nd RIS	*1st RIS*	2nd RIS	*4th LIS*
Pulse	Normal to anacrotic	*Unequal*	Normal to anacrotic	*Brisk,* jerky; systolic rebound

PP, pulse pressure; VPB, ventricular premature beat, SM, systolic murmur; AR, aortic regurgitation; RIS, right intercostal space; LIS, left intercostal space; MR, mitral regurgitation.

pertensive, valvar, pericardial, or pulmonary disease.[13] When it was thought that hypertrophied ventricular muscle caused the obstruction, the terms muscular subaortic stenosis (MSS), idiopathic hypertrophic subaortic stenosis (IHSS), or hypertrophic obstructive cardiomyopathy (HOCM) were applied. When it was later realized that neither obstructive symptoms nor a demonstrable gradient were necessarily present, and, indeed, the existence of true obstruction was doubted, its name was shortened to hypertrophic cardiomyopathy (HCM). Hypertrophic cardiomyopathy is idiopathic and hereditary, but an indistinguishable syndrome can result from chronic left ventricular systolic overloading.

A lively debate has raged over the question of "obstruction."[14,15] There is no doubt that, in most cases, a gradient develops between the body of the left ventricle and the outflow tract; on the basis of this, the "pros" assumed obstruction. But a gradient per se does not prove obstruction, and the "cons" who denied it proposed "cavity obliteration" as the source of the gradient: The catheter in the clamped-down cavity registers a higher pressure than when it is in the noncontractile, subvalvar, aortic vestibule.

Brigden finds the argument "specious."[13] Certainly the combination of angina, syncope or near-syncope on exertion, and exertional dyspnea strongly suggests obstruction; and coexistent mitral regurgitation—which is frequently associated[16,17]—could explain many of the findings that the "cons" use as arguments against obstruction. The demonstration by pulsed Doppler echocardiography that *flow continues in the presence of the gradient*,[18,19] certainly confirms that dynamic obstruction is present, and the cause is apposition of the mitral cusp (systolic anterior motion, or SAM) against the hypertrophied septum.

In HCM, the septum is disproportionately hypertrophied (asymmetric septal hypertrophy—ASH) in over 90% of patients; much less often (2% of 965 cases) the apical region is asymmetrically involved.[20] The hypertrophy is generalized in about 5%,[21] and confined to lateral or mid-regions in about 1% each.

In this syndrome, the left ventricle ejects 70% to 85% of its stroke volume in the first half of systole, compared with the normal 55% to 60%.[22] Symptoms and signs depend on an interplay between the pattern and degree of left ventricular hypertrophy, the degree of subaortic "obstruction," the presence of myocardial ischemia, and the amount of diastolic dysfunction.[23]

SYMPTOMS

In the Hammersmith series, the average age at onset was 29 years, and the mean span to death was 9 years.[24]

Symptoms are notably variable, ranging from symptom-free to total disablement; they are not necessarily proportional to the degree of hypertrophy, and their incidence in the original National Institutes of Health series[25] is listed in Table 20-3. Dyspnea, dizziness, syncope, and angina are common and tend to become worse when the patient is erect, or *following* exertion.[26] The angina is usually due to subendocardial ischemia, secondary to the myocardial hypertrophy, and myocardial infarction—often "silent"—with normal coronary arteries has been reported[27]; but a significant minority (19%) have associated coronary artery disease.[28] Symptoms may be further exaggerated by digitalization, or by any of the other provocateurs listed in Table 20-4.

Table 20–3
Incidence of Symptoms and Signs[25]

Symptoms		Signs	
Dyspnea	69%	Audible S4	89%
Angina	39%	Palpable "A"	70%
Dizziness	34%	Systolic thrill	51%
Syncope	30%	Paradoxic splitting	35%
		Ejection click	10%

Table 20–4
Provocative Agents that Increase Gradient and Ejection Murmur

Postextrasystolic pause[29]
Exercise[30]
Valsalva maneuver[31]
Passive tilting[26]
Digitalis[32]
Isoproterenol[33]
Norepinephrine[22]
Nitroglycerine[34]
Amyl nitrite[35]

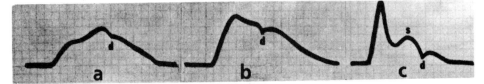

Figure 20–1.   Carotid pulse contour of hypertrophic cardiomyopathy (HCM) compared with normal and with valvar aortic stenosis. **(A)** Severe valvar stenosis: slow upstroke, late summit, poorly formed dicrotic notch (d). **(B)** Normal. **(C)** HCM: rapid upstroke, systolic rebound (s).

In 5% to 10% of patients, especially in those with midventricular hypertrophy, there is progression into a hypokinetic state, with myocardial dilation and development of congestive heart failure.[36] This is sometimes secondary to myocardial infarction, but also occurs in its absence.

SIGNS

The pulse is brisk, jerky, and has a double systolic impact (Fig. 20-1**c**). In normal subjects, as you would expect, the beat ending a postextrasystolic pause shows a rise in left ventricular pressure, arterial systolic pressure, and pulse pressure. But in HCM there is "pressure dissociation": the left ventricular pressure rises all right, but arterial pressures are *lower* than in the beats before the extrasystole (Fig. 20-2). This comparatively weak postextrasystolic beat can be recognized in the pulse, and is as diagnostic as the yield from more sophisticated hemodynamic studies. The gradient that develops is said to depend closely on cycle length, so that in atrial fibrillation a greater gradient may be present at the end of long cycles, whereas little or no gradient is present at the end of short cycles.[37]

A palpable presystolic "A" wave at the apex, corresponding with an exaggerated "A" wave in the apex impulse[38] and an audible S4 (Figs. 20-3, 20-4), are more common than in valvar stenosis. The bifid apical impulse, preceded by the palpable "A" wave, produce a "triple ripple" (Fig. 20-4). On occasion, a third sound may also be palpable, in which case the apical "ripple" becomes quadruple.[39]

An ejection click is rare but occasionally occurs, audible at the apex but not at the base.[40,41]

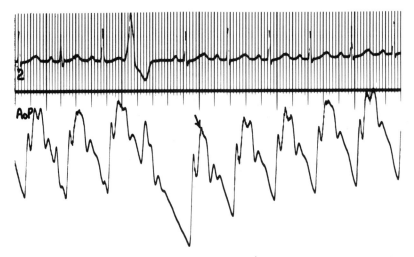

Figure 20–2.   From a 27-year-old woman with hypertrophic cardiomyopathy. The aortic pressure tracing (AoP) is mounted under a simultaneous rhythm strip of lead 2, and the fourth beat is a ventricular extrasystole. In the postectopic beat, the aortic pressure is lower (arrow) than in the sinus beats preceding the extrasystole; and it takes two or three beats to regain the original level of arterial pressure.

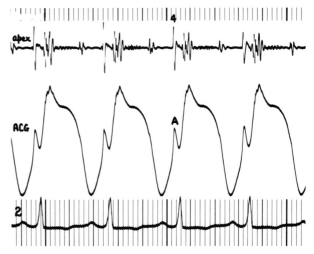

Figure 20–3. From a 22-year-old woman with hypertrophic cardiomyopathy; the giant "A" wave in the apexcardiogram (ACG) is synchronous with an explosive fourth sound (4).

Some observers believe that what is called an ejection click is actually the explosive beginning of the ejection murmur.

The ejection systolic murmur is less rasping than that of valvar aortic stenosis and is seldom well transmitted into the neck; it is usually maximal between the apex and the left lower sternal border, is decreased or abolished by squatting,[42] and there is reason to suspect that it is more an expression of mitral regurgitation than of aortic outflow.[17] During the straining period of a Valsalva maneuver, the murmur gets louder,[43] in contrast with the diminishing murmur of valvar, discrete subvalvar, and supravalvar stenosis. The ejection murmur of HCM may also increase with passive tilting.[44] Of all agents that can be used to provoke a gradient, amyl nitrite is perhaps the

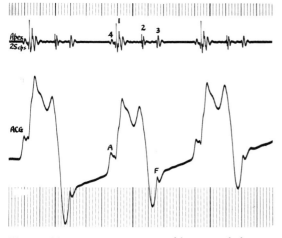

Figure 20–4. From a 35-year-old man with hypertrophic cardiomyopathy. The apexcardiogram (ACG) contains a large, palpable "A" wave corresponding with a fourth sound (4) at the apex, then a bifid systolic impulse, followed by an also palpable rapid filling wave (F) that correlates with the loud third sound (3).

Profile: Hypertrophic Cardiomyopathy

M:F = 2:1
Some familial
Family history of "sudden" death or arrhythmia

Marked variation in severity of symptoms
Dyspnea
Syncope—postural, especially after digitalization
Angina—*after* effort
Unexpected death

Pulse brisk, jerky: double systolic wave
Weaker postextrasystolic beat
Palpable presystolic ("A") wave at apex and double systolic lift ("triple ripple")
Prominent S4
Paradoxical splitting of S2
Systolic thrill and murmur maximal between LLSB and apex
Systolic murmur louder after amyl nitrite, during Valsalva, etc.

(Ejection click and aortic regurgitation rare)

most dependable as well as the safest.[35,45] The mid-diastolic murmur of mitral flow may sometimes be heard.

Left-sided obstruction may be associated with right ventricular outflow tract obstruction as well,[40] in which case right-sided signs are added: Prominent ''a'' wave in the jugular pulse, and thrill and murmur simulating pulmonic stenosis.

Although ventricular tachycardia is the most dreaded arrhythmic complication,[46] atrial fibrillation with the consequent loss of atrial transport function can be devastating in a patient with a stiff, noncompliant left ventricle that depends on a vigorous atrial kick for adequate filling.[13,47,48]

Unexpected death affects a significant minority; in the Hammersmith series of 254 patients, 55% of the 58 who died died suddenly. The most important predictors of it are youth (it rarely happens after the age of 40 years), syncope, and a family history of HCM and sudden death. In adults, non-sustained ventricular tachycardia, recorded by Holter monitoring, is predictive of sudden death,[49] but in infants and children ventricular tachycardia is rare, and their increased risk is unrelated.[50]

REFERENCES

1. Wood P. Diseases of the heart and circulation, ed 3. Philadelphia: JB Lippincott, 1968:391.
2. Williams JCP, et al. Supravalvular aortic stenosis. Circulation 1961;23:1311.
3. Beuren AJ, et al. The syndrome of supravalvular aortic stenosis, peripheral pulmonary stenosis, mental retardation and similar facial appearance. Am J Cardiol 1964;13:471.
4. Beuren AJ, et al. Supravalvular aortic stenosis in association with mental retardation and a certain facial appearance. Circulation 1962;26:1235.
5. Vogel JHK, Blount SG. Clinical evaluation in localizing level of obstruction to outflow from left ventricle: importance of early systolic ejection click. Am J Cardiol 1965;15:782.
6. Perloff JK. The clinical recognition of congenital heart disease, ed 3. Philadelphia: WB Saunders, 1987:95.
7. Taylor AB, et al. Abnormal regulation of circulating 25-hydroxyvitamin D in the Williams syndrome. N Engl J Med 1982;306:972.
8. Logan WFWE, et al. Familial supravalvular aortic stenosis. Br Heart J 1965;27:547.
9. Flaker G, et al. Supravalvar aortic stenosis: a 20-year clinical perspective and experience with patch aortoplasty. Am J Cardiol 1983;51:256.
10. Newfeld EA, et al. Discrete subvalvar aortic stenosis in childhood: study of 51 patients. Am J Cardiol 1976; 38:53.
11. Schneeweiss A, et al. Discrete subvalvar stenosis associated with congenital valvar aortic stenosis: a diagnostic challenge. Am Heart J 1983;106:55.
12. McKenna WJ, Goodwin JF. The natural history of hypertrophic cardiomyopathy. Curr Probl Cardiol 1981;6:5.
13. Brigden W. Hypertrophic cardiomyopathy. Br Heart J 1987;58:299.
14. Criley JM, Siegel RJ. Obstruction is unimportant in the pathophysiology of hypertrophic cardiomyopathy. Postgrad Med J 1986;62:515.
15. Wigle ED, et al. Muscular (hypertrophic) subaortic stenosis (hypertrophic obstructive cardiomyopathy): the evidence for true obstruction to left ventricular outflow. Postgrad Med J 1986;62:531.
16. Wigle ED, et al. Mitral regurgitation in muscular subaortic stenosis. Am J Cardiol 1969;24:698.
17. Kramer DS, et al. The postextrasystolic murmur response to gradient in hypertrophic cardiomyopathy. Ann Intern Med 1986;104:772.
18. Maron BJ, et al. Dynamic subaortic obstruction in hypertrophic cardiomyopathy: analysis by pulsed doppler echocardiography. J Am Coll Cardiol 1985;6:1.
19. Levine RA, Weyman AE. Dynamic subaortic obstruction in hypertrophic cardiomyopathy: criteria and controversy. J Am Coll Cardiol 1985;6:16.
20. Louie EK, Maron BJ. Apical hypertrophic cardiomyopathy: clinical and two-dimensional echocardiographic assessment. Ann Intern Med 1987;106:663.
21. Wigle ED. Hypertrophic cardiomyopathy: a 1987 viewpoint. Circulation 1987;75:311.
22. Krasnow N. Hypertrophic obstructive cardiomyopathy. Am Heart J 1965;69:820.
23. Maron BJ, et al. Hypertrophic cardiomyopathy: interrelations of clinical manifestations, pathophysiology and therapy. N Engl J Med 1987;316:844.
24. McKenna WJ, et al. Arrhythmias in dilated and hypertrophic cardiomyopathy. Med Clin North Am 1984; 68:983.
25. Braunwald E, et al. Idiopathic hypertrophic subaortic stenosis: I. a description of the disease based upon an analysis of 64 patients. Circulation 1964;30(Suppl IV):30.
26. Mason DT, et al. Effects of change in body position on the severity of obstruction to left ventricular outflow in idiopathic hypertrophic subaortic stenosis. Circulation 1966;33:374.
27. Maron BJ, et al. Hypertrophic cardiomyopathy and transmural myocardial infarction without significant atherosclerosis of the extramural coronary arteries. Am J Cardiol 1979;43:1086.
28. Cokkinos DV, et al. Hypertrophic cardiomyopathy and associated coronary artery disease. Texas Heart Institute Journal 1985;12:147.
29. Brockenbrough EC, et al. A hemodynamic technique for the detection of idiopathic hypertrophic subaortic stenosis. 1961;23:189.
30. Whalen RE, et al. Demonstration of the dynamic nature of idiopathic hypertrophic subaortic stenosis. Am J Cardiol 1963;11:8.
31. Marcus FI, et al. The hemodynamic effect of the Valsalva maneuver in muscular stenosis. Am Heart J 1964;67:324.
32. Braunwald E, et al. Studies on digitalis: V. comparison of the effects of ouabain on left ventricular dynamics in valvular aortic stenosis and hypertrophic subaortic stenosis. Circulation 1962;26:166.
33. Braunwald E, Ebert PA. Hemodynamic alterations in idiopathic hypertrophic subaortic stenosis induced by sympathomimetic drugs. Am J Cardiol 1962;19:489.
34. Braunwald E, et al. The circulatory response of patients with idiopathic hypertrophic subaortic stenosis to nitro-

glycerin and the Valsalva maneuver. Circulation 1964; 29:422.

35. Marcus FI, et al. The use of amyl nitrite in the hemodynamic assessment of aortic valvular and muscular subaortic stenosis. Am Heart J 1964;68:468.

36. Fighali S, et al. Progression of hypertrophic cardiomyopathy into a hypokinetic left ventricle: higher incidence in patients with midventricular obstruction. J Am Coll Cardiol 1987;9:288

37. Hancock EW, Eldridge F. Muscular subaortic stenosis: reversibility with varying cycle length. Am J Cardiol 1966;18:515.

38. Wolfe AD. The A wave of the apex cardiogram in idiopathic hypertrophic subaortic stenosis. Br Heart J 1966; 28:179.

39. Schlant RC: Editorial comment. Curr Probl Cardiol 1986;11:581.

40. Goodwin JF, et al. Obstructive cardiomyopathy simulating aortic stenosis. Br Heart J 1960;22:403.

41. Weintraub AM, et al. Poststenotic dilatation of the aorta with muscular subaortic stenosis. Am Heart J 1964; 68:741.

42. de Leon AC: Editorial comment. Curr Probl Cardiol 1981; 6:9.

43. Rosenblum R, Delman AJ. Valsalva's maneuver and the systolic murmur of hypertrophic subaortic stenosis: a bedside diagnostic test. Am J Cardiol 1965;15:868.

44. Pouget JM, et al. Postural hypotension in hypertrophic stenosis. Dis Chest 1966;49:430.

45. Hancock EW, Fowkes WC. Effects of amyl nitrite in aortic valvular and muscular subaortic stenosis. Circulation 1966;33:383.

46. Maron BJ. Prognostic significance of 24 hour ambulatory electrocardiographic monitoring in patients with hypertrophic cardiomyopathy: a prospective study. Am J Cardiol 1981;48:252.

47. Shah PM. Controversies in hypertrophic cardiomyopathy. Curr Probl Cardiol 1986;11:566.

48. Glancy DL, et al. Atrial fibrillation in patients with idiopathic hypertrophic subaortic stenosis. Br Heart J 1970; 32:652.

49. McKenna WJ, et al. Arrhythmias in hypertrophic cardiomyopathy: I. influence on prognosis. Br Heart J 1981; 46:168.

50. McKenna WJ, et al. Arrhythmia and prognosis in infants, children and adolescents with hypertrophic cardiomyopathy. J Am Coll Cardiol 1988;11:147.

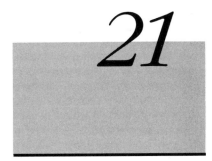

Aortic Regurgitation

Aortic regurgitation* (AR) predominantly affects men, and can result from many diseases (Table 21-1) and mechanisms (Table 21-2).

SYMPTOMS

It is important to realize that compensatory mechanisms are so efficient that patients with severe AR can remain asymptomatic for decades.[14]

Regardless of etiology, the earliest and most common symptoms are palpitation and dyspnea on exertion, but the relentless progression of symptoms in syphilitic AR is twice as rapid as that in rheumatic.[9] Angina occurs in almost half of pa-

---

Note on the Terms "Insufficiency," "Incompetence," and "Regurgitation": These three terms are often used synonymously, but, although they are interdependent, they are not synonyms. The hemodynamic defect is regurgitation, and this is therefore the preferred word unless one is referring specifically to the impaired state of the valvular apparatus, in which case incompetence or insufficiency is appropriate. Naturally enough, the regurgitation that results from the incompetent or insufficient valve is usually implicit in these two terms.

tients with severe AR, and sudden death claims 10%. Less common symptoms include excessive sweating, carotid sheath pain with throbbing and tenderness over carotid arteries, abdominal pain that may simulate a surgical abdomen, "splash" sounds (caused by the vigorous left ventricle or aorta pounding the stomach), and throbbing or pounding sensations anywhere in the body, but particularly in the neck.[15]

PHYSICAL SIGNS

The Murmur

The two most important diastolic murmurs are those of mitral stenosis and of AR. Besides their differences in quality and timing, they offer two other important contrasts: That of mitral stenosis has many mimics, that of AR has few; and in the recognition of subtle mitral stenosis, the murmur plays a modest role, whereas in subtle AR the murmur is the entire cast.

It is sometimes taught that AR is recognized by

Table 21–1
Causes of Aortic Regurgitation

Acquired	Congenital
Rheumatic	With other defects
Syphilitic*	Aortic stenosis
Infective endocarditis[†]	Coarctation of aorta
Ventricular septal defect	Aortic sinus aneurysm, unruptured[6]
Ankylosing spondylitis[1]	Absence of pulmonic valve
Reiter's syndrome[2]	
Dissecting aneurysm	
Marfan's syndrome	
Cystic medionecrosis	Without other defects
Osteogenesis imperfecta[3]	Bicuspid aortic valve
Ehlers-Danlos syndrome[4]	
Giant-cell aortitis[5]	Mechanical equivalents
Hypertension[‡]	Aortico-LV tunnel[7]
Atherosclerosis	Aortic sinus rupture
Fenestration of cusps[§]	Coronary arterio-LV fistula
Exertion, trauma[‖]	

Syphilis as a cause of AR might be thought to be disappearing from the scene; but it accounted for more than two-thirds of the cases in a group of elderly patients as recently as 1966.[8]
[†]In one series of *rheumatic AR*, no less than 22% had a history of infective endocarditis.[9]
[‡]About 6% of *hypertensive* subjects have faint, short murmurs of AR[10]; others have found AR in 9%.[11] The regurgitation associated with hypertension is usually mild or moderate, but in a small percentage it may be severe.[12]
[§]Of hearts examined at autopsy, 72% had some degree of *fenestration* of aortic or pulmonic cusps or both, at times sufficient to permit regurgitation.[13]
[‖]When *exertion* or *trauma* produces AR, there is almost always preexisting disease—rheumatic, syphilitic, infective endocarditis, or Marfan's disease.

---

its peripheral signs; and of course it may happen that way. But if you wait for these signs before making the diagnosis, you will miss half the cases and these the most rewarding—the early cases with trivial leakage—for whom prophylactic treatment offers maximal benefit. *The murmur is the all-important sign*, but it is often not easy to detect: In one series, over half were missed by ward physicians.[8] As with all other auscultatory signs, the first rule is to LISTEN FOR IT; and the way to do this is to follow the "five-step" table in Chapter 18—and press your diaphragm *firmly* with the patient sitting upright and leaning a little forward. Rarely, the murmur is better heard with the patient lying rather than sitting.[16]

The murmur may vary all the way from the shortest, faintest puff to a harsh or musical pandiastolic murmur (Fig. 21-1), accompanied by a thrill, and audible far and wide, including remote and unlikely outposts such as the elbow and the top of the head. Intensity and duration tend to parallel severity, but even serious AR, when accompanied by other signs of rheumatic valvular disease, can be silent.[17] In one important series, the intensity of the murmur did not correlate with the degree of reflux observed at the time of surgery.[18] Having the patient squat may make the faint murmur audible.[19]

Often pandiastolic, the murmur may be shorter both because the leak is slight and because it is severe. When the murmur is musical (Fig. 21-2), one thinks of eversion (Fig. 21-3), perforation or rupture of a cusp[20,21] but this is not necessarily present.[22,23] Musical murmurs may be heard in syphilitic, rheumatic, endocarditic, and traumatic regurgitation.

The shape of the murmur varies. Beginning with S2, it is usually described as decrescendo (Fig. 21-4**A**), but probably always has a short initial crescendo (Figs. 21-4**B–E**). Sometimes it be-

Table 21–2
Mechanisms of Aortic Regurgitation

Deformity of Cusps
Rheumatic
Infective endocarditis
Aortic stenosis
Fenestration
Ankylosing spondylitis
Reiter's syndrome
Bicuspid aortic valve

Enlargement of Ring
Syphilis
Hypertension
Coarctation of aorta
Cystic medionecrosis
Marfan's syndrome
Giant-cell aortitis
Ehlers-Danlos syndrome
Osteogenesis imperfecta

Displacement of Cusps
Dissecting aneurysm
Aortic sinus aneurysm
Ventricular septal defect
Supravalvar aortic stenosis (tethering to constricting ring)

gins late, or at least sounds as though it does (Fig. 21-4**C**). At times there are mid- and late diastolic accentuations (Fig. 21-4**D**), at others just a late

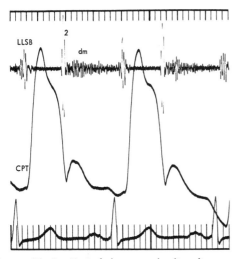

Figure 21–1. Typical decrescendo diastolic murmur (dm) of aortic regurgitation; note that it begins immediately after the second sound (2) and persists until the next first sound. CPT, carotid pulse tracing.

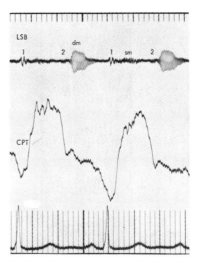

Figure 21–2. Musical decrescendo diastolic murmur (dm); note the "smooth" contour of the recorded murmur, typical of musicality. The summit of the carotid tracing (CPT) is rough and jagged, the so-called carotid "shudder"—visible expression of the palpable thrill. 1, first sound; 2, second sound; sm, systolic murmur.

crescendo imparting a "dumbbell" shape to the murmur (Fig. 21-4**E**).[23]

Usually best heard at Erb's point (3rd left interspace) or at the left lower sternal border, the murmur may be widely transmitted. If it is better heard down the right sternal border, one should think of one of the forms of AR resulting from disease of the aortic root (Table 21-3) rather than rheumatic valvular disease.[24] The combination of hypertension with AR and right-sided transmission suggests aneurysm or dissection of the aorta.

An early diastolic murmur—even in the presence of mitral stenosis and in the absence of other signs of AR—means AR until proven otherwise.[25] In the presence of mitral stenosis it is often tempting to diagnose an early diastolic murmur as a

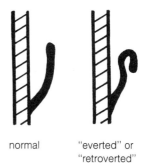

normal   "everted" or "retroverted"

Figure 21–3. Diagrammatic comparison of normal versus everted or retroverted posture of an aortic cusp.

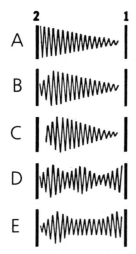

Figure 21–4. Profiles of aortic diastolic murmurs.

Graham Steell murmur; but if you do you will usually be wrong. Of 25 murmurs thought clinically to be Graham Steell murmurs, 18 proved on catheterization to be due to AR.[26] Clinical differentiation between the AR and Graham Steell murmurs is summarized in Chapter 18. In doubtful cases, phonocardiography, by demonstrating whether the murmur begins with A2 or P2, may help to distinguish.[27]

Other Cardiac Findings

You may feel both diastolic and systolic thrills; the apex beat is hyperdynamic and displaced downward and to the left, and a palpable F point (S3) may be felt.

The first heart sound is normal in mild or moderate AR, but may disappear at the apex in severe disease because of premature closure of the mitral

Table 21–3
"Right-Sided" Aortic Diastolic Murmurs

1. Syphilis
2. Dissecting aneurysm
3. Hypertension
4. Atherosclerosis
5. Marfan's syndrome
6. Aortic sinus aneurysm
7. Infective endocarditis
8. VSD with resulting AR

valve. An aortic ejection click is common in moderate or severe AR. The second sound is often loud unless it is diminished by accompanying severe valvular calcific stenosis, and it may have a ringing quality in syphilis, hypertension, or atherosclerosis. A loud third sound is the rule in severe AR; in fact, virtually all patients with free regurgitation have loud aortic systolic murmurs with associated thrills, a ventricular gallop, and an Austin Flint murmur; and the third sound is an index of left ventricular dysfunction, not just a reflection of the hyperdynamic state.[28] Differentiation of the Flint murmur from that of associated mitral stenosis is summarized in Chapter 18; its genesis is probably mitral flow.[29]

Peripheral Signs

Free AR produces a galaxy of peripheral signs that reflect the deranged hemodynamics. Most of these are more intriguing than useful.

The systolic *blood pressure* is normal or high, the diastolic pressure normal or low, and the pulse pressure normal or wide. Severe AR may present with a BP of 280/70 or 120/0 mm Hg—or any points in between!

Perhaps the most valuable single clinical sign in assessing the severity of the regurgitation is *Hill's sign*—a disproportionate elevation of BP in the legs. Normally the systolic BP is 10 or 20 mm higher in legs than arms; in significant AR the leg pressure is over 20 and may be 50 or even 100 mm higher (Hill, 1912). The pressure difference correlates well with severity:[30]

Under 20 mm Hg—hemodynamically insignificant
20–40 mm Hg—mild to moderate regurgitaton
40–60 mm Hg—moderately severe regurgitation
Over 60 mm Hg—severe regurgitation

The *bisferiens pulse* (Fig. 21-5) is of some diagnostic value. It is characteristic of significant AR (Steell, 1894), with or without aortic stenosis. In anemia, hyperthyroidism, and other high-output states, as well as in some healthy people, percussion and tidal peaks may be prominent enough to give a bisferious impression, and in hypertrophic subaortic stenosis and patent ductus a distinct double systolic beat may be felt. Youth, low diastolic BP, large stroke volume, and AR tend to produce bisferiens, whereas advancing age, rise in diastolic pressure, reduction in stroke volume, and aortic

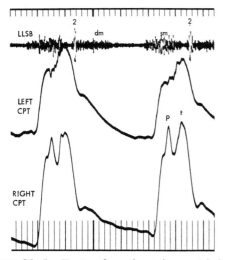

Figure 21–5. Tracing from the right carotid shows typical bisferiens contour; left carotid manifests "shudder." PCG records systolic (sm) and diastolic (dm) murmurs. 2, second sound; p, percussion wave; t, tidal wave.

stenosis tend to oppose its development.[31] Partial compression of the artery proximal to the palpating finger may bring bisferiens to light or accentuate it, and a corresponding double sound may develop as the BP cuff is deflated between systolic and diastolic pressures.[32] Bisferiens may be much better felt in one carotid than the other.

Pulsus alternans (Chapter 4) is common in severe AR.

Corrigan pulse properly refers to the bounding carotid pulse only (Hodgkin, 1829; Corrigan, 1832).

Waterhammer pulse, the "slapping" pulse (Vieussens, 1715), is so called because it is said to be reminiscent of the sharp impact felt on shaking the waterhammer, a Victorian child's toy consisting of a bolus of water in a vacuum tube (Watson, 1843). It is best felt with the flat of the palm pressed against the volar surface of the patient's forearm held aloft. Since the impact retreats sharply as well, the pulse is also called *collapsing*.

Calf sign is a pulse felt when the calf of a raised leg rests on the examiner's palm.

Leg sign: When sitting with legs crossed, the dangling foot jerks forward abnormally with each heart beat.

In *de Musset's sign* the head shakes with each heart beat; it is named after the amorous French poet whose head displayed the sign as he sat writing on the subject in whose pursuit his own aortic valve had lost its competence.

Duroziez' sign: A systolic-diastolic bruit over a major artery; the to-and-fro murmur may have to be worked for by rocking your bell so that the distal rim *partly compresses* the femoral (or other) artery (Duroziez, 1861).

In *"pistol-shot femorals"* the pulse wave creates a sound like a muffled shot when you auscultate *without compressing* the vessel. This sound is obviously the equivalent of a zero diastolic pressure and analogous to the Korotkoff sound.

Traube's sign is a double sound heard with the stethoscope lightly applied over the artery (Traube, 1872)—not to be confused with the double tone associated with bisferiens.

Quincke's pulse, or "capillary pulsation," consisting of alternate flushing and blanching of vascular areas (such as the nailbed or forehead), is a common sign in moderate to severe AR, but is by no means diagnostic of it (Table 21-4). It may be seen in any condition characterized by a high pulse pressure and/or arteriolar dilation, and also seems to be favored by rigid great vessels. It is of greater hemodynamic importance when it is "spontaneous," that is, when you don't have to use nail-bending, skin-scratching, slide-pressing, or trans-illuminating maneuvers to elicit it (Quincke, 1890).

Pulsation of various organs is sometimes seen, including uvula (Muller, 1889), liver (Rosenbach, 1878), spleen (Gerhardt, 1905), or pupil (Landolfi).

Pulsation of visible vessels can also be seen, including retinal arteries and dorsal veins of hand.

In eliciting the above peripheral signs, keep in mind that although they are most florid in AR, most of them can be found, at least in modified form, in other high-output states. And remember that Traube's and the pistol shot signs are present without compressing the artery, whereas Duroziez' murmur and the sounds associated with bisferiens require critical pressure on the artery.

Table 21–4
Causes of "Capillary" Pulsation

Fever, exercise, pregnancy

Hyperthyroidism, anemia

Aortic regurgitation

A-V fistula (PDA, etc.)

Complete A-V block

SUDDEN, SEVERE AR

When severe AR develops abruptly, as from infective endocarditis, there is not time for the left ventricular hypertrophy that characterizes chronic AR to develop; nor are most of the peripheral vascular signs outlined above likely to be present. In fact, the clinical picture is dominated by severe progressive congestive heart failure accompanied by a characteristic clinical profile[35,36]: absent S1 at the apex, visible and palpable double apical impulse in diastole ("double diastolic apex beat"), an early diastolic sound occurring just after S3 and thought to be due to premature closure of the mitral valve, and loud, harsh systolic and diastolic murmurs making the differentiation between systole and diastole difficult.

Apart from these distinctive features, other findings are notable, including the invariable presence of tachycardia, the dominant venous rather than arterial pulsations in the neck,[36] the shorter regurgitant murmur compared with that of chronic AR, and the Austin Flint murmur confined to mid-diastole (because of early mitral closure). Pulsus alternans is common, but the waterhammer pulse, capillary pulsation, Duroziez murmur and the other peripheral signs of chronic AR are absent.

The several causes of acute AR are listed in Table 21-5. A clue to the cause of the sudden catastrophe may be obtained if the patient has a history of hypertension (aortic dissection), if the event interrupted a febrile illness (endocarditis), or if features of Marfan's syndrome are present.

Profile: *Aortic Regurgitation*

M:F = 2 or 3:1
History of RF, syphilis, or endocarditis

Dyspnea, palpitations, "pounding" sensations, angina, carotid sheath pain, excessive sweating, abdominal pain, "splash" sounds, sudden death

Pallor

Peripheral signs: low diastolic BP, wide PP;
  Hill's sign
  de Musset's sign
  Corrigan and waterhammer pulse
  Duroziez' murmur and Traube's double tone
  Pulsus bisferiens and alternans
  "Capillary" pulsation

Hyperdynamic LV impulse, low and wide;
  palpable F-point
Diastolic and systolic thrills
S1—normal or absent
S2—loud, ringing or diminished (with calcific stenosis)
S3—ventricular gallop if severe
Aortic EC common

Early diastolic murmur: maximal at LSB, sometimes RSB; often well heard at apex
Aortic ejection murmur
Austin Flint murmur

Table 21–5
Causes of Acute Aortic Regurgitation

1. Infective endocarditis
2. Rupture of aortic leaflets
   a. Leaflet fenestration
   b. Myxomatous leaflet
   c. Traumatic
3. Prolapse of aortic leaflet
   a. "Normal"
   b. Myxomatous[33]
4. Dissecting aneurysm
5. Behcet's syndrome[34]
6. Surgical—faulty incision[36]

REFERENCES

1. Toone EC, et al. Aortitis and aortic regurgitation associated with rheumatoid spondylitis. Am J Med 1959; 26:255.
2. Rodnan GP, et al. Reiter's syndrome and aortic insufficiency. JAMA 1964;189:889.
3. Criscitiello MG, et al. Cardiovascular abnormalities in osteogenesis imperfecta. Circulation 1965;31:255.
4. Tucker DH, et al. Ehlers-Danlos syndrome with a sinus of Valsalva aneurysm and aortic insufficiency simulating rheumatic heart disease. Am J Med 1963;35:715.
5. Austen WG, Blennerhasset JB. Giant-cell aortitis causing an aneurysm of the ascending aorta and aortic regurgitation. N Engl J Med 1965;272:80.
6. London SB, London RE. Production of aortic regurgitation by unperforated aneurysm of the sinus of Valsalva. Circulation 1961;24:1403.

7. Levy MJ, et al. Aortico-left ventricular tunnel. Circulation 1963;27:841.

8. Bleich A, et al. Aortic regurgitation in the elderly. Am Heart J 1966;71:627.

9. Segal J, et al. A clinical study of one hundred cases of severe aortic insufficiency. Am J Med 1956;21:200.

10. Puchner TC, et al. Aortic valve insufficiency in arterial hypertension. Am J Cardiol 1960;5:758.

11. Barlow J, Kincaid-Smith P. The auscultatory findings in hypertension. Br Heart J 1960;22:505.

12. Waller BF, Roberts WC. Severe aortic regurgitation secondary to systemic hypertension (without aortic dissection). Cardiovasc Rev Rep 1982;3:1504.

13. Friedman B, Hathaway BM. Fenestration of the semilunar cusps, and "functional" aortic and pulmonic valve insufficiency. Am J Med 1958;24:549.

14. Nishimura RA, et al. Chronic aortic regurgitation: indications for operation—1988. Mayo Clin Proc 1988;63:270.

15. Harvey WP, et al. Unusual clinical features associated with severe aortic insufficiency. Ann Intern Med 1957;47:27.

16. Leatham A. Auscultation of the heart. Lancet 1958;2:757.

17. Segal BL, et al. "Silent" rheumatic aortic regurgitation. Am J Cardiol 1964;14:628.

18. Cohn LH, et al. Preoperative assessment of aortic regurgitation in patients with mitral valve disease. Am J Cardiol 1967;19:177.

19. Vogelpoel L, et al. The value of squatting in the diagnosis of aortic regurgitation. Am Heart J 1969;77:709.

20. Stembridge VA, et al. Unusual musical murmurs of anterior cusp aortic regurgitation. Am Heart J 1954;48:163.

21. Groom D, Boone A. The "dove-coo" murmur and murmurs heard at a distance from the chest wall. Ann Intern Med 1955;42:1214.

22. Gelfand D, Bellet S. The musical murmur of aortic insufficiency: clinical manifestations based on a study of 18 cases. Am J Med Sci 1951;221:644.

23. Dressler W, Rubin R. Complex shape and variability of the diastolic murmur of aortic regurgitation. Am J Cardiol 1966;18:616.

24. Harvey WP, Perloff JK. Some recent advances in clinical auscultation of the heart. Prog Cardiovasc Dis 1959;2:97.

25. Brest AN, Udhoji V, Likoff W. A re-evaluation of the Graham Steell murmur. N Engl J Med 1960;263:1229.

26. Runco V, et al. The Graham Steell murmur versus aortic regurgitation in rheumatic heart disease. Am J Med 1961;31:71.

27. Schwab RH, Killough JH. The phonocardiographic differentiation of pulmonic and aortic insufficiency. Circulation 1965;32:352.

28. Abdulla AM, et al. Clinical significance and hemodynamic correlates of the third heart sound gallop in aortic regurgitation. Circulation 1981;64:464.

29. Fortuin NJ, Craige E. On the mechanism of the Austin Flint murmur. Circulation 1972;45:558.

30. Frank MJ, et al: Evaluation of aortic insufficiency: clinical, radiologic, and hemodynamic criteria of severity. Circulation 1963;28:723.

31. Ikram H, et al. The hemodynamic implications of the bisferiens pulse. Br Heart J 1964;26:452.

32. Ciesielski J, Rodbard S. Doubling of the arterial sounds in patients with pulsus bisferiens. JAMA 1961;175:475.

33. Olinger GN, et al. Acute aortic valvular insufficiency due to isolated myxomatous degeneration. Ann Intern Med 1978;88:807.

34. Comess KA, et al. Acute, severe, aortic regurgitation in Behcet's syndrome. Ann Intern Med 1983;99:639.

35. Wigle ED, Labrosse CJ. Sudden severe aortic insufficiency. Circulation 1965;32:708.

36. Morganroth J, et al. Acute severe aortic regurgitation: pathophysiology, clinical recognition, and management. Ann Intern Med 1977;87:223.

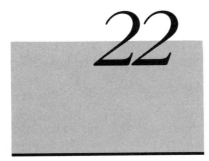

Mitral Stenosis

Mitral stenosis may be concealed under a quarter of a dollar.

Osler

On the rare occasions when narrowing of the mitral valve is not due to *rheumatic* mitral stenosis (MS), it may be *congenital* (''funnel'' and ''diaphragm'' types), or caused by exuberant vegetations in the course of *infective endocarditis* on an otherwise only incompetent valve, or by *amyloid* infiltration. Left ventricular inflow tract obstruction, however, can result from other lesions originating both above and below the mitral orifice. An *atrial myxoma* or *massive atrial thrombus* may occlude the valve orifice, and, below the valve, hypertrophy of ventricular muscle (*obstructive cardiomyopathy*, either primary or secondary to the LV hypertrophy of aortic stenosis, coarctation, etc.) can obstruct inflow.

RHEUMATIC MITRAL STENOSIS

In the Western world, rheumatic MS has a bias for women, whom it affects three or four times more often than men, with onset of symptoms at an aver-age of about 30 years,[1] two decades after the initial attack of rheumatic fever; an average of 7 more years is then required to produce total disability.[2] Half the patients with mitral stenosis give no history of an attack of rheumatic fever.

In other climates and races the disease may show different proclivities; in India, for example, it prefers men and develops rapidly to produce serious pulmonary hypertension and great incapacity at an earlier age, but with low incidence of atrial fibrillation and embolism.[3]

PATHOPHYSIOLOGY

The train of trouble in MS stems from a two-fold resistance to blood flow: Primarily at the mitral orifice and secondarily in the pulmonary arteriolar bed.[4] Mitral narrowing becomes significant when the valve area is reduced to 25% or less of normal, and pulmonary arteriolar resistance when it increases to five times normal.[5] The sequence of important hemodynamic events in the natural history of MS is as follows:

Valve narrows from normal size (4–5 cm²) to less than 25%
↓
Left atrial pressure rises to maintain mitral flow
↓
Pulmonary venous and capillary pressures rise   → Pulmonary edema, hemoptysis
↓
Arteriolar changes develop increasing pulmonary vascular   → Protects against pulmonary edema
resistance and pulmonary artery pressure   and hemoptysis
↓
RV hypertrophy and failure; cardiac output and O₂ saturation fall

---

The high pulmonary vascular resistance saves the patient from drowning but imposes a low cardiac output; instead of hemoptysis, orthopnea, paroxysmal dyspnea, and pulmonary edema, she suffers venous and hepatic distention, peripheral edema, and fatigue.[1]

The incidence of clinical findings in large series of patients with "pure" MS is remarkably consistent (Table 22-1).

SYMPTOMS

Dyspnea is the earliest and most common symptom, secondary to the raised left atrial/pulmonary vein pressure and consequently noncompliant lungs. In its most florid form, frank *pulmonary edema* develops and may be lethal.

Hemoptysis in MS takes five forms[1]:

1. *"Pulmonary apoplexy"*: sudden, unexpected, profuse; often provoked by exertion or pregnancy; a relatively early symptom, not in itself so serious as it is alarming,
2. *Blood-stained sputum* associated with attacks of dyspnea due to acute pulmonary congestion,
3. *Blood-streaked sputum* associated with attacks of bronchitis,
4. *Pink, frothy sputum* due to pulmonary edema, and
5. *Frank hemoptysis* from pulmonary infarction.

Angina, indistinguishable from that of ischemic heart disease (brought on by effort, relieved by nitroglycerin, etc.) occurs in 12% to 16%, but only in patients who have developed significant pulmonary hypertension. The cause of the pain is uncertain: It may be due to reduced perfusion of the right ventricular myocardium because of the high intracavitary pressure,[8] or it may be that the lowered left ventricular output starves the coronary circulation.

Systemic embolism occurs in 14% to 16% of patients with pure stenosis, and atrial fibrillation

Table 22–1
Incidence (%) of Selected Clinical Findings Among Patients with Mitral Stenosis "Pure" Enough to be Submitted to Valvotomy

Author	No. Cases	History of Rheumatic Fever	Hemoptysis	Angina	Systemic Embolism	RV Lift	Closing Snap	Opening Snap	Atrial Fibrillation
Wood[1]	150	60	50	12	14	79	90	83	41
Goodwin[6]	70	47	48	16	16	85	80	84	55
Schrire[7]	356	44	49	14	14	70	50+	85	22

is present in more than half of these.[1,6] There is a definite relationship between the size of the left atrial appendage and the incidence of embolism, though the size of the appendage is not itself related to the overall size of the left atrium or to the degree of stenosis.[9]

An occasional patient develops *hoarseness* from impingement by the enlarging left atrium on the recurrent laryngeal nerve.

PHYSICAL SIGNS

If you see a freckle-faced, red-haired young woman sitting in an outpatient department waiting to see a cardiologist, you can be reasonably sure she has mitral stenosis. If her family name is O'Reilly, or something equally Irish, you have further confirmation. She may show the malar flush that has earned the designation, *mitral facies.* Mild *peripheral cyanosis* is not uncommon, with cold fingers and toes.

A *right ventricular lift* is found in 70% to 85% of patients with "pure" MS. Its presence usually indicates tight stenosis, pulmonary hypertension, and the need for valvotomy.[10] It can be seen and felt, and, to elicit the sign, Dressler recommends applying the heel of the hand "with considerable pressure to the precordial area close to the lower half of the sternum." Associated tricuspid regurgitation, which causes precordial retraction in systole, may diminish or eliminate the lift. A *diastolic thrill* is often palpable at the apex.

The *opening snap* (OS), discussed in detail in Chapter 12, is illustrated in Figures 22-1 to 22-3. It is audible in about 85% of patients with stenosis "pure" enough to warrant valvotomy, but is a sign of leaflet pliancy. Factors that reduce the incidence or intensity of a snap include significant mitral insufficiency,[1] rigidity and calcification of the valve,[11–14] high pulmonary vascular resistance,[1,15,16] and massive thrombus in the left atrium.[17]

An early OS may be confused with the second component of a widely split S2. Having the patient stand may clarify the issue: On standing, the interval between A2 and P2 narrows, whereas the S2–OS interval widens.[18] But the surest means of distinction is to hear all three transients—A2, P2, and OS. In Figure 22-2 the two components of S2 (A,P) separate and make it clear that the final transient is an OS.

An elevated left atrial pressure causes the mitral valve to:

1. Open earlier—which brings OS closer to S2, ie, shortens the 2–OS interval (measured from onset of A2 to onset of OS), and
2. Close later—which delays M1, ie, lengthens the Q–1 interval (measured from onset of QRS to onset of M1).

In general, the 2–OS interval by itself is an unreliable guide to the severity of the stenosis,[19] but a 2–OS interval of 0.07 second or less usually indicates significant stenosis; at times this degree of shortening develops only after exercise.

Figure 22–1. From a 35-year-old woman with pure mitral stenosis. A2 (A) and the opening snap (os) are conspicuous, and the snap is followed by a middiastolic murmur (mdm) that fades before gathering intensity in late diastole (psm). The presystolic murmur ends in a much accentuated first sound ("closing snap"); the barely visible lower tip of its excursion in the PCG is indicated by S1.

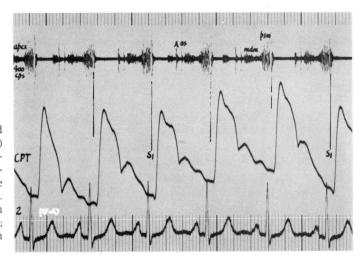

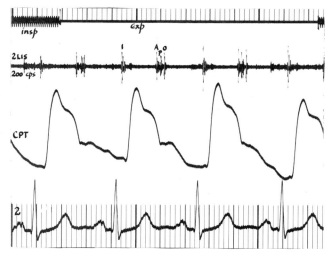

Figure 22–2. From the same patient as in Figure 22–1. The three transients A2 (A), P2 (P), and the opening snap (O) are discretely audible. 2LIS, 2nd left interspace; 1, first heart sound; CPT, carotid pulse tracing.

The Q–1 and 2–OS intervals have been combined to produce a formula (Wells' index[20]: Q–1 minus 2–OS) to predict the severity of the stenosis. Unfortunately, because of other variables, the index is not dependable; at times it has correlated well with the severity found at surgery,[21] but on the whole is a better predictor of the diastolic gradient across the valve.[22] Other investigators[23] have found that neither the 2–OS interval alone nor the Wells' index is a good guide to severity.

The OS is the trademark but not the monopoly of MS, because one may be heard in a number of conditions associated with exuberant flow across the atrioventricular valves.[24]

The *closing snap* (or accentuated S1) is one of the most important clues to MS (Figs. 22-1, 22-4, 22-6); at its most typical it feels and sounds like a

small metallic hammer-tap within the chest. It is present in from 50% to 90% of patients with pure stenosis (Table 22-1). Factors that may reduce the intensity of the closing snap include: A rigid, calcified valve; associated significant mitral regurgitation; aortic regurgitation; pulmonary hypertension; congestive failure; atrial fibrillation; and lengthened cycles.

During atrial fibrillation, the short diastoles sometimes end with an obviously split S1; this is the two-fold result of (1) delaying M1, and (2) intensifying T1. Normally M1 occurs slightly before T1; in MS, because of the abnormally high pressure in the left atrium, mitral closure is delayed, and this delay is further enhanced by short diastoles—which give even less time for left atrial decompression. Thus M1 may occur an apprecia-

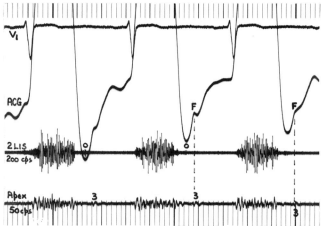

Figure 22–3. Illustrates the relationship of the diastolic transients to events in the apexcardiogram (ACG). The opening snap (o)—best seen in the high-frequency (200 cps) PCG—coincides with the O-point, and the third sound (3)—best seen in the low-frequency (50 cps) PCG—with the F-point.

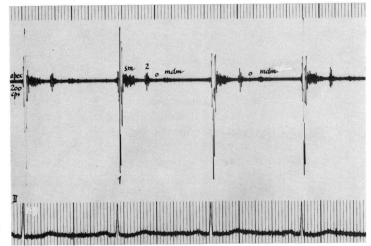

Figure 22–4. From a 55-year-old man with mitral stenosis, showing the greatly accentuated first sound (1)— "closing snap"—followed by a short, decrescendo systolic murmur (sm). Opening snap (o) and mid-diastolic murmur (mdm) are faintly recorded.

ble time *after* T1, with audible and obvious splitting. Knowledge of these time relationships is important if you have a phonocardiograph (PCG) available and wish to measure the Q–1 interval.

In patients with pulmonary hypertension, you may hear a pulmonic ejection sound and murmur.

The *diastolic murmur* is always present except in those rare cases of "silent" or "murmurless" stenosis. Be sure to listen for it precisely at the apex beat, aware that it may be sharply localized— remember Osler's quarter! The murmur always begins an appreciable interval after S2. It may be a short, mid-diastolic (Fig. 22-5**A**), or just a late diastolic (presystolic) murmur (Fig. 22-5**B**); or the two may combine to form a long decrescendo-crescendo murmur (Fig. 22-5**C**); or the mid-diastolic and presystolic elements may be separated by a silent interval (Fig. 22-5**D**); or it may be a long, low-pitched murmur rumbling its way through diastole without much variation in intensity (Fig. 22-5**E**). On the other hand, the long murmur may begin loudly or show presystolic accentuation.

Factors that influence the form of the murmur include:

1. The two periods of rapid ventricular filling, that is, "mid" diastole (right after the A-V valve opens) and presystole (during atrial contraction). It was naturally thought that the presystolic component was due to atrial contraction, but careful timing has demonstrated that the maximal moment of the presystolic murmur occurs after atrial contraction is over; some claim that the major mechanism is the effect of closing leaflets

that narrow the inlet in the face of the still oncoming stream.[25] This could explain why a presystolic murmur is still heard even during atrial fibrillation at the end of the shorter cycles, though others have cast doubt on this interpretation,[26] and for the moment the explanation is not entirely clear. Moreover, presystolic accentuation of the murmur is not diagnostic of MS, because the diastolic flow murmurs of atrial septal defect and of mitral regurgitation may manifest a similar accentuation at the end of short cycles.[27]

2. The size of the stenosed orifice, and hence the balance between stenosis and incompetence, affects the onset and length of the murmur. If the murmur begins loudly and ends sooner, the orifice is large (long diameter greater than 2 cm) and regurgitation is the dominant lesion; if it be-

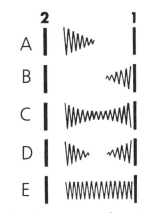

Figure 22–5. The various configurations of the diastolic murmur that may be heard in mitral stenosis. 2, second sound; 1, first sound.

gins quietly and lasts longer, the orifice is small (less than 1.5 cm) and stenosis is the dominant lesion.[28] Thus, the most important gauge of severity is not the loudness but the length of the murmur, and this can best be evaluated in the longer cycles during atrial fibrillation.

When you hear an early diastolic murmur in a patient with MS, it is almost always due to an associated aortic regurgitation[29]; but in a few patients, when significant pulmonary hypertension develops, the so-called *Graham Steell murmur* may appear—the early diastolic murmur of pulmonic regurgitation. It is well heard down the left sternal border and is therefore easily mistaken for an associated aortic regurgitation.[30]

The following *systolic murmurs* are commonly encountered in mitral stenosis:

1. Pansystolic (or sometimes shorter) murmur of mitral regurgitation (Fig. 22-3),
2. Pansystolic murmur of secondary tricuspid regurgitation,
3. Pulmonic ejection murmur secondary to pulmonary hypertension,
4. Aortic ejection murmur of aortic stenosis or regurgitation, and
5. Unexplained short apical murmur in the proved absence of mitral regurgitation (Fig. 22-4). Of 22 less-than-pansystolic, apical murmurs in MS, 14 had no regurgitation at surgery,[31] and Schrire[32] found "immaterial" apical systolic murmurs in 28 (8%) of 356 patients with pure MS.

When you remember that the murmurs of tricuspid regurgitation and AS may be well heard at the apex, and that of mitral regurgitation may project itself loudly to the LSB and base, it is clear that the systolic murmur in MS can pose a knotty problem. Keep in mind the important caveat: *in mitral disease a systolic murmur at the apex does not necessarily make the diagnosis of mitral regurgitation*; it *may* mean mitral regurgitation, but it may also represent tricuspid regurgitation, pulmonary hypertension, or an associated aortic lesion; or it may have no clinical importance.

MITRAL STENOSIS AND PREGNANCY

With its predilection for women, MS is much the most common valvular lesion encountered in pregnancy. The increased hemodynamic load imposed by pregnancy creates a unique threat for the mother and may seriously aggravate her respiratory symptoms. Most maternal deaths have occurred in patients who have been correctly but dangerously classified according to the New York Heart Association classification as class I or II because they are virtually symptom-free in early pregnancy[33]— only to develop fatal pulmonary edema when the hemodynamic load peaks in the third trimester or during delivery.

LUTEMBACHER'S SYNDROME

This is the combination of a congenital atrial septal defect (ASD) with acquired MS. About 4% of patients with secundum ASDs acquire MS, while less than 1% of women with MS have an ASD.[34] If the stenosis is significant, the septal defect provides a safety valve—a second exit—which lightens the load of the left atrium and the pulmonary circulation, so the symptoms and signs of the MS are mitigated. The symptoms of pulmonary congestion are uncommon and late to develop, and fatigue is a more common complaint than the breathless states of pure MS.

But improvement in the MS scenario is at the expense of aggravating the manifestations of the ASD, since the augmented left-to-right shunt accelerates the march towards atrial fibrillation and right ventricular failure, and the associated valvular involvement increases the risk of infective endocarditis.

In the Lutembacher syndrome, the jugular "a" wave is prominent, as are the right ventricular and pulmonary artery impulses; but the loud first sound, opening snap, and diastolic murmur that are the rule in MS are now the exception--because the overloaded right ventricle now forms the apex and at the same time mitral flow is reduced because of the double run-off from the left atrium.[34] On the other hand, if pulmonary hypertension develops, the left-to-right shunt is decreased, and mitral signs may predominate.

MITRAL MIMICS

All that rumbles is not mitral stenosis.

There are, indeed, numerous conditions that can closely simulate the murmur of MS (Table 22-2). Anything that produces exuberant flow

Table 22–2
Causes of Mid-Diastolic Rumbles

1. Inflow Tract Obstruction
   a. At valve
      Mitral stenosis
      Tricuspid stenosis
      Atrial tumors or thrombi
   b. Below valve
      Obstructive cardiomyopathy
         Primary
         Secondary to ventricular hypertrophy

2. High Flow Across A-V Valve
   Mitral regurgitation   ASD, APVR
   Tricuspid regurgitation   Anemia, thyrotoxicosis, etc.
   VSD, PDA, other A-V fistulas

3. A-V Valve Deformity Without Stenosis
   Valvulitis (Carey Coombs)

4. Enlarged Ventricle
   Ischemic heart disease   Cardiomyopathy
   Hypertension   Complete A-V block, etc.

5. Semilunar Valve Regurgitation
   Austin Flint murmur—left- and right-sided

ASD, atrial septal defect; VSD, ventricular septal defect; APVR, anomalous pulmonary venous return; PDA, patent ductus arteriosus.

across the A-V valves will produce a mid-diastolic rumble. Enlargement of the ventricular chamber leaves the valve relatively narrow ("relative stenosis") and may result in a mid-diastolic flow murmur. And then, in the presence of associated aortic valve incompetence, the *Austin Flint murmur* may develop, supposedly due to the mitral leaflet fluttering in the regurgitant aortic current. The Flint murmur may be associated with a thrill and have an intensity up to grade 6/6; it may be mid-diastolic or presystolic; and its quality cannot be distinguished from that of the mitral stenotic murmur. The differentiation, therefore, can be extremely difficult.[35] Helpful pointers are presented in Table 22-3.

Besides true murmurs that imitate the rumbles of MS, there are also deceptive sounds that are not murmurs. One of the most difficult distinctions is between a resonant third heart sound and a short mid-diastolic rumble. According to Leatham,[36] the normal S3 gets louder with inspiration in 30% and louder with expiration in 70%; he attributes this to

Table 22–3
Mitral Stenosis Versus Austin Flint Murmur

	Mitral Stenosis (with AR)	**Austin Flint Murmur**
Sex preference	More often women	More often men
Hemoptysis	Common	Uncommon
Atrial fibrillation	Common	Uncommon
Opening and closing snaps	No snaps	No snaps
Third sound	No S3	S3 commonly heard and felt
Amyl nitrite	Increases murmur	Decreases murmur
Calcification	Mitral valve	Ascending aorta (if syphilitic AR)

the respective dominance of right or left ventricular sounds. When both are audible, it is particularly difficult to distinguish the sound from a short rumble. Again, variations in the first sound, or the combination of S4 with S1, can create the illusion of a crescendo presystolic murmur,[37] and the combination of S3 + S4 can simulate a rumble.

THE MISSED MITRAL

Much labor is lost ... through persisting in the effort to time instead of learning to know it [the murmur of mitral stenosis] as one learns to know a dog's bark.

Lewis

But don't wait to hear the bark before you suspect it.

Example   A busy surgeon visited several medical Meccas in search of relief from a disabling atrial paroxysmal tachycardia from which he had suffered for 15 years. He was repeatedly told he had no heart disease. On examination, he had a thick chest wall through which nothing abnormal could be felt. The first clue to abnormality was a clipped first sound—louder, sharper, and shorter than normal. This led to an intensive murmur hunt, and, finally, after walking him briskly up three flights of stairs, an unmistakable grade 1/6 late diastolic rumble came to light. This could not be recorded on the PCG, but the loud tapping S1 showed up well (Fig. 22-6); notice that although nothing suspi-

cious was palpable to the hand, the sharp systolic tap that couldn't be felt left a clear imprint (s) on the apexcardiogram.

The first point that this case illustrates and emphasizes is the importance of paying close attention to the quality of S1. Mitral stenosis can easily be missed if you focus your attention predominantly on the search for murmurs. Let the sharp voice of valve closure ("closing snap") speak its message to your fingers. The second point to note is the value of exercise in bringing out the latent murmur (see Table 18-2).

There are numerous overlooked clues and neglected details of technique that may allow MS to escape notice (Table 22-4).

In an adult, unless she has an ultra-thin chest wall, pulsation in the pulmonic area is most unusual; therefore, if you see or feel pulsation it alerts you to the probability of a dilated pulmonary artery, and one of the common causes of this in the adult is the pulmonary hypertension secondary to MS. Similarly the detection of a RV impulse (anterior lift at left lower sternal border), an accentuated P2, or a pulmonic ejection click may direct your thoughts toward pulmonic hypertension and so to MS as the cause.

The low-frequency vibrations of the murmur may be felt more easily than heard; and since the hand covers a much larger area than the stethoscope, you may detect the localized vibrations more readily with your larger hand than with your smaller bell.

When you begin to listen, it is the sounds that

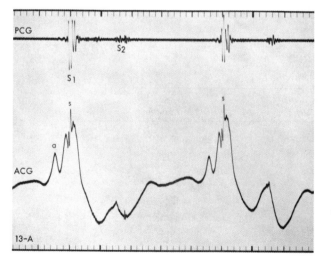

Figure 22–6. From a middle-aged surgeon with "missed" mitral stenosis. Note the abnormally loud S1 (closing snap) and the corresponding sharp impact (s) recorded in the ACG.

Table 22–4
Reasons for Missing Mitral Stenosis

Not Seeing:

RV impulse

PA pulsation

Not Feeling:

RV impulse	Accentuated P2
PA pulsation	Diastolic thrill
Tapping S1	

Not Recognizing:

Closing snap	Ectopic P2
Opening snap	Pulmonic ejection click
Accentuated P2	

Not Hearing *mitral diastolic murmur because of:*

   a. Not using bell

   b. Not using bell properly

   c. Not exercising patient

   d. Not turning on left side

   e. Not making exhale

   f. Forgetting Osler's quarter

   g. Not using amyl nitrite

   h. "Silent" stenosis

Inadequate Warm-up

---

tell you more *about the valve* than the murmur—the murmur just tells you that blood passing into the ventricle is producing turbulence, and there are numerous causes of this that are not MS (Table 22-3). But the sounds tell you how the valve itself is behaving—if it's diseased it opens with a snap and closes with a snap. If you hear P2 where you shouldn't ("ectopic" P2)—at the apex or to the right of the sternum—it alerts you to pulmonary hypertension.

When you seek the murmur, it may elude you because you don't use the bell or you don't use it properly (ie, you press it too hard). On the other hand, judicious pressure can be quite revealing. If you *think* you hear a low diastolic rumble, it can often be negatively confirmed by pressing with the bell, whereupon the supposed rumble disappears behind the dermal diaphragm. The barely audible murmur of MS has been aptly described as "something going on" in diastole, and, indeed, it is often so elusive that this is its best description. In such cases, when pressure with the bell clearly reduces the situation to "nothing going on," the previous impression of "something" is confirmed.

The murmur may also escape you because you don't exercise the patient or turn her on her left side, or make her blow her breath out; or because you forget Osler's quarter—how localized the murmur can be—and you don't listen precisely at the left ventricular apex; or because you don't use amyl nitrite, which may be more effective than exercise in bringing it to light; or because the stenosis may be truly murmurless.

And of course you may miss any or all of the above signs by simply not allowing enough time for "warm-up" (Chapter 6).

Profile: Mitral Stenosis

History of rheumatic fever in only about 50%

F:M = 3 or 4:1

Dyspnea, orthopnea (due to pulmonary congestion)

Tiredness (due to low cardiac output)

Hemoptysis (5 types)

Angina

Mitral facies, peripheral cyanosis, cold extremities—in minority

RV impulse, PA pulsation—seen and felt

Tapping S1, accentuated P2—felt and heard

Opening snap, closing snap, pulmonic ejection click and murmur

Mid, late, or mid-through-late diastolic thrill and murmur

(No S3 and no LVH)

REFERENCES

1. Wood P. An appreciation of mitral stenosis. Br Med J 1954;1:1051 and 1113.

2. Selzer A, Cohn KE. Natural history of mitral stenosis: a review. Circulation 1972;45:878.

3. Sen PK, et al. Mitral stenosis in the young. Dis Chest 1966;49:384.

4. Lewis BM, et al. Clinical and physiological correlations in patients with mitral stenosis. Am Heart J 1952;43:2.

5. Gorlin R, Gorlin SG. Hydraulic formula for calculation of the area of the stenotic mitral valve, other cardiac valves and central circulatory shunts. Am Heart J 1951; 41:1.

6. Goodwin JF, et al. Mitral valve disease and mitral valvotomy. Br Med J 1955;2:573.

7. Schrire V, Barnard CN. The pre-operative assessment of mitral-valve disease. S Afr Med J 1964;38:721.
8. Ross RS. Right ventricular hypertension as a cause of precordial pain. Am Heart J 1961;61:134.
9. Somerville W, Chambers RJ. Systemic embolism in mitral stenosis: relation to size of the left atrial appendix. Br Med J 1964;2:1167.
10. Dressler W, et al. Physical sign of tight mitral stenosis: aid in selection of patients for valvulotomy. JAMA 1954;154:49.
11. Wynn A. Gross calcification of the mitral valve. Br Heart J 1953;15:214.
12. Belcher JR. The influence of mitral regurgitation on the results of mitral valvotomy. Lancet 1956;2:7.
13. Turner RWD, Fraser HRL. Mitral valvotomy: a progress report. Lancet 1956;2:525 and 587.
14. Leo TF, Hultgren HN. Phonocardiographic characteristics of tight mitral stenosis. Medicine 1959;38:85.
15. Evans W, Short DS. Pulmonary hypertension in mitral stenosis. Br Heart J 1957;19:457.
16. McKinnon J, et al. Mitral stenosis with very high pulmonary vascular resistance and atypical features. Br Heart J 1956;18:449.
17. Surawicz B, Nierenberg MA. Association of "silent" mitral stenosis with massive thrombi in the left atrium. N Engl J Med 1960;263:423.
18. Surawicz B. Effect of respiration and upright position on the interval between the two components of the second heart sound and that between the second sound and the mitral opening snap. In: McKusick VA, ed. Symposium on cardiovascular sound. II. Clinical aspects. Circulation 1957;16:422.
19. Ebringer R, et al. Hemodynamic factors influencing opening snap interval in mitral stenosis. Br Heart J 1970;32:350.
20. Wells BG. The assessment of mitral stenosis by phonocardiography. Br Heart J 1954;16:261.
21. Craige E. Phonocardiographic studies in mitral stenosis. N Engl J Med 1957;257:650.
22. Wells BG. Prediction of mitral pressure gradient from heart sounds. Br Med J 1957;1:551.
23. Rackley CE, et al. Phonocardiographic discrepancies in the assessment of mitral stenosis. Arch Intern Med 1968; 121:50.
24. Millward DK, et al. Echocardiographic studies to explain opening snaps in presence of nonstenotic mitral valves. Am J Cardiol 1973;31:64.
25. Fortuin NJ, Craige E. Echocardiographic studies of genesis of mitral diastolic murmurs. Br Heart J 1973;35:75.
26. Tavel ME, Bonner AJ. Presystolic murmur in atrial fibrillation: fact or fiction? Circulation 1976;54:167.
27. Bonner AJ, et al. "Presystolic" augmentation of diastolic heart sounds in atrial fibrillation. Am J Cardiol 1975; 37:427.
28. Nixon PGF. Clinical assessment of mitral orifice in patients with regurgitation. Br Med J 1960;2:1122.
29. Runco V, et al. Basal diastolic murmurs in rheumatic heart disease: intracardiac phonocardiography and cineangiography. Am Heart J 1975;75:153.
30. McArthur JD, et al. Reassessment of Graham Steell murmur using platinum electrode technique. Br Heart J 1974;36:1023.
31. Mounsey P, Brigden W. The apical systolic murmur in mitral stenosis. Br Heart J 1954;16:255.
32. Schrire V. The relation of the apical systolic murmur to mitral valve disease. Am Heart J 1964;68:305.
33. Szekely P, et al. Pregnancy and the changing pathology of rheumatic heart disease. Br Heart J 1973;35:1293.
34. Perloff JK. The clinical recognition of congenital heart disease, ed 3. Philadelphia: WB Saunders, 1987:300–302.
35. Segal JP, et al. The Austin Flint murmur: its differentiation from the murmur of rheumatic mitral stenosis. Circulation 1950;18:1025.
36. Leatham A, et al. Auscultatory and phonocardiographic findings in healthy children with systolic murmurs. Br Heart J 1963;25:451.
37. Alimurung MM, et al. Variations in the first apical sound simulating the so-called "presystolic murmur of mitral stenosis." N Engl J Med 1949;241:631.
38. Rabbino MD, et al. The clinical recognition of "silent" mitral stenosis. Dis Chest 1965;47:608.
39. Ongley PA, et al. The diastolic murmur of mitral stenosis. N Engl J Med 1955;253:1049.

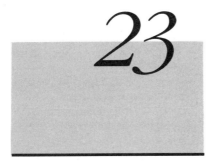

23

Mitral Regurgitation

The architecture of mitral incompetence[1] is more complex than that of mitral stenosis. Regurgitation may result from defective function of leaflets, papillary muscles, or chordae tendineae; or from enlargement of the orifice. The many causes of mitral valve incompetence are listed in Table 23-1.

Formerly, rheumatic disease was regarded as the most common cause of mitral incompetence, but in recent decades, rheumatism has been supplanted by mitral valve prolapse (MVP) and ischemic heart disease.[2] Of 97 mitral valves removed because of severe pure mitral regurgitation and reported in 1982, 62% were replaced because of severe prolapse, 30% for papillary muscle dysfunction, 5% for infective endocarditis, and only 3% for rheumatic involvement.[3] Bacterial endocarditis plays an important role both as a cause of incompetence and as a complication of other pathologic processes. Seven of 33 patients[1] and four of 23[4] with pure mitral regurgitation gave a history of bacterial endocarditis. Many of the other causes of incompetence are important because of their severity and because some are more amenable to curative surgery than the rheumatic.[5]

Early in the 20th century, leading cardiologists, including Mackenzie, Steell, Lewis, and Cabot, made light of the mitral systolic murmur, regarding it as unimportant except as a stimulus to search for an associated diastolic murmur.[6] In fact, Cabot stated: ''The diagnosis of mitral regurgitation without stenosis is never justified.'' Times have changed. We now can diagnose pure mitral regurgitation with confidence at the bedside.

Nixon[7] stressed the paradox that although mitral regurgitation is a systolic phenomenon, no systolic event has proved useful in assessing its severity. Diastolic events, on the other hand, are of great value. Based on 400 carefully studied mitral patients, he divided those disabled by their disease into three categories: Severe obstruction, severe incompetence, and the rigid valve.[7–9] The distinctive clinical features are set out in Table 23-2.

SYMPTOMS

Mitral regurgitation may remain asymptomatic for many years. When it is the result of leaflet prolapse

Table 23–1
Causes of Mitral Valve Regurgitation

Congenital	Acquired
Isolated	Chronic
Prolapsing leaflet	**Ischemic heart disease**
Cleft leaflet	**Rheumatic**
Anomalous chordal insertion	**Bacterial endocarditis**
Ebstein-type anomaly of mitral valve	**Dilation of left ventricle**
Dilation of mitral annulus	Submitral aneurysms
Part of a syndrome	Papillary muscle dysfunction
Endocardial cushion defect	Left atrial tumor
Ostium primum	Marfan's syndrome
A-V communis	Ehlers-Danlos syndrome
Corrected transposition	Acute
Endocardial fibroelastosis	Ruptured chorda tendinea
Dilation of left atrium or ventricle	Ruptured papillary muscle
Associated with coarctation, patent ductus, etc.	Perforated leaflet (endocarditis)
	Premature beats

Table 23–2
Mitral Syndromes (after Nixon)

Valve Diameter	Palpable F-point	OS	S3	Diastolic Murmur	
Severe Obstruction					
1.5 cm	Never	Usually	Never	Begins at OS, rumbles at constant intensity through diastole	
Severe Incompetence					
2.0 cm	Always	Usually	Always	Begins loudly or accentuates at S3 and fades rapidly	
The Rigid Valve					
1.5–2.0 cm	Seldom	Seldom	Seldom	Begins at OS but waxes louder at S3, then wanes throughout diastole	

Look back at the pressure curves sketched in Figure 12-2. In MS, the pressure difference between atrium and ventricle persists throughout diastole—that is why the murmur persists; in MR, atrial and ventricular pressures start far apart but rapidly close to equalize in the period of "stasis"—that is why the diastolic flow murmur of MR is short-lived and quickly wanes: Its contour matches that of the narrowing pressure difference.

(see Chapter 24), atypical chest discomfort is common, and there may be a family history of the disease.

An onset with tiredness, rather than shortness of breath, suggests mitral regurgitation rather than stenosis. Palpitation is also a more common complaint, probably not because arrhythmias are more common, but because the more active left ventricle makes itself more annoyingly felt; but palpitation due to frequent extrasystoles was the presenting symptom in 15 of 30 patients with pure mitral regurgitation.[10] The development of atrial fibrillation may also be responsible.

When the incompetent valve results from the ravages of ischemic disease (ischemic cardiomyopathy), obviously angina may be a prominent symptom. When the left ventricle fails, dyspnea and orthopnea develop, whereas concomitant right ventricular failure results in edema. When regurgitation develops acutely, dyspnea, pulmonary edema, and the symptoms of congestive heart failure rapidly supervene.

SIGNS

Although heart failure may be postponed for decades, the enlarging left atrium may engender atrial fibrillation, which in turn may precipitate failure (see Chapter 38).

The pulse is quick and vigorous and has earned recognition as a "small waterhammer pulse."[11] The apex beat is dynamic and enlarged, and a diffuse parasternal lift may result from the systolic

filling of the left atrium. A rapid filling wave (F-point) may be palpable, accompanied by a third sound (Fig. 23-1). The intensity of the first sound is widely reputed to be diminished, but this may be as much that it is unnoticed, swamped by the overwhelming murmur, as that it is subdued. It is often erroneously reported as "replaced by" the murmur, but careful auscultation and phonocardiography show it to be of normal intensity in the majority of patients with pure regurgitation—it was normal in 25 of 33 patients.[1]

The opening snap was formerly regarded as a sign of pure mitral stenosis[12]; it was not heard in any of 18 patients[13] or of 30 patients[10] with pure mitral regurgitation. It was present, however, in four of Perloff's 33 patients, and Nixon regarded it as common in severe regurgitation (Fig. 23-2; also see Fig. 23-5). In cases with the largest orifices, where the leaflets are usually healthy though separated by dilation of the A-V ring, an opening snap is the rule rather than the exception. If the snap is absent in the presence of severe incompetence, the orifice is likely to measure 2 to 2.5 cm, and the aortic cusp is probably immobilized by fibrosis spreading from the commissural adhesions.[7,8]

A loud third sound (Figs. 23-1, 23-2) is evidence that there is no tight stenosis and indicates that the regurgitation is important. One was heard in 15 of 30 patients,[10] 14 of 18,[13] and 26 of 33.[1] The sound decreases with amyl nitrite and increases with pressor amines.[1]

The second sound was widely split in 14 and fixed in six of 33 cases.[1] All patients with fixed

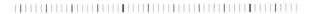

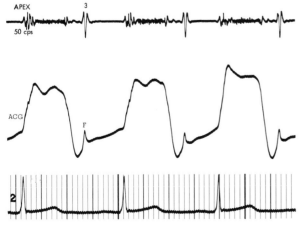

Figure 23-1. From a 12-year-old girl with pure mitral regurgitation. Note the pansystolic murmur and the F-point, like an accusatory finger pointing at the extremely loud S3 (3).

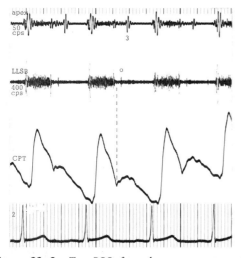

Figure 23-2. Two PCGs from the same youngster illustrating the loud S3 in the low-frequency record and the opening snap (o) in the high-frequency tracing. The dashed line (up from the dicrotic notch of the carotid curve) gives the timing of A2; the opening snap occurs 0.09 and S3 0.15 seconds after A2. The pansystolic murmur is evident in both tracings.

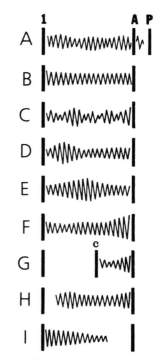

Figure 23-3. Diagrammatic depiction of the nine configurations of the mitral regurgitant murmur alluded to in text.

splitting were in right ventricular failure. Abnormally wide splitting is supposedly due to early closure of the aortic valve, presumably as a result of shortened left ventricular ejection, thanks to the double run-off.

The systolic murmur assumes many shapes and sizes (Fig. 23-3 **A–I**). It is usually pansystolic (Fig. 23-3 **A–F**; Figs. 23-1, 23-2). It may be of even intensity ("plateau"), spilling beyond A2 (Fig. 23-3A), or stopping at A2 (Fig. 23-3D); it

may be of uneven, varying intensity (Fig. 23-3C), or may show early (Fig. 23-3D), mid (Fig. 23-3E), or late (Fig. 23-3F) systolic accentuation. It may vary from time to time and beat to beat in the same patient. It is often loud and associated with a thrill: one was palpable in 12 of 23 cases,[4] and in 30 of 33 cases.[1] The murmur tends to radiate in one or

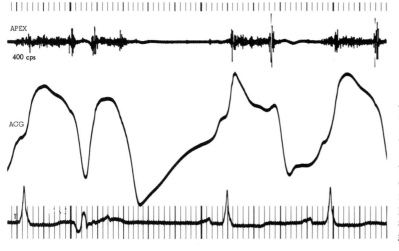

Figure 23-4. Tracings are from a 28-year-old man with pure rheumatic mitral regurgitation. The PCG, taken at the apex, documents the pansystolic murmur. The second beat is a ventricular extrasystole; note that the murmur is no louder after the long postectopic cycle than after the shorter cycles. ACG, apexcardiogram.

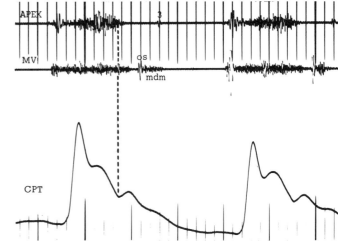

Figure 23–5. Simultaneous recording of two phonocardiograms in a 55-year-old woman with pure mitral regurgitation. The upper tracing recorded externally at the cardiac apex, the lower trace from inside the heart with the phonocatheter at the mitral valve (MV). The vertical dashed line indicates the moment of aortic valve closure (A2); note that the murmur continues briefly beyond A2. The intracardiac lead also records an opening snap (os) and a short mid-diastolic flow murmur (mdm). The apical tracing records a third sound (3) approximately 0.17 second after A2.

more of three directions: (1) left axilla and angle of left scapula; (2) left sternal border, base of heart and neck; and (3) spine, neck to sacrum. Unlike ejection and stenotic murmurs, it tends to get *louder* when heart failure sets in.

When the murmur is transmitted to the base of the heart, it may be difficult to distinguish it from the murmur of aortic stenosis. In this situation, a premature beat or the varying cycles in atrial fibrillation may be helpful. The regurgitant murmur is no louder after a long cycle than after a short cycle (Fig. 23-4), whereas the murmur of aortic stenosis is intensified after a long diastole (see Figure 19-6).

On occasion, the regurgitant murmur is less than pansystolic: It may be confined to late systole, with or without an introductory midsystolic click (Fig. 23-3**G**). The late murmur usually characterizes mild regurgitation, but it may sometimes be severe,[14] and some are associated with other lesions of serious import (eg, Marfan's syndrome or dangerous arrhythmias).[15] A late systolic "whoop" or "honk" may be present.[16,17] In some patients with papillary muscle dysfunction, the murmur is said to begin late, a short silent period corresponding to the isovolumic phase of left ventricular systole separating its onset from the first sound (Fig. 23-3**H**); rarely, it may take the form of a short decrescendo murmur (Fig. 23-3**I**). Or there may be no murmur at all.

Atrial and ventricular pressures may not equalize until slightly after semilunar valve closure; the regurgitant murmur may therefore continue into early diastole (Fig. 23-3**A**), and perhaps be mistaken for a short early diastolic murmur of aortic regurgitation. In Figure 23-5, two phonocardiograms are simultaneously recorded—one is external at the apex, the other intracardiac at the mitral valve—in a patient with mitral regurgitation. The external tracing shows the systolic murmur stopping at S2 and it records an S3; the intracardiac tracing shows that the murmur continues beyond S2 and it records an opening snap followed by a short diastolic murmur. The systolic murmur, third sound, and diastolic flow murmur are all diminished with inhalation of amyl nitrite.[11]

Mitral regurgitation may be as *silent* as the proverbial nun. Flint (1859) recognized that mitral regurgitation could present with a diastolic and no systolic murmur. At times the murmur may diminish or disappear with onset of atrial fibrillation or congestive failure, but at other times its silence is mysterious. The murmurless rheumatic heart may quite fail to suggest valvular heart disease at the bedside, and one entertains the diagnosis of cardiomyopathy or ischemic heart disease. In these silent cases the clue to the underlying mitral incompetence may lie in disproportionate enlargement of the left atrium on x-ray[18] or in subtle signs of left ventricular hypertrophy in the electrocardiogram.[19]

DECEPTIONS

Pure MR can misleadingly present a picture suggesting right ventricular hypertrophy and/or pulmonary hypertension when hemodynamic studies prove that neither exists:

SIGN	SUGGESTS	BUT IS DUE TO
Anterior lift,	Right ventricular hypertrophy,	Systolic ballooning of left atrium lifting heart forward.
Pulmonary artery pulsation and accentuated P2,	Pulmonary hypertension,	Anterior displacement of heart by large left atrium holding right ventricle and pulmonary artery close to anterior chest wall.

Compare the similar false impression of right ventricular and pulmonary arterial overactivity that may result from skeletal contours that artificially approximate the heart to the anterior chest wall—straight back syndrome and pectus excavatum. And on the other side of the coin, genuine right ventricular hypertrophy and pulmonary hypertension may, as a result of the retrograde effects of raised left atrial pressure, dominate the clinical picture of MR, and so lead you astray.[20]

Profile: Mitral Regurgitation

Tiredness—rather than shortness of breath
Palpitations—with arrhythmias

LV impulse with palpable diastolic filling wave (F-point, S3)

RV impulse may be simulated

Apical systolic thrill—may radiate to base of heart and neck, or to back of chest

S2 often widely split

Opening snap

Loud S3

(Normal S1 in most)

Pansystolic murmur, high-pitched, usually maximal at apex, usually radiating to axilla, often to back, sometimes to base of heart and neck; decreases with inspiration, with amyl nitrite; increases with phenylephrine

Mid-diastolic, decrescendo apical murmur, beginning loudly at S3

Signs of pulmonary hypertension may supervene.

REFERENCES

1. Perloff JK, Harvey WP. Auscultatory and phonocardiographic manifestations of pure mitral regurgitation. Prog Cardiovasc Dis 1962;5:172.
2. Silverman ME, Hurst JW. The mitral complex. Am Heart J 1968;76:399.
3. Waller BF, et al. Etiology of isolated, severe, chronic, pure mitral regurgitation: analysis of 97 patients over 30 years of age having mitral valve replacement. Am Heart J 1982;104:276.
4. Ross J, et al. Clinical and hemodynamic observations in pure mitral insufficiency. Am J Cardiol 1958;2:11
5. Menges H, et al. The clinical diagnosis and surgical management of ruptured chordae tendineae. Circulation 1964;30:8.
6. Vander Veer J. Mitral insufficiency: historical and clinical aspects. Am J Cardiol 1958;2:5.
7. Nixon PGF, et al. The opening snap in mitral incompetence. Br Heart J 1960;22:395.
8. Nixon PGF. Phases of diastole in various syndromes of mitral valvular disease. Br Heart J 1963;25:393.
9. Nixon PGF. The diagnosis of the mitral lesion in patients with regurgitation. Postgrad Med J 1964;40:136.
10. Brigden W, Leatham A. Mitral incompetence. Br Heart J 1953;15:55.
11. Reicheck N, et al. Clinical aspects of rheumatic valvular disease. Prog Cardiovasc Dis 1973;15:491.
12. Wood P. An appreciation of mitral stenosis. Br Med J 1954;1:1051.
13. Hubbard TF, et al. A phonocardiographic study of the apical diastolic murmurs in pure mitral insufficiency. Am Heart J 1959;57:223.
14. Linhart JW, Taylor WJ. The late apical systolic murmur. Am J Cardiol 1966;18:164.
15. Hancock EW, Cohn K. The syndrome associated with mid systolic click and late systolic murmur. Am J Med 1966;41:183.
16. Leighton RF, et al. Mild mitral regurgitation. Am J Med 1966;41:168.
17. Leon DF, et al. Late systolic murmurs, clicks, and whoops arising from the mitral valve. Am Heart J 1966;72:325.
18. Schrire V, et al. Silent mitral incompetence. Am Heart J 1961;61:723.
19. Aravanis C. Silent mitral insufficiency. Am Heart J 1965;70:620.
20. Bentivoglio L, et al. The paradox of right ventricular enlargement in mitral insufficiency. Am J Med 1958;24:193.

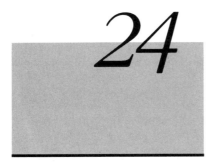

24

Mitral Regurgitant Syndromes

MITRAL VALVE PROLAPSE (MVP)

This fashionable syndrome has acquired so many names in the past two or three decades that Abrams[1] was able to list no less than 17 sobriquets in 1988, including "click-murmur syndrome," "billowing mitral leaflet syndrome," "floppy valve syndrome," and "Barlow's syndrome." The epithets prolapsing, billowing, floppy, and flail are often used as though they were synonymous and interchangeable; but Barlow[2] is at pains to point out that they represent differing patterns of abnormality.

Furthermore, all MVP does not have the same pathologic basis.[3,4] The idiopathic form results from loss of collagen in the cusps and chordae; accordingly, some cases are seen in the company of connective tissue diseases such as Marfan's syndrome, osteogenesis imperfecta, Ehlers-Danlos syndrome, and pseudoxanthoma elasticum. Secondary forms of MVP may result from ischemic disease, cardiomyopathy, or chordal rupture. In one series of 134 patients with prolapsing leaflets, 11% were secondary to chordal rupture.[5]

Incidence

MVP has been reported in from 2% to 21% of healthy young women and in 5% to 15% of various populations; but its real incidence is uncertain because many of the owners of prolapsing valves are unaware of them, are completely free of symptoms, and are never examined. Moreover, the exact prevalence is virtually impossible to assess because it necessarily varies greatly depending on the population explored, the diagnostic tool employed, and the criteria accepted for "prolapse." Accepting the echocardiogram as the standard for diagnosis may lead to including valves that should be regarded as within normal range[6]; in Oakley's words, "echo only" MVP may be a variant of normal—a phenomenon as transient as youth.[7]

In the Framingham study, evidence of prolapsing leaflets was found in 2.5% of men and 7.6%

of women.[8] Among these men, prolapse was detected in 2% to 4% in all decades, whereas women showed a striking and progressive decrease in frequency with advancing years: From 17% in the '20s, to only 1% in the '80s.[8] Among over 1000 young women, 74 (6.3%) had midsystolic clicks or late systolic murmurs, and of these, 60 had prolapse confirmed by echocardiogram.[9] In another population of 100 presumed healthy young women in California, evidence of mitral valve abnormality was found in no less than 28; of these, 21 had MVP.[10]

Many claims have been made for an association with other abnormalities, so that in 1987 Levy and Savage[11] were able to report nearly 50 claimed associations, including connective tissue disorders, congenital heart diseases, conduction disturbances, cardiomyopathies, and neuroendocrine, metabolic, psychiatric, and hematologic disorders. Barlow[12] published a similar list of 47 entities "causing or associated with" MVP. Certainly there is a higher incidence of MVP in patients with Marfan's syndrome, but most of the other claimed associations are doubtful—certainly their sparse correlation does not contribute to the overall incidence of the syndrome.

At times a familial tendency surfaces.[13,14]

Symptoms

The frequency with which the common symptoms associated with MVP are encountered varies with the observer, and one must keep in mind that all the symptoms are nonspecific, and that in some controlled studies,[15,16] these symptoms are just as common in those without as in those with MVP. It is probable that the majority of subjects with MVP have no symptoms at all.[1]

The most common symptom is atypical (ie, nonanginal) *chest pain*, reported in 35% to 72% of cases.[13,17] It is variably described as "sharp" or "jabbing,"[17] but may last for hours and be called "burning" or "pressure."[18] It is usually unrelated to activity and may be greatly improved by reassurance that it is benign. It is often attributed to ischemia of a papillary muscle or abnormal tugging on the ventricular wall,[19] but in some subjects it may have an esophageal origin.[20]

Palpitations are reported in nearly 50% of patients with MVP. Dyspnea was present in 38% of Jeresaty's series, *fatigue* in 47%, and *lighthead-*

edness in 28%.[13] Minor neurologic symptoms (lightheadedness, dizziness, paresthesiae) are not uncommon complaints, but serious ones (syncope, hemiparesis, transient ischemic attacks) are rare. Orthostatic hypotension may be the cause of dizziness or syncope in some cases.[21]

Physical Signs

The classical signs of MVP are the nonejection (ie, mid- or late systolic) click and mid–late systolic murmur at the cardiac apex (Table 24-1). In most cases, the click ushers in the murmur.[22] These physical findings are, however, by no means constant: In the Framingham study,[15] only half of the subjects with clicks had prolapsing leaflets by echocardiography, and on routine examination only a minority of those with echo-documented MVP had physical findings to match. Moreover, any combination—click or no click, early, mid-, late, or pansystolic murmur—may be encountered in MVP; and the murmur sometimes assumes the character of a "honk" or "whoop."[23] Jeresaty[24] reported that 16% of 207 patients with proven MVP had neither click nor murmur ("silent" prolapse).

Furthermore, although click and murmur are presumptive evidence of MVP, they may be found in an occasional normal person, in ischemic heart disease with papillary muscle dysfunction, and in mitral regurgitation of rheumatic origin.[25]

Various maneuvers and pharmacologic agents produce characteristic changes in click and murmur that may prove helpful in establishing the diagnosis (Fig. 24-1, Table 24-2).[26,27] Maneuvers and agents that increase left ventricular volume (squatting, inducing bradycardia, beta blockers, and pressor agents) reduce redundancy of the leaflets and delay the click and onset of murmur. Conversely, those that cause a reduction in left ven-

---

Table 24–1

Relationship of Auscultatory Findings to Type of Regurgitation

Regurgitation	Murmur	Click	S1
Early	Pansystolic	0	Loud
Mid–late	Mid–late	+	Normal
Flail	Pansystolic	0	Soft

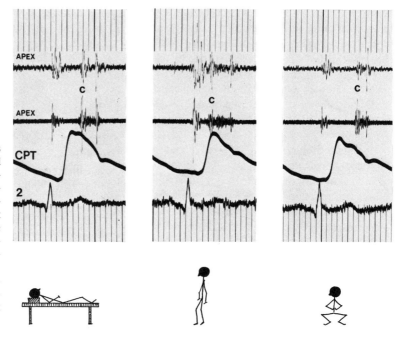

Figure 24–1. Effect of various postures on the murmur and click of MVP: On sitting and standing, the click moves earlier towards S1 and the murmur lengthens; with squatting, the click moves later towards S2 and the murmur is postponed and shortened. (Reproduced with permission from Epstein EJ, Coulshed N. Phonocardiogram and apexcardiogram in systolic click–late systolic murmur syndrome. Br Heart J 1973;35:260.)

tricular volume (standing, inducing tachycardia, the Valsalva maneuver, and amyl nitrite) advance click and murmur to an earlier point in systole. Things that increase systolic blood pressure, such as squatting, handgrip, and pressor agents, make the systolic murmur louder.

Since the murmur of both MVP and hypertrophic cardiomyopathy may be increased on standing and decreased by squatting, the differential diagnosis may be difficult; additional maneuvers may prove helpful (Table 24-2).

You should give special attention to the first heart sound (see Table 24-1), because its intensity may afford an important clue to prognosis[28]: A loud S1 signals early prolapse—usually associated with pansystolic murmur and no click; whereas a reduced or absent S1 suggests a flail valve—associated with more severe regurgitation and a greater likelihood of progressive deterioration.[29]

A diastolic sound, occurring earlier than an opening snap, and an early diastolic murmur simulating aortic regurgitation may be heard in a few patients.[30]

There is said to be a statistical relationship between underdevelopment of breast tissue (hypomastia) and MVP.[31]

Complications

People with MVP may lead long, uncomplicated lives, but serious complications do develop, including progressive deterioration of the regurgitation,[16,32] ruptured chorda,[33] infective endocarditis, hemiparesis, and sudden death. Complications are more likely to affect patients with redundant leaflets, and several studies suggest that the prognosis in general may not be as rosy as usually depicted.[33–35]

Arrhythmias

There is widespread belief that both ventricular and supraventricular arrhythmias are common in

Table 24–2
Maneuvers/Agents Affecting Mid–Late Click/Murmur

Makes Them Earlier	*Makes Them Later*
Inspiration	Handgrip
Tilting to 45°	Squatting
Standing	Propranolol
Valsalva maneuver	Phenylephrine
Amyl nitrite	
Isoproterenol	

MVP.[36,37] Ventricular extrasystoles have been reported variously in between 58% and 89% of patients, and atrial extrasystoles in 35% to 90%.[38] Because of the occasional sudden death, one assumes that serious ventricular arrhythmias occur, and certainly intractable ventricular tachycardia and fibrillation have been reported.[39–41] Others have reported bradyarrhythmias, sometimes life-threatening.[36]

However, it may not be MVP itself that favors the development of arrhythmias, since they have been found with similar frequency in significant mitral regurgitation without MVP; and it may be regurgitation that is the partner in crime and not the prolapse.[42] Others doubt that arrhythmias are any more frequent in MVP than in the general population.[43]

Infective Endocarditis

If you have MVP, the risk of developing infective endocarditis is approximately five times greater than if you do not, and men with MVP have at least twice the risk of women.[44] It has been calculated that the chances of a person without MVP developing infective endocarditis is about one in 22,000 per annum, whereas with MVP the risk is about one in 2000. Both sex and age appear to alter the incidence of endocarditis: In one series, nine of 11 patients with endocarditis under the age of 20 were women, whereas over the age of 50 years 68% of the patients were men.[4]

Sudden Death

Although sudden death is a well documented outcome, it is comparatively rare. In one forensic series there were about 100 sudden deaths from ischemic heart disease for every one from MVP.[3]

Cerebroretinal Events

Strokes, transient ischemic attacks, and visual disturbances have all been reported; when faced with any such symptoms in youth, one should certainly think of and exclude MVP.[45]

RUPTURED CHORDAE TENDINEAE

Chordae may rupture in many circumstances[46–50]: As a result of infective endocarditis, active or healed; but rheumatic disease, without superimposed infective endocarditis, may also cause chordal rupture. Occasionally it complicates hypertrophic cardiomyopathy; rarely it results from trauma. A surprising proportion of ruptures (46% in one series of 39) is "spontaneous" (idiopathic).[51]

Diagnosis

Chordal rupture may present as abrupt worsening of previous cardiovascular symptoms, or as sudden and unexpected exertional dyspnea or pulmonary edema. It should be suspected when severe mitral regurgitation develops suddenly; or when severe regurgitation is associated with slight if any left atrial enlargement, sinus rhythm, and a loud fourth heart sound gallop, in contrast with the usual severe mitral regurgitation of rheumatic origin with great left atrial enlargement, atrial fibrillation, and a third sound gallop.[50] With chordal rupture, atrial fibrillation and left atrial enlargement are conspicuously absent, though an S3 is common.[51] There is usually a large "a" wave in the neck, a systolic thrill at the apex, and a loud (grade 4/6) pansystolic murmur whose intensity diminishes in late systole.[52] In a few cases, chordal rupture may result in only minor prolapse and regurgitation, and the patient may remain asymptomatic.[5]

Remember that this, like other forms of mitral regurgitation, can closely mimic aortic stenosis.

PAPILLARY MUSCLE SYNDROMES

Papillary muscle syndromes are varied,[53–57] but take two main forms: (1) rupture, and (2) dysfunction without rupture.

During the earliest moments of left ventricular systole, pressure in the ventricle rises and the mitral valve closes, but there is no shortening of the myocardial fibers—isovolumetric phase (Fig. 24-2). Then the myocardium, including papillary muscles, shortens and initiates the ejection phase. The unruptured but noncontracting muscle therefore functions adequately during the isovolumetric phase; but, when the rest of the myocardium contracts while the papillary muscles fail to shorten, the leaflets tethered to the noncontracting muscles evert into the atrium and permit regurgitation. The murmur of dysfunction without rupture, therefore, begins *after* the first sound (Fig. 24-2), whereas that associated with rupture (which permits the unanchored cusp to leak from the start of systole) is pansystolic.[53] Useful as this distinction may

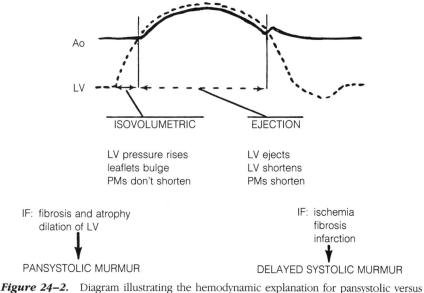

Ao

LV

| ISOVOLUMETRIC | EJECTION |

LV pressure rises
leaflets bulge
PMs don't shorten

LV ejects
LV shortens
PMs shorten

IF: fibrosis and atrophy
dilation of LV

IF: ischemia
fibrosis
infarction

PANSYSTOLIC MURMUR

DELAYED SYSTOLIC MURMUR

Figure 24–2. Diagram illustrating the hemodynamic explanation for pansystolic versus delayed systolic murmur in papillary muscle dysfunction. Ao, aortic pressure curve (solid line); LV, left ventricular curve (dashed line).

sometimes be, it is not reliable, because some hearts, with dysfunction only, may present with pansystolic murmurs.[55,57]

Rupture

The chief cause of rupture is myocardial infarction; rare causes are trauma, myocardial abscess,[58] and polyarteritis.[59] Papillary muscle rupture is most often seen with inferolateral or inferoposterior myocardial infarction, which is often small and often only subendocardial.[60,61] Rupture may occur from the 1st to the 28th day after infarction; in the Mayo series, nine of the 17 happened on the 4th or 5th day.[61]

Clinically, the picture is one of the sudden massive mitral regurgitation, with rapidly developing pulmonary edema, shock, and death. Rapid clinical diagnosis is of paramount importance because the patient's best hope lies in prompt surgery.

Dysfunction

Papillary muscle dysfunction is usually associated with ischemic heart disease, and results from myocardial infarction or from ischemia without infarction. Fibrosis, fibroelastosis, and dilation or aneurysm of the left ventricle may impair papillary

muscle function. Blunt trauma to the chest wall can result in localized papillary muscle necrosis and dysfunction.[62] The dysfunctioning muscle may be *noncontracting*, as in acute infarction or ischemia; *strictured*, as with old infarction or congenital syndromes; or *undermined*, as in ventricular dilation or aneurysm.

Clinically, the primary manifestation of papillary muscle dysfunction is mitral regurgitation. The murmur may develop only during anginal attacks and disappear as the angina subsides.[63] The murmur may be loud enough to produce a thrill, and a soft mid-diastolic murmur may accompany it. With a noncontracting papillary muscle, the murmur is often delayed and diamond-shaped, in contrast with the level, pansystolic murmur of rheumatic mitral regurgitation; the murmur may radiate to the left axilla, or sometimes to the aortic area, and simulate aortic stenosis.[64] Papillary muscle dysfunction can produce only intermittent bouts of valvular regurgitation with pulmonary edema.[65]

MISCELLANEOUS REGURGITANT SYNDROMES

Left atrial tumors more often produce mid-diastolic murmurs and simulate mitral stenosis, but occasionally the dominant apical murmur may be pansystolic. Left atrial myxoma[66] and primary sarcoma[67] may each present the picture of pure mitral regurgitation with congestive heart failure and constitutional symptoms, including clubbing.

In *Marfan's syndrome*, involvement of the mitral apparatus with resulting regurgitation is the most common intracardiac lesion,[68–72] and may be responsible for rapidly progressive heart failure and death.

A variety of lesions account for the valvular incompetence associated with congenital lesions. In endocardial cushion defects, not only the cleft leaflet but also abnormal papillary muscles, short chordae, and abnormal tendinous insertions may contribute to severe incompetence. In fibroelastosis, undersized leaflets, inadequate papillary muscles, abnormal origins of papillary muscles, shortened and thickened chordae, and dilation of the left ventricle all may play a role.[73]

REFERENCES

Mitral Valve Prolapse

1. Abrams J. Mitral valve prolapse: a plea for unanimity. Am Heart J 1976;92:413.
2. Barlow JB, Pocock WA. Billowing, floppy, prolapsed or flail mitral valves. Am J Cardiol 1985;55:501.
3. Davies MJ, et al. The floppy mitral valve: study of incidence, pathology, and complications in surgical, necropsy, and forensic material. Br Heart J 1978;40:468.
4. Baddour LM, Bisno AL. Mitral valve prolapse: multifactorial etiologies and variable prognosis. Am Heart J 1986;112:1359.
5. Grenadier E, et al. The prevalence of ruptured chordae tendineae in the mitral valve prolapse syndrome. Am Heart J 1983;105:603.
6. Warth DC, et al. Prevalence of mitral valve prolapse in normal children. J Am Coll Cardiol 1985;5:1173.
7. Oakley CM. Mitral valve prolapse: harbinger of death or variant of normal? Br Med J 1984;288:1853.
8. Savage DD, et al. Mitral valve prolapse in the general population: I. epidemiological features: the Framingham study. Am Heart J 1983;106:571.
9. Procacci PM, et al. Prevalence of clinical mitral-valve prolapse in 1169 young women. N Engl J Med 1976;294:1086.
10. Markiewicz W, et al. Mitral valve prolapse in one hundred presumably healthy young females. Circulation 1976;53:464.
11. Levy D, Savage D. Prevalence and clinical features of mitral valve prolapse. Am Heart J 1987;113:1281.
12. Barlow JB, Pocock WA. The mitral valve prolapse enigma—two decades later. Modern Concepts of Cardiovascular Disease 1984;53:13.
13. Jeresaty RM. Mitral valve prolapse-click syndrome. Prog Cardiovasc Dis 1973;15:623.
14. Hunt D, Sloman G. Prolapse of the posterior leaflet of the mitral valve occurring in 11 members of a family. Am Heart J 1969;78:149.
15. Savage DD, et al. Mitral valve prolapse in the general population: 2. clinical features: the Framingham study. Am Heart J 1983;106:577.
16. Hickey AJ, Wilchen DEL. Age and the clinical profile of idiopathic mitral valve prolapse. Br Heart J 1986;55:582.
17. Malcolm AD, et al. Clinical features and investigative findings in presence of mitral leaflet prolapse: study of 85 consecutive patients. Br Heart J 1976;38:244.
18. Tommaso CL, Gardin JM. Mitral valve prolapse: clinical perspectives. Primary Cardiology 1980;(Dec):65.
19. Pocock WA, Barlow JB. Etiology and electrocardiographic features of the billowing posterior mitral leaflet syndrome: analysis of a further 130 patients with a late systolic murmur or nonejection systolic click. Am J Med 1971;51:731.
20. Koch KL, et al. Esophageal dysfunction and chest pain in patients with mitral valve prolapse: a prospective study utilizing provocative testing during esophageal manometry. Am J Med 1989;86:32.
21. Santos AD, et al. Orthostatic hypotension: a commonly unrecognized cause of symptoms in mitral valve prolapse. Am J Med 1981;71:746.
22. Barlow JB, et al. Late systolic murmurs and non-ejection ("mid-late") systolic clicks: an analysis of 90 patients. Br Heart J 1968;30:203.
23. Perloff JK, et al. New guidelines for the clinical diagnosis of mitral valve prolapse. Am J Cardiol 1986;57:1124.
24. Jeresity RM, et al. "Silent" mitral valve prolapse: analysis of 32 cases. Am J Cardiol 1975;35:146.
25. Steelman RB, et al. Midsystolic clicks in arteriosclerotic heart disease: a new facet in the clinical syndrome of papillary muscle dysfunction. Circulation 1971;44:503.
26. Fontana ME, et al. Postural changes in left ventricular and mitral valve dynamics in the systolic click-late systolic murmur syndrome. Circulation 1975;51:165.
27. Devereux RB, et al. Mitral valve prolapse. Circulation 1976;54:3.
28. Perloff JK, Roberts WC. The mitral apparatus: functional anatomy of mitral regurgitation. Circulation 1972;46:227.
29. Tei C, et al. The correlates of an abnormal first heart sound in mitral valve prolapse syndromes. N Engl J Med 1982;307:334.
30. Wei JY, Fortuin NJ. Diastolic sounds and murmurs associated with mitral valve prolapse. Circulation 1981;63:559.
31. Rosenberg CA, et al. Hypomastia and mitral valve prolapse: evidence of a linked embryologic and mesenchymal dysplasia. N Engl J Med 1983;309:1230.
32. Kolibash AJ, et al. Evidence for progression from mild to severe mitral regurgitation in mitral valve prolapse. Am J Cardiol 1986;58:762.
33. Naggar CZ, et al. Frequency of complications of mitral valve prolapse in subjects aged 60 years and older. Am J Cardiol 1986;58:1209.
34. Nishimura RA, et al. Echocardiographically documented mitral-valve prolapse: long-term follow-up of 237 patients. N Engl J Med 1985;313:1305.
35. Duren DR, et al. Long-term follow-up of idiopathic mitral valve prolapse in 300 patients: a prospective study. J Am Coll Cardiol 1988;11:42.
36. de Maria AN, et al. Arrhythmias in the mitral valve prolapse syndrome: prevalence, nature, and frequency. Ann Intern Med 1976;84:656.
37. Winkle RA, et al. Arrhythmias in patients with mitral valve prolapse. Circulation 1975;52:73.
38. Kligfield P, et al. Arrhythmias and sudden death in mitral

valve prolapse in 1169 young women. Am Heart J 1987; 113:1298.

39. Ritchie JL, et al. Refractory ventricular tachycardia and fibrillation in a patient with the prolapsing mitral leaflet syndrome: successful control with overdrive pacing. Am J Cardiol 1976;37:314.

40. Winkle RA, et al. Life-threatening arrhythmias in the mitral valve prolapse syndrome. Am J Med 1976;60:961.

41. Wei JY, et al. Mitral-valve prolapse syndrome and recurrent ventricular tachyarrhythmias: a malignant variant refractory to conventional drug therapy. Ann Intern Med 1978;89:6.

42. Kligfield P, et al. Complex arrhythmias in mitral regurgitation with and without mitral valve prolapse: contrast to arrhythmias in mitral valve prolapse without mitral regurgitation. Am J Cardiol 1985;55:1545.

43. Savage DD, et al. Mitral valve prolapse in the general population: 3. dysrhythmias: the Framingham study. Am Heart J 1983;106:582.

44. MacMahon SW, et al. Risk of infective endocarditis in mitral valve prolapse with and without precordial systolic murmurs. Am J Cardiol 1986;58:105.

45. Wolf PA, Sila CA. Cerebral ischemia with mitral valve prolapse. Am Heart J 1987;113:1308.

Ruptured Chordae

46. Osmundson PJ, et al. Ruptured mitral chordae tendineae. Circulation 1961;23:42.

47. Menges H, et al. The clinical diagnosis and surgical management of ruptured chordae tendineae. Circulation 1964; 30:8.

48. Childress RH, et al. Mitral insufficiency secondary to ruptured chordae tendineae. Ann Intern Med 1966;65: 232.

49. Sanders CA, et al. Severe mitral regurgitation secondary to ruptured chordae tendineae. Circulation 1965;31:506.

50. Roberts WC, et al. Ruptured papillary muscle after acute myocardial infarction. Am Heart J 1966;33:58.

51. Sanders CA, et al. Diagnosis and surgical treatment of mitral regurgitation secondary to ruptured chordae tendineae. N Engl J Med 1967;276:943.

52. Ronan JA, et al. The clinical diagnosis of acute severe mitral insufficiency. Am J Cardiol 1971;27:284.

Papillary Muscle Syndromes

53. Burch GE, et al. Clinical manifestations of papillary muscle dysfunction. Arch Intern Med 1963;112:112.

54. Phillips JH, et al. The syndrome of papillary muscle dysfunction: its clinical recognition. Ann Intern Med 1963;59:508.

55. Orlando MD, et al. Mitral regurgitation caused by infarcted papillary muscle: report of 15 cases. Circulation 1964;30:111.

56. Robinson JS, et al. Ruptured papillary muscle after acute myocardial infarction. Am Heart J 1965;70:233.

57. Sudrann R, Tesluk H. Differentiation of dysfunction from rupture of papillary muscle. California Medicine 1966; 105:38.

58. Hackel DB, Kaufman N. Papillary muscle rupture due to a myocardial abscess. Ann Intern Med 1952;38:824.

59. Askey JM. Spontaneous rupture of a papillary muscle of the heart. Am J Med 1950;9:528.

60. Vlodaver Z, Edwards JE. Rupture of ventricular septum or papillary muscle complicating myocardial infarction. Circulation 1977;55:815.

61. Nishimura RA, et al. Papillary muscle rupture complicating acute myocardial infarction: analysis of 17 patients. Am J Cardiol 1983;51:373.

62. Schroeder JS, et al. Papillary muscle dysfunction due to non-penetrating chest trauma. Br Heart J 1972;34:645.

63. Holmes AM, et al. Transient systolic murmurs in angina pectoris. Am Heart J 1968;76:680.

64. Burch GE, et al. The syndrome of papillary muscle dysfunction. Am Heart J 1968;75:399.

65. Brody W, Criley JM. Intermittent severe mitral regurgitation: hemodynamic studies in a patient with recurrent acute left-sided heart failure. N Engl J Med 1970;283: 673.

Miscellaneous

66. Wittenstein GJ, et al. ''Myxoma'' of the left atrium simulating pure mitral insufficiency. Surgery 1959;45:981.

67. Raftery EB, et al. Primary sarcoma of the left atrium. Br Heart J 1966;28:287.

68. Miller R, et al. Mitral insufficiency simulating aortic stenosis. N Engl J Med 1959;260:1210.

69. Bowers D. An electrocardiographic pattern associated with mitral valve deformity in Marfan's syndrome. Circulation 1961;23:30.

70. Segal B, et al. Mitral regurgitation in a patient with the Marfan syndrome. Dis Chest 1962;41:457.

71. Raghib G, et al. Marfan's syndrome with mitral insufficiency. Am J Cardiol 1965;16:127.

72. Bowden DH, et al. Marfan's syndrome: accelerated course in childhood associated with lesions of mitral valve and pulmonary artery. Am Heart J 1965;69:96.

73. Moller JH, et al. Endocardial fibroelastosis: a clinical and anatomic study of 47 patients with emphasis on its relationship to mitral insufficiency. Circulation 1964; 30:759.

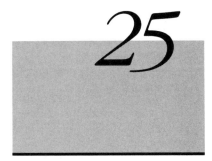

25

Tricuspid Disease

TRICUSPID STENOSIS

The causes of obstruction to tricuspid flow are listed in Table 25-1. As tricuspid stenosis (TS) is found 3.3 to 10 times more frequently at autopsy than it is diagnosed in life among those with rheumatic valvular disease, one must conclude that the majority are clinically missed: So LOOK FOR IT! It can be elusive, even at catheterization[7]; yet with care the diagnosis may be made at the bedside even before a transvalvar gradient is detectable.[8]

Bousvaros[9] summarizes the importance of not missing the diagnosis: (1) Its signs may mimic heart failure and so give a false impression of the severity of associated valvular involvement[2]; (2) its presence may preclude improvement following otherwise successful mitral or aortic surgery[10,11]; (3) its murmur may be mistaken for aortic or pulmonic regurgitation; and (4) failure to suspect it at the bedside may result in missing it at catheterization.[12]

Rheumatic Tricuspid Stenosis

Rhematic TS is thoroughly feminine—of 123 patients, 103 were women.[7–9,12–17] It is almost invariably accompanied by mitral stenosis and often by aortic involvement[12,15,16]; only rarely is it an isolated lesion.[2,16,18]

Symptoms

The most common symptoms are dyspnea and edema, and there is a striking lack of paroxysmal symptoms, such as pulmonary apoplexy or edema,[12] unless the associated mitral stenosis is very severe.[15] In fact, TS affords a measure of protection against the pulmonary hazards of mitral stenosis. The patient may be aware of the venous pulsations in her neck from the large ("giant") "a" waves; indeed, the earliest symptom may be "fluttering" in the neck on effort.[2] Hepatic pain on exertion is an occasional complaint.[17]

Table 25–1

Causes of Right Ventricular Inflow Tract Obstruction

Valvar	Supravalvar	Subvalvar
Congenital[1]	RA thrombus	Mural thrombus
Rheumatic	RA myxoma[5]	Fibroma of RV
Systemic lupus[2]	RA sarcoma	Obstructive CMP
Endocardial fibroelastosis[3]	Leiomyosarcoma of IVC[6]	Primary
Endomyocardial fibrosis[4]	Metastatic malignancy	Secondary
Carcinoid disease		

CMP, cardiomyopathy; IVC, inferior vena cava; RA, right atrial; RV, right ventricle.

Signs

In patients with sinus rhythm, the giant, "flicking" "a" waves, best seen in the external jugulars at the root of the neck and invariably visible with the patient sitting,[19] are accentuated by inspiration and may be palpable. Careful inspection of the internal jugular may detect that the "v" wave is small with gentle, almost imperceptible, "y" descent.

The "suffusion sign" suggests TS: On lying flat, the patient's face becomes quickly suffused and cyanotic with scalp veins prominent and dilated.[20] The arterial pulse is small, and at least half the patients have atrial fibrillation. A diastolic thrill at the left lower sternal border (LLSB) or over the midprecordium is palpable in the majority—11 of 12 in Killip's series[16]—although it was reported in only about one-third of a series of Egyptian cases,[19] and its intensity increases with inspiration. There is often little or no right ventricular lift, but hepatic pulsation—presystolic in sinus rhythm, systolic in atrial fibrillation—may be palpable. Note that presystolic hepatic pulsation, like the jugular giant "a" wave, occurs in other conditions, including heart failure, pulmonic stenosis, pulmonary hypertension, pericardial effusion, and interatrial shunts.[21]

An opening snap at the left or right sternal border may be heard,[22] but is uncommon[12]; when present it becomes louder with inspiration. The tricuspid opening snap usually falls a little later than the mitral, and apparently does not always indicate a diseased tricuspid valve.[23] The first sound is accentuated and often split, and its second, louder component may intensify with inspiration.[2] The second sound sometimes doesn't split—presumably because of underfilling of the right ventricle with consequently shortened ejection and earlier P2. An atrial sound may be heard over the jugulars.

Murmurs

The diastolic murmur is best heard parasternally at the 4th or 5th left interspace, or between the LLSB and the apex. Its territory overlaps with that of the almost invariably associated mitral murmur; but some find a relatively "silent" area between the peak point of each murmur,[8] and recommend listening first at the apex and "inching" towards the LLSB—the mitral murmur fades before the tricuspid murmur swells. The tricuspid murmur gets louder with inspiration (one of Carvallo's signs), whereas the mitral murmur softens. The tricuspid murmur changes its complexion with the rhythm: In atrial fibrillation it is mid-diastolic but is higher-pitched than the mitral mid-diastolic murmur, and sounds more superficial and scratchy, so that it is easily mistaken for the murmur of semilunar regurgitation—especially that of pulmonic regurgitation not secondary to pulmonary hypertension. Note also that pure tricuspid regurgitation may produce an indistinguishable diastolic flow murmur.[17] In sinus rhythm the mid-diastolic murmur is not heard,[9,12] and instead there is a presystolic murmur. Because the right atrium starts contracting just before the left, this murmur has a slightly earlier onset than that of mitral stenosis during sinus rhythm; also, it wanes before S1, even with a normal P–R interval, and thus is diamond-shaped.[7–9]

Signs of Rivera-Carvallo

In tricuspid disease, inspiration may intensify the first sound, the opening snap, the diastolic murmur of tricuspid stenosis, and the pansystolic murmur of tricuspid regurgitation (Fig. 25-1). The intensification may last for several cycles or may be confined to one or two cycles at the start of inspiration.[12] Carvallo himself recommends held inspiration ("postinspiratory apnea"), but the involuntary Valsalva that results may actually decrease the loudness of tricuspid sounds and murmurs,[12]

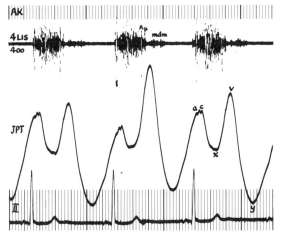

Figure 25–1. From a 24-year-old woman with mitral and tricuspid regurgitation. The PCG at the 4th left interspace (4LIS) records the pansystolic murmur of tricuspid regurgitation and the subsequent mid-diastolic murmur (mdm) of tricuspid flow. The second sound (A,P) is persistently split. The jugular pulse shows the "x" descent failing to develop fully because of the TR, and instead the "v" wave builds up to an unusually tall peak.

and during atrial fibrillation, inspiratory augmentation is less reliable because of varying cycle lengths.[7]

Marked thinning and dilation of the right atrial wall (atrium papyraceum or "paper-thin" atrium)[24] alters the typical response to respiration: Deep inspirations may be required before augmentation occurs (Carvallo's sign of the repeated maneuver), and with extreme thinning and dilation, the sign may disappear—instead of getting louder, all the sounds decrease on held inspiration (Carvallo's paradoxic sign). In the presence of significant tricuspid stenosis, the systolic murmur of associated tricuspid regurgitation may behave paradoxically (ie, become softer with inspiration).[17]

But remember: Although the intensification of a murmur with inspiration is a strong clue to a right-sided origin, lack of loudening is not against it.

TRICUSPID REGURGITATION

Isolated organic tricuspid regurgitation (TR) is uncommon,[25] but is sometimes seen in congenital conditions (especially Ebstein's disease), carcinoid disease, and infective endocarditis. In Ebstein's

Profile: *Tricuspid Stenosis*

F:M = 5:1
Virtually all have significant MS, many have aortic disease

Dyspnea, edema, etc.
Relative lack of paroxysmal pulmonary symptoms
Fluttering in neck, especially on exertion
Hepatic pain on exertion, jaundice—uncommon

Giant, "flicking" "a" wave in jugular pulse with small "v" and gentle "y" descent
Small arterial pulse; often atrial fibrillation
Diastolic thrill at LLSB or midprecordium*
Hepatic pulsation—presystolic in sinus rhythm, systolic in atrial fibrillation
OS at LSB in minority*
S1 accentuated, split*
S2 may not split
MDM (in atrial fibrillation)* or presystolic murmur* (in sinus rhythm) at LLSB or toward apex

*Intensified on inspiration

Signs of associated mitral and aortic disease

disease, however, there is usually an associated atrial septal defect; in carcinoid there is almost always involvement of the pulmonic valve and often of the mitral; and in infective endocarditis other valves are usually involved.[26] Rheumatic involvement is never limited to the tricuspid valve.

On the other hand, TR is usually an isolated valvular lesion when it is due to anterior chest trauma (steering-wheel injuries, kick by horse, etc.).[27,28] Tricuspid regurgitation may complicate acute inferior infarction, presumably thanks to involvement of the papillary muscles.[29,30] Rupture of the papillary muscles of the right ventricle has been reported as a complication of external cardiac massage.[31]

The tricuspid valve is structurally more prone to leak than the mitral,[32] and causes of TR are listed in Table 25-2. Some degree of TR is extremely common in all forms of congestive heart failure, and valvular incompetence may come and go with *atrial fibrillation*.[39] Even a single, long

Table 25-2
Causes and Mechanisms of Tricuspid Regurgitation

Causes	Mechanism
Functional	
Secondary to right ventricular failure (mitral stenosis, pulmonary embolism, etc.)	Valve ring dilation
Secondary to atrial fibrillation	Inadequate valve closure
Organic	
Rheumatic	
Infective endocarditis	
Myocardial infarction	Papillary muscle dysfunction or rupture[33]
Carcinoid disease	Endocardial fibrosis
Endomyocardial fibrosis	
Congenital	Ebstein's anomaly, shortened chordae, bicuspid valve[34]
Traumatic	Ruptured papillary muscle,[35] ruptured chorda,[36] leaflet destruction,[37] dilation of ring[38]

diastole, with overfilling of the right ventricle, may induce one-stroke incompetence.

Traumatic TR may be remarkably well tolerated, with survival for decades,[26,27,40] and in congenital TR, even massive incompetence (in the absence of Ebstein's anomaly) may show remarkable improvement as time passes.[41]

Rheumatic Tricuspid Regurgitation

Rheumatic TR also favors women, in a ratio of 2 to 1.[42,43] In an autopsied series of 90 patients with rheumatic aortic and/or mitral valvular disease, TR—either rheumatic or functional incompetence secondary to congestive failure—was found in 28.[44] The diagnosis is often missed clinically: Of 146 patients with mitral stenosis, 60 (41%) had associated TR, of whom only 14 (23%) were recognized clinically.[42] But it is important not to miss the diagnosis, because the systolic murmur of TR may be prominent at the apex and so masquerade as mitral regurgitation in patients with pure mitral stenosis.[45,46]

Mitral stenosis is as inseparable a companion of TR as it is of tricuspid stenosis,[42,43] and latent TR may be unmasked by the hemodynamic changes following a successful mitral valvotomy.[47] In patients with TR, dyspnea is almost universal, but the venous distention is pronounced out of proportion to the dyspnea, and orthopnea is often absent or suprisingly mild; many patients can lie flat for prolonged periods. Persistent and resistant hepatomegaly, edema, and ascites are common. The combination of cyanosis with jaundice ("icterocyanosis") is uncommon but rather diagnostic when seen. A precordial see-saw movement is characteristic[48]—in systole the lower part of the right chest lifts massively forward while the left side retracts. There is sometimes a systolic thrill in the lower sternal-xiphoid region. Atrial fibrillation is usually present—it complicated 120 out of 136 cases.[39,42,43]

Venous and Hepatic Pulsations

Venous pulsations play a cardinal role in tricuspid diagnosis. In atrial fibrillation the normal a-c-v sequence in the jugular pulse is replaced by an entirely systolic "cv" complex. This powerful systolic wave (Lancisi's sign), reducing or eliminating the negative "x" descent, is readily seen, increases with inspiration, and is easily palpable; it is transmitted far and wide to peripheral and varicose veins[43,49] and of course to the liver. Systolic sounds (venous "pistol-shot" sounds), thrills, and murmurs can sometimes be detected over the femoral veins.[50] In the rare case in sinus rhythm with both TS and TR, both presystolic and systolic pulsations may be seen and felt in veins and liver.[51]

When TR is not accompanied by stenosis, e.g., in functional TR, the "v" wave may tower over the "a" wave and be followed by a sharp diastolic collapse ("y" descent) (Fig. 25-1); but when both stenosis and regurgitation are present, the "v" component of the systolic complex occurs later after the "c," and is followed by a more gradual "y" descent.

In distinguishing between true hepatic systolic pulsation and transmitted pulsation from the abdominal aorta, an extrasystole may be helpful: Apparently the premature beat produces a true hepatic venous pulse ("cannon wave" in the liver) but doesn't raise a forceful enough aortic pulse to be transmitted.[52]

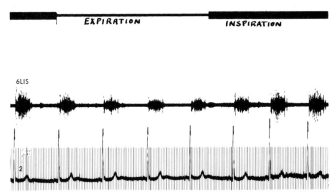

Figure 25–2. From the same patient as in Figure 25–1. The pansystolic murmur at the left lower sternal border in the 6th intercostal space (6LIS) is clearly much louder during inspiration than expiration.

Murmurs

The murmur of TR, organic or functional, is pansystolic and high-pitched (Fig. 25-1; Fig. 25-2); it is only moderately loud (grade 2–4/6), is usually maximal at the LLSB or over the xiphoid, and is often well heard at the apex but is poorly transmitted to the left axilla. Most important, it is usually intensified by inspiration (Fig. 25-2)—as in 33 of 42 cases.[43] Being a regurgitant murmur, it is usually not influenced by cycle length (Fig. 25-3), but sometimes it behaves like an ejection murmur and becomes louder after a long diastole and softer after a short.[53] The murmur with these characteristics is often known as Carvallo's murmur, the presence of which is a reliable index of TR, but its absence certainly does not exclude it.[54]

In functional TR secondary to emphysematous cor pulmonale, the murmur may be maximal lower down over the free edge of the liver.[55] Tricuspid regurgitation may be murmurless when the regurgitation is gross with virtually identical right atrial and ventricular pressure curves.[36] Apart from the diastolic murmur of associated tricuspid stenosis, a diastolic tricuspid flow murmur (Fig. 25-1), analogous to that of mitral regurgitation, may result from pure TR.[43]

Mild to moderate TR can be a difficult clinical diagnosis, and more sophisticated noninvasive studies may be needed to uncover it.[56]

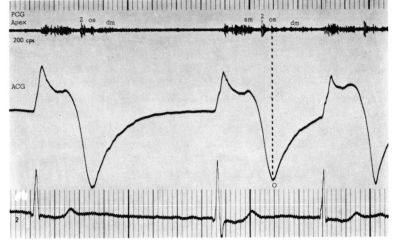

Figure 25–3. From a 47-year-old man with tricuspid regurgitation (TR), mitral stenosis, and atrial fibrillation. Note that the systolic murmur (sm) of TR is no louder after the long cycle than after the short. The opening snap (os) synchronizes with the O point in the apexcardiogram (ACG). In the phonocardiogram (PCG), 2 represents the second heart sound, and dm is diastolic murmur.

Profile: *Tricuspid Regurgitation*

F:M = 2:1

Dyspnea, but mild orthopnea
Persistent hepatomegaly, edema, ascites
Cyanosis with jaundice—rare but indicative

See-saw precordium
Atrial fibrillation in most
Systolic ("cv") jugular pulse—Lancisi's sign—
    with sharp diastolic ("y") collapse
Widespread systolic venous pulsation, sounds,
    thrills, murmurs

Systolic hepatic pulsation
Pansystolic murmur (with occasional thrill) at
    LLSB–xiphoid region, intensified by
    inspiration
Diastolic flow murmur—occasional

Signs of associated mitral and aortic disease

EBSTEIN'S ANOMALY

In 1866, Ebstein[57] described displacement into the
right ventricle of the attachments of the tricuspid
valve; this displacement is often accompanied by
redundancy and deformity of the valve cusps with
resulting regurgitation. It is always associated with
a patent foramen ovale or atrial septal defect,
rarely with a ventricular septal defect and/or
pulmonic stenosis,[58] or with mitral valve prolapse.[59,60] The anomaly is uncommon, accounting
for less than 0.5% of all congenital heart disease.[61]
It affects men and women with equal frequency,[62]
and there is some reason to believe that the maternal intake of lithium during the first trimester
may be causative in some cases.[63] Rarely, a familial tendency is evident.[61,64] Most patients died in
their teens; among 121 patients with the anomaly,
the mortality under 1 year was 23%, and by the
20th year, 69%.[59] In the experience at the Mayo
Clinic, however, most patients have attained early
adulthood.[65] About 5% reach the half century,[66]
and a few live even to old age; the oldest reported
survivor died at 85 years.[67]

The outlook ranges from the development of

cyanosis and heart failure with death in infancy,
to survival to a ripe old age without serious symptoms; this is because the anatomy and physiology
are very variable. To understand the extreme variability of clinical presentation, it is necessary to
appreciate the anatomic and pathophysiologic
diversity.

Structure and Function

The anterior leaflet is large, deformed, and abnormally adherent to the ventricular wall, but is usually attached to the annulus; the posterior and septal leaflets are displaced downward into the right
ventricle (Fig. 25-4). This distal displacement of
the valve divides the ventricle into two chambers;
the upper forms a common cavity with the atrium
and is said to be "atrialized," whereas the lower,
encroached on by the displaced valve, is the functioning ventricle but has a reduced capacity, varying with the level to which the valve is displaced
and the extent to which the leaflets are plastered
against the ventricular wall. Its efficiency as a
pump depends on several variables: Its size; the
volume of regurgitation through the tricuspid
valve; the presence or absence of pulmonic valve
stenosis; the quality of the ventricular muscle,
which may be substandard; and the success of the
atrium in propelling blood through the valve into
the lower ventricular chamber. In turn, the atrial
success depends on a number of variables: The
smaller the pumping ventricle, the greater the resistance to diastolic filling; the presence or absence
of narrowing of the tricuspid orifice; and contrac-
tility and distensibility of the atrialized ventricular
segment, which is abnormally thin and muscularly
deficient. The atrium contracts first and then the
upper and lower ventricular segments contract in
unison, so the atrialized segment is relaxed when
the atrium contracts and is therefore distended,
sometimes aneurysmally, by atrial contraction;
then, as the atrium relaxes, the ventricle contracts
and the atrialized segment ejects its blood backward into the atrium proper; pressure is raised
above left atrial pressure, and blood flows through
the attendant defect in the atrial septum to produce
a right-to-left shunt and the predictably consequent
cyanosis. Meanwhile, the starved and foreshort-
ened distal segment does its best to feed the pulmonary circulation.

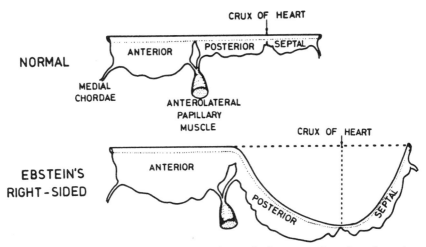

Figure 25–4. The usual disposition of the Ebstein displacement: The enlarged anterior leaflet remains attached at the normal level, whereas posterior and septal leaflets sag downwards with maximal displacement at their shared commissure. (Reproduced with permission from Anderson KR, et al. Morphologic spectrum of Ebstein's anomaly of the heart: a review. Proc Mayo Clin 1979;54:174.)

Diagnostic and Surgical Risks

Because of the dangers inherent in cardiac catheterization and palliative surgery, the clinical diagnosis of Ebstein's anomaly becomes especially important—to protect the patient from potentially dangerous interventions. Of 363 catheterized patients, 13 died, six suffered cardiac arrest, and 90 developed paroxysmal tachycardia; and of the 57 who were taken to surgery, 54% died.[62] In another series of autopsied patients, the cause of death was surgery in 25% and complications of catheterization in 8%; congestive heart failure accounted for death in 21%, and sudden death for another 19%.[68] Fortunately, the diagnosis can almost always be established with reasonable certainty from the clinical picture aided by noninvasive studies.

Clinical Findings

The incidence of various symptoms and signs as reported in several series of Ebstein patients is summarized in Tables 25-3 and 25-4.

Cyanosis and heart failure usually develop in infancy. The cyanosis may improve—as pulmonary vascular resistance regresses—for several months, but gradually reappears and becomes gross between 2 and 5 years. Some children are asymptomatic at first, but 80% to 85% eventually become cyanotic; the depth of cyanosis, however, does not necessarily parallel the degree of disablement.

In the severe cases, pulses are weak, the pulse pressure low. The heart is enlarged both to the left and right of sternum, but there is no right ventricular lift.

Table 25–3
Frequency of Selected Symptoms in Ebstein's Anomaly

	Total Cases	Dyspnea	Cyanosis	Facial Erythema	Tachy	Syncope	Squatting
Schiebler[69]	23	18	15	10	7	5	5
Vacca[70]	86	68	69	—	18	6	—
Genton[66]	17	15	12	9	—	—	—
Kumar[71]	55	34	38	16	15	5	17
Bialostozky[72]	65	33	30	—	—	22	4
Giuliani[65]	67	40	41	—	—	—	—

Table 25–4
Frequency of Selected Signs in Ebstein's Anomaly

	Total cases	SM	Gallops	Thrill	DM	Split S1	Clubbing
Schiebler[69]	23	23	18	15	11	11	6
Vacca[70]	86	74	44	—	33	—	—
Genton[66]	17	14	12	7	8	—	6
Kumar[71]	55	48	42	28	34	—	—
Bialostozky[72]	65	56	65	34	16	—	27

On auscultation, the first heart sound is widely split, and its second component—presumably related to tricuspid valve closure—is louder than the first,[73] has a clicking quality, and loudens with inspiration; some call it the "sail sound."[74] At times, the first sound has three audible components; the second and third are presumably related to tricuspid closure.[75] Delayed tricuspid closure may be due to the large size and increased excursion of the voluminous anterior leaflet rather than to the associated right bundle-branch block (RBBB).[76]

The second sound is persistently split, as expected with the almost invariable RBBB, although in the cases with "type B" preexcitation it may present paradoxical splitting.[75] A triple rhythm is due to an early diastolic sound higher and sharper than the usual S3,[75] which is perhaps an opening snap of the tricuspid valve. Sometimes a fourth sound produces a quadruple rhythm.

The pansystolic murmur of TR is present in almost all cases, with a thrill in about half of them, at the LLSB or inside the apex. Also at the LLSB a mid-diastolic or presystolic, often "scratchy,"[61,77] murmur is reported in from 35% to 80% of cases. In the occasional acyanotic adult patient, the defect is readily mistaken for rheumatic heart disease. In perhaps 5% to 10%, no murmurs are audible.

Complications

Paroxysmal tachycardia complicates about 30% of cases. Patients with Ebstein's disease are predisposed to circus-movement tachycardia by having more than their fair share of accessory pathways. In a series of 21 investigated patients who suffered from paroxysms of tachycardia, 30 accessory pathways were found (26 atrioventricular and four Mahaim tracts); eight of the 21 patients had multiple pathways, and 25 of the 26 A-V pathways were right-sided.[78]

Some children develop a cerebral abscess,[79] and a few die suddenly.[66,70,71] Infra-Hisian complete A-V block has been reported.[80] Among the long-lived survivors, coronary disease may be the eventual cause of death.[68]

REFERENCES

Tricuspid Stenosis

1. Paul MH, Lev M. Tricuspid stenosis with pulmonary atresia. Circulation 1960;22:198.
2. Gibson, R, Wood P. The diagnosis of tricuspid stenosis. Br Heart J 1955;17:553.
3. Dennis JL, et al. Endocardial fibroelastosis. Pediatrics 1953;12:130.
4. Davies JNP, Ball JD. The pathology of endomyocardial fibrosis in Uganda. Br Heart J 1955;17:337.
5. Lyons HA, et al. Right atrial myxoma. Am J Med 1958; 25:321.
6. Hoffbrand AV, Lloyd-Thomas HG. Leiomyosarcoma of the inferior vena cava leading to obstruction of the tricuspid valve. Br Heart J 1964;26:709.
7. Sanders CA, et al. Tricuspid stenosis: a difficult diagnosis in the presence of atrial fibrillation. Circulation 1966; 33:26.
8. de Brito AHX, et al. Early stages of tricuspid stenosis. Am J Cardiol 1966;18:57.
9. Bousvaros GA, Stubington D. Some auscultatory and phonocardiographic features of tricuspid stenosis. Circulation 1964;29:26.
10. Lowther CP, Turner RWD. Deterioration after mitral valvotomy. Br Med J 1962;1:1027.
11. Watson H, Lowe KG. Severe tricuspid stenosis revealed after aortic valvotomy. Br Heart J 1962;24:241.
12. Perloff JK, Harvey WP. Clinical recognition of tricuspid stenosis. Circulation 1960;22:346.
13. Wood P. Diseases of the heart and circulation. Philadelphia: JB Lippincott, 1956:42–57.
14. Yu PN, et al. Clinical and hemodynamic studies of tricuspid stenosis. Circulation 1956;13:680.

15. Goodwin JF, et al. Rheumatic tricuspid stenosis. Br Med J 1957;2:1383.
16. Killip T, Lukas DS. Tricuspid stenosis: clinical features in twelve cases. Am J Med 1958;24:836.
17. Kitchin A, Turner R. Diagnosis and treatment of tricuspid stenosis. Br Heart J 1964;26:354.
18. Sapirstein W, Baker CB. Isolated tricuspid-valve stenosis. N Engl J Med 1963;269:236.
19. El-Sherif N. Rheumatic tricuspid stenosis: a hemodynamic correlation. Br Heart J 1971;33:16.
20. Levine SA. Some clues in cardiovascular diagnosis from simple inspection. South Med J 1961;54:732.
21. Grishman A, et al. Presystolic pulsations of the liver in the absence of tricuspid disease. Am Heart J 1950;40:731.
22. Kossman CE. The opening snap of the tricuspid valve: a physical sign of tricuspid stenosis. Circulation 1955;11:378.
23. Luisada AA, et al. Double (mitral and tricuspid) opening snaps in patients with valvular lesions. Am J Cardiol 1965;16:800.

Tricuspid Regurgitation

24. Rivera-Carvallo JM, Ramirez-Jaime MH. Atrium papyraceum: the clinical diagnosis of the paper-thin right atrium. Am J Cardiol 1965;16:369.
25. Ahn AJ, Segal BL. Isolated tricuspid insufficiency. Prog Cardiovasc Dis 1966;9:166.
26. Glancy DL, et al. Isolated organic tricuspid valve regurgitation: causes and consequences. Am J Cardiol 1969;46:989.
27. Marvin RF, et al. Traumatic tricuspid insufficiency. Am J Cardiol 1973;32:723.
28. Croxson MS, et al. Traumatic tricuspid regurgitation: long-term survival. Br Heart J 1971;33:750.
29. Zone DD, Botti RE. Right ventricular infarction with tricuspid insufficiency and chronic right heart failure. Am J Cardiol 1976;37:445.
30. McAllister RG, et al. Tricuspid regurgitation following inferior myocardial infarction. Arch Intern Med 1976;136:95.
31. Gerry JL, et al. Rupture of the papillary muscle of the tricuspid valve. Am J Cardiol 1977;40:825.
32. Hollman A. The anatomical appearance in rheumatic tricuspid valve disease. Br Heart J 1957;19:211.
33. Eisenberg S, Suyemoto J. Rupture of a papillary muscle of the tricuspid valve following acute myocardial infarction. Circulation 1964;30:588.
34. Barritt DW, Urich H. Congenital tricuspid insufficiency. Br Heart J 1956;18:133.
35. Osborn JR, et al. Traumatic tricuspid insufficiency: hemodynamic data and surgical treatment. Circulation 1964;30:217.
36. Brandenberg RO, et al. Traumatic rupture of the chordae tendineae of the tricuspid valve. Am J Cardiol 1966;18:911.
37. Shabetai R, et al. Successful replacement of the tricuspid valve 10 years after tricuspid insufficiency. Am J Cardiol 1966;18:916.
38. Salzer J, et al. Isolated tricuspid insufficiency. Am J Cardiol 1966;18:921.
39. Muller O, Shillingford J. Tricuspid insufficiency. Br Heart J 1954;16:195.
40. Morgan JR, Forker AD. Isolated tricuspid insufficiency. Circulation 1971;43:559.
41. Boucek RJ, et al. Spontaneous resolution of massive congenital tricuspid insufficiency. Circulation 1976;54:795.
42. Sepulveda G, Lukas DS. The diagnosis of tricuspid insufficiency: clinical features in 60 cases with associated mitral valve disease. Circulation 1955;11:552.
43. Salazar E, Levine HD. Rheumatic tricuspid regurgitation: the clinical spectrum. Am J Med 1962;33:111.
44. Hansing CE, Rowe GG. Tricuspid insufficiency: a study of hemodynamics and pathogenesis. Circulation 1972;45:793.
45. Schilder DP, Harvey WP. Confusion of tricuspid insufficiency with mitral insufficiency: a pitfall in the selection of patients for mitral surgery. Am Heart J 1957;54:352.
46. Uricchio JF, et al. Tricuspid regurgitation masquerading as mitral regurgitation in patients with pure mitral stenosis. Am J Med 1958;25:224.
47. Mounsey P. Tricuspid insufficiency following successful mitral valvotomy. Br Heart J 1959;21:123.
48. Dressler W. Pulsations of the chest wall as diagnostic signs. Modern Concepts of Cardiovascular Disease 1957;26:421.
49. Brickner PW, et al. Pulsating varicose veins in functional tricuspid insufficiency. Circulation 1962;25:126.
50. Hultgren HN. Venous pistol shot sounds. Am J Cardiol 1962;10:667.
51. Calleja JB, et al. Pulsations of the liver in heart disease. Am J Med 1961;30:202.
52. Terry RB. Coupled hepatic pulsations in tricuspid insufficiency. Am Heart J 1959;57:158.
53. McMichael J, Shillingford JP. The role of valvular incompetence in heart failure. Br Med J 1957;1:537.
54. Cha SD, et al. Intracardiac phonocardiography in tricuspid regurgitation: relation to clinical and angiographic findings. Am J Cardiol 1981;48:578.
55. Verel D, et al. Tricuspid insufficiency in cor pulmonale. Br Heart J 1962;24:441.
56. DePace NL, et al. Tricuspid regurgitation: Noninvasive techniques for determining causes and severity. J Am Coll Cardiol 1984;3:1540.

Ebstein's Anomaly

57. Schiebler GL, et al. Ebstein's anomaly of the tricuspid valve: translation of original description and comments. Am J Cardiol 1968;22:867.
58. DeLeon AC, et al. Congenital pulmonic stenosis complicating Ebstein's anomaly of the tricuspid valve. Am J Cardiol 1964;14:695.
59. Cabin HS, Roberts WC. Ebstein's anomaly of the tricuspid valve and prolapse of the mitral valve. Am Heart J 1981;101:177.
60. Roberts WC, et al. Prolapse of the mitral valve (floppy valve) associated with Ebstein's anomaly of the tricuspid valve. Am J Cardiol 1976;38:377.
61. Simcha A, Bonham-Carter RE. Ebstein's anomaly: clinical study of 32 patients in childhood. Br Heart J 1971;33:46.
62. Watson H. Natural history of Ebstein's anomaly of the tricuspid valve in childhood and adolescence: an international co-operative study of 505 cases. Br Heart J 1974;36:417.
63. Nora JJ, et al. Lithium, Ebstein's anomaly, and other congenital heart defects. Lancet 1974;2:594.
64. Donegan CC, et al. Familial Ebstein's anomaly of the tricuspid valve. Am Heart J 1968;75:375.

65. Giuliani ER, et al. The clinical features and natural history of Ebstein's anomaly of the tricuspid valve. Mayo Clin Proc 1979;54:163.

66. Genton E, Blount SG. The spectrum of Ebstein's anomaly. Am Heart J 1967;73:395.

67. Seward JB, et al. Ebstein's anomaly in an 85-year-old man. Mayo Clin Proc 1979;54:193.

68. Cabin HS, et al. Ebstein's anomaly in the elderly. Chest 1981;80:212.

69. Schiebler GL, et al. Clinical study of twenty-three cases of Ebstein's anomaly of the tricuspid valve. Circulation 1959;19:165.

70. Vacca JB, et al. Ebstein's anomaly: complete review of 108 cases. Am J Cardiol 1958;2:210.

71. Kumar AE, et al. Ebstein's anomaly: clinical profile and natural history. Am J Cardiol 1971;28:84.

72. Bialostozky D, et al. Ebstein's malformation of the tricuspid valve: a review of 65 cases. Am J Cardiol 1972;29:826.

73. Crews TL, et al. Auscultatory and phonocardiographic findings in Ebstein's anomaly: correlation of first sound with ultrasonic records of tricuspid valve movement. Br Heart J 1972;34:681.

74. Fontana ME, Wooley CF. Sail sound in Ebstein's anomaly of the tricuspid valve. Circulation 1972;46:155.

75. Pocock WA, et al. Mild Ebstein's anomaly. Br Heart J 1969;31:327.

76. Willis PW, Craige E. First heart sound in Ebstein's anomaly: observations on the cause of wide splitting by echophonocardiographic studies before and after operative repair. J Am Coll Cardiol 1983;2:1165.

77. Nadas AS. Pediatric cardiology. Philadelphia: WB Saunders, 1963:497.

78. Smith WM, et al. The electrophysiologic basis and management of symptomatic recurrent tachycardias in patients with Ebstein's anomaly of the tricuspid valve. Am J Cardiol 1982;49:1223.

79. Kilby R, et al. Ebstein's malformation: a clinical and laboratory study. Medicine 1956;35:161.

80. Price JE, et al. Ebstein's disease associated with complete atrioventricular block. Chest 1978;73:542.

Pulmonic/Pulmonary Disease

PULMONIC VALVE STENOSIS

As we enter the territory in which congenital lesions predominate, Table 26-1 lists the percentage incidence of the eight most common congenital anomalies encountered in several large series.

Pulmonic stenosis is almost a congenital monopoly, and ranks third or fourth, accounting for 7% or 8% of all congenital heart disease. Of these, the great majority are valvar, a minority are supravalvar, and only a few subvalvar. Isolated valvar pulmonic stenosis affects males and females equally, and rarely it is familial.[8,9] Acquired stenosis is a rarity (Table 26-2), but may result from rheumatic disease, malignant carcinoid syndrome, right ventricular hypertrophy secondary to a ventricular septal defect,[10] etc.

Pulmonic stenosis is the most common cardiac anomaly in Noonan's syndrome[19]; it was found in over 60% of one series of 206 patients.[20]

Usually there is a history of a murmur being heard during the first few days of life.[21] Most patients survive to adulthood, and mild stenosis is compatible with long and asymptomatic life[22]; but patients with right ventricular systolic pressures over 80 mm Hg are likely to suffer progressive disability. Important symptoms are fatigue, dyspnea, cyanosis (from a right-to-left shunt through a foramen ovale), angina, syncope, and congestive failure. In one series of 50 patients, the incidence of various symptoms was as follows:[23]

Fatigue, 54%,
Dyspnea, 52%,
Cyanosis, 30%,
Epistaxis, 18%,
Clubbing, 16%, and
Heart failure, 12%.

One-quarter of the patients had no symptoms at all, but one should be aware that the asymptomatic patient with significant stenosis may deteriorate rapidly.[21] Some patients are aware of vigorous pulsation in the neck, due to giant ''a'' waves (see below). Failure is a grim prognostic sign at any age, but particularly so in infancy,[24] and is the most frequent cause of death. Sudden, unexpected death also occurs in a significant minority.[25]

Table 26-1
Percentage Incidence of Most Common Congenital Diseases

Author	No. Patients	VSD	TET	PDA	PS	ASD	COA	AS	TGA
Gasul[1]	1943	18%	13%	11%	8%	8%	6%	3%	4%
Schrire[2] (all ages)	1439	22	12	16	9	17	6	4	—
Nadas[3] (children)	3786	20	15	12	12	10	5	6	4
Keith[4] (children)	1866	22	11	17	7	7	6	4	8
Wood[5] (all ages except infancy)	900	12	11	15	12	21	9	3	1
Kjellberg[6] (mainly children)	342	16	11	22	9	9	8	4	3
Abbott[7] (all autopsied)	1000	6	11	10	3	3	8	2	5

VSD, ventricular septal defect; TET, tetralogy of Fallot; PDA, patent ductus arteriosus; PS, pulmonic stenosis; ASD, atrial septal defect; COA, coarctation of aorta; AS, aortic stenosis; TGA, transposition of great arteries.

Table 26–2
Causes of Pulmonic Stenosis

Congenital
Valvar
Supravalvar (pulmonary artery stenosis or coarctation)
Subvalvar (infundibular)

Acquired
Valvar
    Rheumatic
    Infective endocarditis
    Atherosclerosis
    Malignant carcinoid[11]
    Myxoma of pulmonic valve[12]

Supravalvar
    Extrinsic pressure by
        Aortic aneurysm[13]
        Intrapericardial tumor[14]
        Mediastinal tumor[15]
        Rheumatic pericarditis
    Intrinsic obstruction by
        Organized embolus or thrombus
        Tumor invasion

Subvalvar
    Infundibular hypertrophy
        Idiopathic
        Secondary to pulmonary hypertension, Valvar
            pulmonic stenosis, etc.
        Tumor of right ventricle[16,17]
        Anomalous muscle bundle[18]
        Organized mural thrombus

Physical Findings

Inspection and Palpation

Prominent or giant "a" waves in the jugular pulse are seen only in moderately severe or severe stenosis (Fig. 26-1). A systolic thrill is often palpable in the neck, especially in the suprasternal notch. In mild cases there is no abnormal precordial pul-

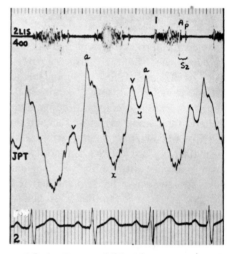

Figure 26–1. From a child with severe pulmonic stenosis (gradient across pulmonic valve 140 mm). The jugular tracing contains a sharp, giant "a" wave and vibrations of the transmitted thrill. The PCG shows a high-frequency, somewhat musical, diamond-shaped murmur going up to and slightly beyond A2. The second sound (AP) is widely and fixedly split, its components being approximately 0.09 second apart.

sation; on the other hand, poststenotic dilation of the pulmonary artery may occur with only mild stenosis, and then pulmonary artery pulsation is evident at the left upper sternal border. At the left border, a sustained right ventricular lift is seen and felt in moderate and severe stenosis,[26] with its magnitude usually proportional to the severity of the stenosis, and a presystolic "A" wave may develop. In adults it is surprising how often the maximal precordial impulse occupies the area generally allotted to the *left* ventricular apex.[27] A systolic thrill is felt at the left upper sternal border in 80% to 90%.[23]

Auscultation

Those who have studied the auscultatory findings in pulmonic stenosis and carefully compared them with phonocardiographic records are in good agreement over the following findings[28–33]: A pulmonic ejection click, best heard at the left upper sternal border and fading or disappearing with inspiration (Fig. 26-2), is audible in the majority of cases, occurring 0.10 to 0.11 second after the Q wave in the electrocardiogram (ECG).[34] Earlier observers found it commonly in mild and seldom in severe stenosis,[28,31] but later workers have found it to be as common in severe cases.[33] In mild stenosis it occurs later (up to 0.15 second after the onset of the QRS in a simultaneous ECG),

whereas in severe cases it falls earlier, approaching S1 so that it can easily be missed and mistaken for a component of S1; it may masquerade simply as an abnormally loud S1 at the left sternal border during expiration.

The characteristic respiratory behavior of the pulmonic ejection click is neatly explained[35]: The click demonstrably occurs at the moment of maximal "doming" of the valve. During inspiration, the pulmonic valve is maintained in the "domed" posture by the increased venous return to the right heart; thus there is no slack permitting further movement with ventricular systole, and no click. During expiration, on the other hand, the semilunar cusps "relax," and slack is available for vigorous doming with ventricular contraction, producing a click.

The second sound is abnormally widely split (Fig. 26-2) even in mild cases; with increasing severity splitting becomes wider, P2 fainter, and A2 more obscured by the murmur (Fig. 26-3, Tables 26-3, 26-4). To dodge this obscuration of A2, listen *away from* the point of maximal murmur intensity (Fig. 26-3); A2 is always audible, clearly heard at the apex. Pulmonic stenosis is the only condition in which P2 is both soft and separated in expiration from A2 by more than 0.05 second. The degree of splitting ranges between 0.05 and 0.11 second,[28,30,32] and in some patients the splitting may be fixed.[36] In some mild cases, P2 may

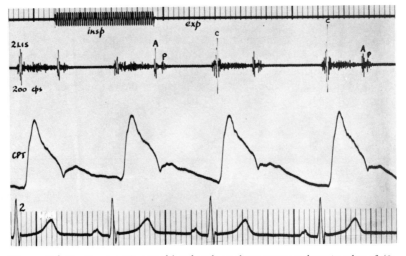

Figure 26–2. From a 10-year-old girl with gradient across pulmonic valve of 40 mm. There is persistent splitting of S2 (0.04–0.06 second), typical of mild pulmonic stenosis. Note the loud, early ejection click (c), which disappears during inspiration.

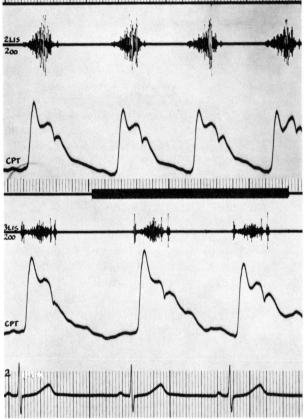

Figure 26–3. From an 11-year-old boy with moderately severe pulmonic stenosis. In upper tracing, the murmur is recorded at its maximum in the 2nd left interspace (2LIS), clearly peaks in the second half of systole, and obscures the aortic sound. Lower tracing shows the value of recording (or listening) where the murmur is not so loud; in the 3rd interspace (3LIS) the persistent splitting of S2 is obvious and ranges from 0.06 to 0.08 second.

sound abnormally loud.[37] Normal splitting generally—but not absolutely—excludes pulmonic stenosis.[38]

In the severer cases, a fourth sound appears; but an audible third sound casts doubt on the "purity" of the pulmonic stenosis, and alerts you to the possibility of associated atrial septal defect and/or anomalous pulmonary venous return.[29]

Murmurs

The crescendo-decrescendo ejection murmur is usually heard at or shortly after birth. In most mild cases it is usually grade 1–3/6, and in moderate or severe cases grade 3–6/6. It radiates to the neck (Fig. 26-1), left shoulder, and back. As severity increases, the murmur peaks later and lasts longer

Table 26–3
Auscultatory Findings in Pulmonic Stenosis

	Mild (<60*)	Moderate (60–100*)	Severe (120–200*)
Murmur Peak	Mid-systole	Beyond mid-systole	End quarter systole
Murmur Duration	Not beyond A2	Often beyond A2	Well beyond A2
A2	Clearly heard	Always audible	Partly obscured by murmur
P2	Normal or loud	Softer than normal	Very soft or inaudible

*Right ventricular pressure in mm Hg.

Table 26-4
The A2-P2 Interval* in Pulmonic Stenosis

Author	No. Cases	Mild	Moderate	Severe
Crevasse[29]	10	3–6	6–10	10–14
Yahini[31]	32	4–6	5–10	6–14
Vogelpoel[32]	43	2–9	5–12	6–12
Dimond[30]	21	3–5	4–8	5–12
Gamboa[33]	50	5.6–7.4	5.4–12.5	8.4–17.7
Leatham[28]	44	3–6	5–14	

*Expressed in hundredths of a second.

(Figs. 26-3, 26-4). With severe congestive failure the murmur may dwindle to insignificance or disappear.

With severe stenosis, a presystolic murmur may appear at the left sternal border, attributed to forceful atrial systole raising right atrial pressure above pulmonic diastolic pressure, and so forcing a modicum of blood through the stenosed pulmonic orifice.[32] Rarely, there is an early diastolic murmur of associated pulmonic regurgitation, and this suggests the possibility of calcific pulmonic stenosis.[39]

A cyanotic patient with signs of severe pulmonic stenosis but with no more than a slight right ventricular lift, little or no evidence of right ven-

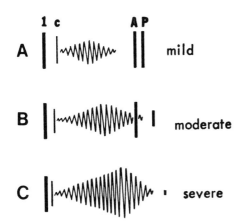

Figure 26–4. Diagram of the behavior of the ejection click, murmur, and components of S2 in mild, moderate, and severe pulmonic stenosis.

tricular hypertrophy in the ECG, and paradoxical splitting of S2, has pulmonic stenosis with underdevelopment of the right ventricle and hypoplasia of the tricuspid ring.[40]

Muscle-Bound Ventricle

The muscular hypertrophy necessary to overcome valvular obstruction has its own drawbacks: When the obstruction is surgically relieved, a postoperative infundibular stenosis may take its place—the hypertrophied outflow tract clamps down in systole and substitutes infundibular for valvular stenosis. This may happen in up to 77% of cases,[41] and the prognosis may be seriously prejudiced by the resulting systemic hypotension and right ventricular failure. It is therefore important to recognize the "muscle-bound" right ventricle that will give postoperative trouble, and two clinical findings are helpful:[32]

1. In the jugular pulse a slow "y" descent and shallow or absent "y" trough reflect much increased resistance to right ventricular filling, and
2. Paradoxical softening of the pulmonic ejection murmur during the tachycardia following amyl nitrite administration signals the inability of the stiff right ventricle to increase its output during tachycardia.

Clinical Assessment of Severity

Studies have repeatedly demonstrated that the clinical appraisal of the degree of aortic stenosis is unreliable, whereas that of pulmonic stenosis is reasonably accurate. In general, the earlier the ejection click, the longer the murmur and the later its peak intensity, and the wider the splitting of the second sound, the more severe the stenosis. The degree of splitting (A2–P2 interval: Table 26-4) is helpful,[28,29] but murmur length (Fig. 26-4, Table 26-3) is better[32] because the timing of pulmonic closure may be influenced by the degree of poststenotic dilation of the pulmonary artery, which is *not* related to the severity of stenosis (compare the mechanism of the delayed P2 in idiopathic dilation, Chapter 11). The most accurate assessment probably takes into account all three auscultatory signs: Time of ejection click, width of S2 splitting, and duration and timing of peak intensity of the murmur.[33]

INFUNDIBULAR PULMONIC STENOSIS

Though of great practical importance, the distinction between valvar and infundibular stenosis is difficult. Note the following points[32]:

1. Infundibular pulmonic stenosis is rare as an isolated lesion; it is much more often accompanied by a ventricular septal defect. Of 215 patients operated on for pulmonic stenosis with intact ventricular septum, only 17 (8%) were infundibular.[42]
2. There is no pulmonic ejection click, or click-like S1, so common in valvar pulmonic stenosis.
3. For a given severity of stenosis, splitting of S2 is even wider in infundibular than in valvar stenosis.
4. Location of the maximal murmur is seldom of differential aid; in infundibular stenosis it *may* be maximal in the 4th interspace, but more often occupies the 3rd.

PULMONARY ARTERY STENOSIS

Several classifications of congenital pulmonary artery (PA) stenoses are available[43-46]; a practical one is as follows[43]:

1. Single, central stenosis (affecting main PA),
2. Stenosis at bifurcation,
3. Multiple peripheral (or "segmental") stenoses, and
4. Combined central and peripheral stenoses.

One-half of the cases, in one series 72 (62%) of 117,[46] is complicated and more or less masked by associated defects, the most common being valvar pulmonic stenosis, ventricular septal defect, and tetralogy; atrial septal defect and patent ductus are less often found. Pulmonary artery stenoses are well recognized as part of the rubella syndrome, along with valvar pulmonic stenosis, patent ductus, cataracts, and deafness.[47,48] Congenital stenoses do not get worse as the victim ages.[49] Organized embolus or thrombus can produce an acquired form of PA stenosis.[50]

A history of hemoptysis suggests the diagnosis of pulmonary arterial stenosis,[21] as does a history of maternal rubella during the first trimester—infection after the 16th week does not result in congenital cardiovascular defects.[51] The patient may be aware of exaggerated pulsation in the neck.

Physical signs depend, as in valvar stenosis, on the severity of obstruction as well as on the associated lesions. Many features may mimic valvar stenosis: Cyanosis, giant "a" waves in the jugular pulse, presystolic hepatic pulsation, signs of right ventricular hypertrophy, and ejection murmurs are common to both, but several differences may be expected. There will be no ejection click, P2 is normal or loud,[52] the murmurs are widespread, and may be detectable even in the right axilla.

The murmurs may be ejection, pansystolic, to-and-fro, or continuous, and may be widely disseminated—equally well heard parasternally, in both axillae, in the back and in the neck. Loudness of the murmurs parallels the severity of the arterial narrowing, with one important exception: Pinpoint stenosis may be associated with a deceptively soft murmur in the newborn, and may produce congestive heart failure and early death.

The murmurs may be readily missed unless the lung fields are carefully examined; one should pay special attention to the right side, since left-sided murmurs are more readily attributable to commonly associated lesions, such as pulmonic stenosis and patent ductus. Auscultation in axillae and over the back should be part of the routine cardiovascular examination.[53]

A continuous murmur, though uncommon,[21] is more likely to be heard when the stenoses are multiple and bilateral. It was present in five of nine patients,[46] two of 11 with central stenoses, and seven of seven with peripheral[54]; on the other hand, it was found in none of 84 patients, although it was specifically sought.[44] In the rubella syndrome, a continuous murmur is usually due to an associated patent ductus and not to the arterial stenoses.[21] On occasion, its source may be continuous systolic/diastolic flow across the constriction, but it may sometimes be due to dilated, tortuous bronchial arteries supplying the deprived lung.[55]

You should think of PA stenoses when an early diastolic murmur is associated with valvar pulmonic stenosis; when a tetralogy is associated with a continuous murmur; and if a continuous or ejection murmur persists after ligation of a patent ductus.[46,55]

It is important not to overlook an associated PA stenosis when it complicates another defect that is to be tackled surgically; its presence may prohibit surgery or greatly increase its risks.

PULMONIC REGURGITATION

Usually an incidental finding, incompetence of the pulmonic valve sometimes assumes hemodynamic significance. Its various causes are listed in Table 26-5.

Physical signs include PA pulsation, diastolic thrill, pulmonic ejection click, and an ejection murmur—all at the left upper sternal border. Depending on the individual circumstances, S2 is quite variable[59]: It may be single (Fig. 26-5) (P2 absent with absent pulmonic valve), P2 may be loud (pulmonary hypertension, idiopathic dilation of PA), or delayed, producing wide splitting (right ventricular diastolic overload; dilation of PA; right bundle-branch block) or fixed splitting (dilation of PA).

The diastolic murmur varies with the type of regurgitation (for review, see Chapter 18). With pulmonary hypertension (Graham Steell type) the murmur is high-pitched and early, usually beginning with pulmonic closure, though there are exceptions that begin later. It is therefore easily confused with the commoner murmur of aortic regurgitation (for differentiating points, see Chapter 18). With organic regurgitation, congenital or acquired, the murmur is more likely to begin later and be lower pitched, so that it simulates a tricuspid diastolic murmur.[60-62] The phonocardiogram is invaluable for precisely timing the onset of the murmur—beginning with A2, with P2, or after P2.[63] Both types are usually loudest at the 2nd and 3rd left spaces; but either may be maximal at the 4th interspace—which further invites confusion

Table 26-5
Causes of Pulmonic Regurgitation

Congenital
Abnormalities of cusps
    Absence of valve (almost always associated with VSD
      or TET)
    Hypoplasia of cusp(s)
    Bicuspid valve[56]
    Quadricuspid valve, supernumerary cusp
    Associated with pulmonic stenosis
Idiopathic dilation of pulmonary artery

Acquired
Functional
Pulmonary hypertension
    Primary
    Secondary
Organic
Infective endocarditis (usually solitary valve involvement[57])
Rheumatic (rare: other valves always involved)
Postvalvotomy (virtually all cases)
Cusp prolapsed through VSD[58]
Pulmonary arteritis, syphilis, etc.
Pulmonary artery aneurysm
Fenestration of cusps
Carcinoid syndrome
Trauma

with the murmurs of aortic regurgitation or tricuspid flow. In rheumatic mitral disease it is important not to confuse the murmurs of pulmonic and aortic regurgitation, since pulmonic regurgitation is no

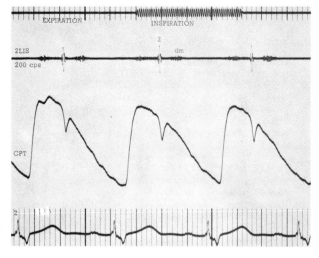

Figure 26-5. From a 10-year-old child 4 years after surgery for pulmonic stenosis. The ECG shows surgically induced RBBB, and the PCG illustrates the single second sound (absent P2) with the typically delayed diastolic murmur (dm) of postoperative pulmonic regurgitation.

contraindication to mitral surgery, whereas aortic regurgitation may be. Among 25 patients with mitral stenosis in whom the diagnosis of a Graham Steell murmur was entertained, 18 turned out to have aortic regurgitation.[61]

In the presence of mitral disease, an early basal diastolic murmur means aortic regurgitation until proved otherwise.

The reason for the late onset of the diastolic murmur of organic pulmonic regurgitation is uncertain: It may be that the relatively small diastolic PA/RV gradient (compared with that in pulmonary hypertension) favors delay; some observers have attributed it to a "right-sided Austin Flint" mechanism.[64]

IDIOPATHIC DILATION OF PULMONARY ARTERY

This comparatively benign affair gains importance because of its easy confusion with atrial septal defect or pulmonic valve disease. There is precordial pulsation in the pulmonic area, often an ejection click, an ejection systolic murmur maximal in the same area, never louder than grade 3/6, but sometimes accompanied by a thrill, and wide splitting, sometimes fixed, of S2.[65] As many as 28% may have a soft delayed diastolic murmur of mild pulmonic regurgitation.[62] Cardiac catheterization and angiography are necessary to exclude more serious defects and clinch the diagnosis.

REFERENCES

Pulmonic Valve Stenosis

1. Gasul BM, et al. Heart disease in children: diagnosis and treatment. Philadelphia: JB Lippincott, 1966.
2. Schrire V. Experience with congenital heart disease at Groote Schuur Hospital, Cape Town: an analysis of 1439 patients studied over an eleven-year period. S Afr Med J 1963;37:1175.
3. Nadas AS. Pediatric cardiology. Philadelphia: WB Saunders, 1963.
4. Keith J, et al. Heart disease in infancy and childhood. New York: Macmillan, 1958.
5. Wood P. Diseases of the heart and circulation. Philadelphia: JB Lippincott, 1956
6. Kjellberg SR, et al. Diagnosis of congenital heart disease. Chicago: Year Book Publishers, 1955.
7. Abbott ME. Atlas of congenital cardiac disease. New York: American Heart Association, 1936.
8. McCarron WE, Perloff JK. Familial congenital valvular pulmonic stenosis. Am Heart J 1974;88:357.
9. Klinge T, Laursen HB. Familial pulmonary stenosis with underdeveloped or normal right ventricle. Br Heart J 1975;37:60.
10. Watson H, et al. Spontaneous evolution of ventricular septal defect into isolated pulmonary stenosis. Lancet 1969;2:1225.
11. Thorson A, Nordenfelt O. Development of valvular lesions in metastatic carcinoid disease. Br Heart J 1959;21:243.
12. Cotton RW, et al. A myxoma of the pulmonary valve causing severe stenosis in infancy. Am Heart J 1963;66:248.
13. Schrire V, et al. Aneurysm of the ascending aorta obstructing right ventricular outflow and producing severe "pulmonary stenosis." Am Heart J 1963;65:396.
14. Waldhausen JA, et al. Pulmonic stenosis due to compression of the pulmonary artery by an intrapericardial tumor. J Thorac Cardiovasc Surg 1959;37:679.
15. Babcock KB, et al. Acquired pulmonic stenosis: report of a case caused by mediastinal neoplasm. Circulation 1962;26:931.
16. Gottsegen G. et al. Right ventricular myxoma simulating pulmonic stenosis. Circulation 1963;27:95.
17. Pund EE, et al. Primary cardiac rhabdomyosarcoma presenting as pulmonic stenosis. Am J Cardiol 1963;12:249.
18. Lucas RV, et al. Anomalous muscle bundle of the right ventricle: hemodynamic consequences and surgical considerations. Circulation 1962;25:443
19. Pearl W. Cardiovascular anomalies in Noonan's syndrome. Chest 1977;71:677.
20. Van der Hauwaert LG, et al. Cardiovascular malformations in Turner's and Noonan's syndrome. Br Heart J 1978;40:500.
21. Perloff JK. The clinical recognition of congenital heart disease, ed 3. Philadelphia: WB Saunders, 1987:188–207
22. Wild JB, et al. Three patients with congenital pulmonic valvular stenosis surviving more than 75 years. Am Heart J 1957;53:393.
23. Silverman BK. Pulmonic stenosis with intact ventricular septum. Am J Med 1956;20:53.
24. Levine OR, Blumenthal S. Pulmonic stenosis. Circulation 1965;31,32(Suppl III):33.
25. Lambert EC, et al. Sudden unexpected death from cardiovascular disease in children. Am J Cardiol 1974;34:89.
26. Schmidt RE, Craige E. Precordial movements over the right ventricle in children with pulmonic stenosis. Circulation 1965;32:241.
27. Holt JH, Eddleman EE. The precordial movements in adults with pulmonic stenosis. Circulation 1967;35:492.
28. Leatham A, Weitzman D. Auscultatory and phonocardiographic signs of pulmonic stenosis. Br Heart J 1957;19:303
29. Crevasse L, Logue RB. Valvular pulmonic stenosis: auscultatory and phonocardiographic characteristics. Am Heart J 1958;56:898.
30. Dimond EG, Benchimol A. Phonocardiography in pulmonic stenosis: special correlation between hemodynamics and phonocardiographic findings. Ann Intern Med 1960;52:145.
31. Yahini JH, et al. Pulmonic stenosis: a clinical assessment of severity. Am J Cardiol 1960;5:744.
32. Vogelpoel L, et al. The preoperative recognition of the "muscle-bound" right ventricle in pulmonic stenosis with intact ventricular septum. Br Heart J 1964;26:380.

33. Gamboa R, et al. Accuracy of the phonocardiogram in assessing severity of aortic and pulmonic stenosis. Circulation 1964;30:35.

34. Waider W, Craige E. First heart sound and ejection sounds. Am J Cardiol 1975;35:346.

35. Hultgren HN, et al. The ejection click of valvular pulmonic stenosis. Circulation 1969;40:631.

36. Singh SP. Unusual splitting of the second heart sound in pulmonic stenosis. Am J Cardiol 1970;25:28.

37. Gasul BM, et al. Heart disease in children. Philadelphia: JB Lippincott, 1966:770.

38. Stern J, Delman AJ. Normal splitting of the second heart sound in significant valvular pulmonic stenosis. Am Heart J 1968;76:13.

39. Alday LE, Moreyra E. Calcific pulmonic stenosis. Br Heart J 1973;35:887.

40. Williams JCP, et al. Underdeveloped right ventricle and pulmonic stenosis. Am J Cardiol 1963;11:458.

41. Johnson AM. Hypertrophic infundibular stenosis complicating simple pulmonary valve stenosis. Br Heart J 1959;21:429.

42. Brock R. The surgical treatment of pulmonic stenosis. Br Heart J 1961;23:337.

Pulmonary Artery Stenosis

43. Franch RH, Gay BB. Congenital stenosis of the pulmonary artery branches: a classification with post-mortem findings in two cases. Am J Med 1963;35:512.

44. D'Cruz IA, et al. Stenotic lesions of the pulmonary arteries: clinical and hemodynamic findings in 84 cases. Am J Cardiol 1964;13:441.

45. Delaney TB, Nakas AS. Peripheral pulmonic stenosis. Am J Cardiol 1964;13:451.

46. Oram S, et al. Post valvular stenosis of the pulmonary artery and its branches. Br Heart J 1964;26:832.

47. Rowe, RD. Maternal rubella and pulmonary artery stenoses: report of 11 cases. Pediatrics 1963;32: 180.

48. Venables AW. The syndrome of pulmonary stenosis complicating maternal rubella. Br Heart J 1965;27:49.

49. Eldredge WJ, et al. Observations on the natural history of pulmonary artery coarctations. Circulation 1972;45: 404.

50. Dimond EG, Jones TR. Pulmonary artery thrombosis simulating pulmonic valve stenosis with patent foramen ovale. Am Heart J 1954;47:105.

51. Miller E, et al. Consequences of confirmed maternal rubella at successive stages of pregnancy. Lancet 1982;2: 781.

52. Perloff JK, LeBauer EJ. Auscultatory and phonocardiographic manifestations of isolated stenosis of the pulmonary artery and its branches. Br Heart J 1969;31:314.

53. Rios JC, et al. Congenital pulmonary artery branch stenosis. Am J Cardiol 1969;24:318.

54. Baum D, et al. Congenital stenosis of the pulmonary artery branches. Circulation 1964;29:680.

55. Lees MH, Dotter CT. Bronchial circulation in severe multiple peripheral pulmonary artery stenosis. Circulation 1965;31:759.

Pulmonary Regurgitation

56. Ford AB, et al. Isolated congenital bicuspid pulmonary valve. Am J Med 1956;20:474.

57. Levin HS, et al. Pulmonic regurgitation following staphylococcal endocarditis. Circulation 1964;30:411.

58. Gould L, Lyon AF. Prolapse of the pulmonic valve through a ventricular septal defect. Am J Cardiol 1966; 18:127.

59. Jacoby WJ, et al. The second heart sound in congenital pulmonary valvular insufficiency. Am Heart J 1965;69: 603.

60. Bousvaros GA, Deuchar DC. The murmur of pulmonary regurgitation which is not associated with pulmonary hypertension. Lancet 1961;2:962.

61. Runco V, et al. The Graham Steell murmur versus aortic regurgitation in rheumatic heart disease. Am J Med 1961; 31:71.

62. Brayshaw JR, Perloff JK. Congenital pulmonary insufficiency complicating idiopathic dilation of the pulmonary artery. Am J Cardiol 1962;10:282.

63. Schwab RH, Killough JH. The phonocardiographic differentiation of pulmonic and aortic insufficiency. Circulation 1965;32:352.

64. Sloman G, Wee KP. Isolated congenital pulmonary valve incompetence. Am Heart J 1963;66:532.

Idiopathic Dilation of Pulmonary Artery

65. Karnegis JN, Wang Y. The phonocardiogram in idiopathic dilatation of the pulmonary artery. Am J Cardiol 1964;14:75.

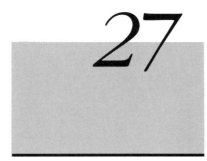

Coarctation of the Aorta

In youthful hypertension, feel for the femorals!

Coarctation of the aorta presents a paradox, and an unfortunate one: It is a life-threatening anomaly that requires early diagnosis to ensure timely surgical therapy before permanent damage is done; yet, despite remarkably specific physical findings, it is one of the most commonly overlooked diagnoses.

Coarctation is one of the more common congenital lesions, ranking sixth in most large series and accounting for approximately 7% of all congenital heart lesions (Table 27-1). It is two or three times more common in men than women; but it has a predilection for women with gonadal aplasia and the webbed-neck syndrome (most of whom have a male chromatin pattern), in whom coarctation is far the most common cardiovascular ab-

normality. In one series of 27 such patients, it complicated eight.[6] Coarctation occasionally shows a familial tendency.[7–9]

The clinical picture varies greatly: From death in a few hours after birth to 90 years of symptom-free life[10]; but then, we are dealing with a variety of syndromes under one name.

CLASSIFICATION

Most coarctations are situated close to the ductus arteriosus (''juxtaductal'') and are usually distal to the left subclavian artery. A clinicopathologic classification divides the coarctation syndromes into four varieties[11]:

PATHOLOGIC	CLINICAL
Postductal (''adult''): 83%; localized constriction beyond ductus (Fig. 27-1**A**)	*Usual*: without disability in childhood *Unusual*: heart failure in infancy
Preductal (''infantile''): 17%; diffuse narrowing proximal to ductus (Fig. 27-1**B**)	*Usual*: heart failure in infancy *Unusual*: survival to adulthood

Table 27–1
Congenital Cardiovascular Lesions Associated with Coarctation

	Tawes[1]	Becker[2]	Liberthson[3]	Hesslein[4]	Glancy[5]
Total	119	100	234	97	84
Bicuspid AV	32(27%)	46	—	—	—
Tubular HYPO	—	49	—	—	—
AS	—	37	33(14%)	31	9
Shunts	—	49	—	—	—
PDA	—	—	40(17%)	58	8
VSD	—	—	18(8%)	53	7
ASD/APVR	—	—	—	32	—
Mitral VD	—	26	6(2.5%)	24	6
Parachute MV	—	—	—	18	—
Small LV	—	—	—	8	—
Transpositions	—	13	—	—	—

HYPO, hypoplasia; AS, aortic stenosis; PDA, patent ductus arteriosus; VSD, ventricular septal defect; ASD/APVR, atrial septal defect/anomalous pulmonary venous return; VD, valve disease; MV, mitral valve; LV, left ventricle.

In rare cases, the coarctation may be proximal to the origin of both subclavian arteries.[12]

In *postductal* coarctation the strain falls on the left ventricle in proportion to the severity of the aortic constriction—and left ventricular hypertrophy results.

Preductal narrowing is usually not severely obstructive, so the left ventricle is not greatly taxed; but the right ventricle pumps blood not only into the lungs but down the descending aorta as well via the ductus (Fig. 27-1**B**), and right ventricular hypertrophy results. Both situations are modified by the presence and severity of additional defects. Virtually all, postductal and preductal, who develop symptoms in the first few months of life have associated patent ductus, and half of them have additional major cardiac anomalies, such as ventricular septal defect, transposition of the great arteries, or atrial septal defect.[13,14] Congenital bicuspid aortic valves have been found in as many as 85% of coarctations,[15] although others have found them in only 27% of 119 children dying with coarctation.[1]

From a purely clinical standpoint, one can also separate four syndromes with important therapeutic implications[16]:

1. Severe overwhelming failure with death a few hours or days after birth,
2. Severe heart failure in infancy, difficult to control and requiring early surgery for survival,
3. Less severe failure in infancy, more easily controlled, with marked spontaneous improvement after the first few months (presumably thanks to collaterals opening up), and
4. (The largest group) No symptoms in childhood, often chance discovery in adolescence or adulthood.

COARCTATION IN INFANCY

In the early months, the diagnosis may be difficult or impossible by clinical examination. In excellent hands, 11 out of 15 fatal cases escaped premortem diagnosis.[9] The main camouflages that obscure the issue are:

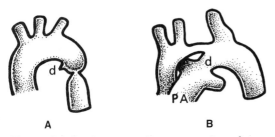

Figure 27–1. Diagrammatic representation of postductal (**A**) and preductal (**B**) coarctation. d, ductus; PA, pulmonary artery.

1. Intracardiac L-to-R shunt: lessens hypertension in arms,
2. Patent ductus distal to coarct: supplies abundant blood to legs with good femoral pulses, and
3. Proximal obstruction (MS or AS): lessens effect of distal obstruction.

Of 30 babies in early trouble with coarctation, 22 had complicating intracardiac defects as well; and all who died in infancy with complicating lesions showed evidence of *right* ventricular hypertrophy.[9]

The mode of presentation among 181 infants and children reported from London[17] varied markedly with the child's age, and is summarized in Table 27-2, where the incidence of the two most common symptoms is contrasted with the absence of symptoms at various ages up to 14 years.

The infant typically presents with respiratory distress, sometimes associated with frank cyanosis, rapidly progressing to severe heart failure—coarctation is the most common cause of heart failure in the first month of life. In preductal lesions the lower limbs are cyanosed, since the pulmonary artery discharges its unoxygenated blood down the aorta (Fig. 27-1**B**). Attacks of abdominal pain indicate spasmodic closure of the ductus and are as serious as the development of failure; they call for prompt surgical relief of the coarctation.[18]

CLASSICAL COARCTATION

Surgical repair should usually be undertaken before the age of 6 years,[13] and therefore early diagnosis is vitally important for optimal therapy. Despite this and the fact that remarkably specific physical findings prevail, coarctation is notorious for going unrecognized. For example, in a series of 65 patients, the diagnosis before referral was made in only 14%,[19] and in another cohort of 119 patients with ages ranging from 3 to 56 years, the diagnosis was made by ''chance'' in two-thirds.[20]

Excluding the severe syndromes of infancy, most patients enjoy a symptom-free youth and develop into sturdy adults; about a quarter show exceptional development of the upper half of the body, with broad shoulders and heavy musculature. More are diagnosed at the time of an unsuspecting physical examination than present to the physician for symptoms related to the coarctation.[15,19,20] Symptoms, when they arise, result from:

1. Lower limb starvation: coldness, numbness, ''heaviness'' of legs and feet; intermittent claudication, cramps in legs, and
2. ''Top-heavy'' circulation: headaches, epistaxis, vertigo, CVA; dyspnea, palpitations, LV failure, angina.

The incidence of symptoms in one series[20] is listed in Table 27-3. In patients over 40 years, there is marked increase in symptoms due to left ventricular strain and cerebral hypertension, but little increase in those due to impoverished peripheral blood flow.[20]

PERIPHERAL SIGNS

One may first suspect coarctation on inspection if, in a well developed youth, the suprasternal notch and carotids pulsate prominently—''carotid swell.''[21] A systolic thrill in the suprasternal notch

Table 27–2
Symptomatology Versus Age in Coarctation

	Age			
	1–6 Days	*1–4 Weeks*	*4 Weeks–1 Year*	*1–14 Years*
Total	55	44	44	38
CHF*	46(84%)	37(84%)	20(45%)	1(3%)
Cyanosis	15(27%)	7(16%)	2(1%)	0
No symptoms	4(7%)	6(14%)	22(50%)	37(97%)

*Congestive heart failure.

Table 27–3
Symptoms in 119 Patients[20]

Dyspnea	29%
Claudication, cold feet, etc.	18%
Headache	17%
Palpitations	10%
Angina	7%
Cerebrovascular accident	4%

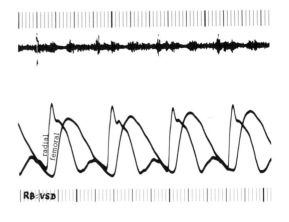

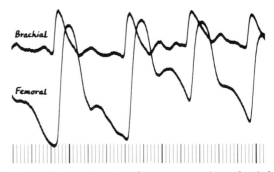

Figure 27–2. Top: Simultaneous recording of radial and femoral pulses in a patient with coarctation, demonstrating the lag in femoral rise and peak. Bottom (for comparison): Simultaneous brachial and femoral tracings from a patient with a ventricular septal defect.

is common, carotid thrills less so. But the diagnostic sign par excellence is the *pulse and pressure differential between arms and legs*. Normally the peak of the femoral pulse wave seems to occur almost simultaneously with the peak of brachial or radial pulse wave (Fig. 27-2**A**), whereas to the appreciative finger in the presence of coarctation there is a recognizable lag in the arrival of the femoral pulse wave (Fig. 27-2**B**); and the systolic pressure in the legs is at least several millimeters higher than in the arms.

Although accurate blood pressure readings in all four limbs are an essential part of every workup for coarctation, suspicion of the diagnosis can be quickly confirmed or allayed by simply feeling the femoral pulse: In significant coarctation it is almost always weak as well as late. Many a curable coarctation has been missed through failure to palpate femoral pulses; thus it is imperative not to omit this simple act.

But don't imagine that a bounding femoral excludes the diagnosis: The hemodynamics of coarctation can be masked, especially in the early years, by associated lesions, notably a patent ductus arteriosus.[8,9]

Although the detection of hypertension in the arms is often the first clue, coarctation cannot be excluded by a normal blood pressure, especially in youth. In fact, the blood pressure was normal in 85% of patients under 1 year and in 60% between 5 and 10 years; and in the first decade the blood pressure is seldom more than 150/90.[6] The blood pressure tends to increase up to the age of 17 or 18 years and then levels off at an average of 190/105.[22] In infants, the flush method for determining (mean) pressures is invaluable (see Chapter 5).

Taking the leg pressures can be troublesome. If you can feel a dorsalis pedis or posterior tibial pulse, the following simple procedure makes life much easier for you and the patient. Have the patient lie comfortably on his back with one leg bent at the knee. Apply the cuff snugly to that thigh and inflate the cuff while you feel one of the pulses at the ankle. If by this palpatory method the pressure is obviously equal to or higher than the arm reading, coarctation is excluded without further fuss.

With exercise the systolic blood pressure normally rises; in coarctation this response is exaggerated.

In most patients the blood pressure is similar in the two arms; if the right is higher than the left by only 10 to 20 mm Hg, it may have no added significance. But if the pressure in the right arm exceeds that in the left by more than 20 mm Hg, it indicates either (1) coarctation proximal to the left subclavian artery, or (2) stenosis of the left subclavian. If the left exceeds the right, it indicates an anomalous right subclavian originating from the aorta below the coarctation.

Rarely, both subclavians arise below the coarctation, and then all four limbs have low blood pressure. You suspect the diagnosis in such cases when universally weak limb pulses are found in company with vigorous carotid and temporal pulses.[7]

Other important peripheral signs include the detection of pulsating dilated collateral vessels in the interscapular area, in the axillae, and in intercostal spaces anteriorly. Having the patient stand with head and arms hanging down—in the toe-touching position—favors their recognition over the back.[23]

The blanching time (time required for normal color to return after firm pressure on skin) is normally about 1.3 seconds in the toes, but averages over 3 seconds in the presence of coarctation.[24]

The eye-grounds characteristically reveal "corkscrew" tortuosity of the retinal arteries, with little or no signs of hypertensive retinopathy.[25]

THE HEART

The precordium manifests a left ventricular impulse, usually not widely displaced. A systolic thrill is sometimes felt over the upper chest, and an aortic ejection click is common, especially

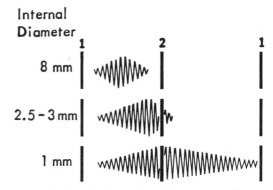

Figure 27–3. Configuration of the murmurs of coarctation related to degree of lumen narrowing.

when a bicuspid aortic valve or aortic stenosis is associated. A2 is usually accentuated.

The duration and timing of the murmur due to the coarctation itself depend on the degree of narrowing (Fig. 27-3). These murmurs are best heard over the spine between the scapulae, with the patient lying prone, pillow under chest, and arms at sides. They may also be well heard anteriorly, usually maximal over the left upper chest.

Aortic ejection murmurs are heard in many patients (Fig. 27-4), and actual aortic or subaortic stenosis occurs in 5% to 10%.[22,26,27] The murmur of aortic regurgitation develops in 10% to 25% of cases.[22,27,28] An apical mid-diastolic murmur has been reported in about 35%.[21,29] When there is a

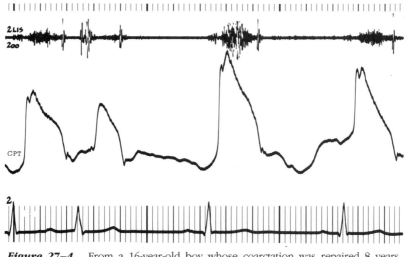

Figure 27–4. From a 16-year-old boy whose coarctation was repaired 8 years earlier. The ejection murmur persists and shows the characteristic amplification at the end of the longer postextrasystolic cycle.

coexisting patent ductus, its classic continuous murmur may be modified into separate systolic and diastolic elements.[21] Some authors deny that collaterals cause continuous murmurs[27]; others claim continuous murmurs that can be obliterated by compression of collateral channels.[21,30] The numerous murmurs that may accompany coarctation are listed in Table 27-4.

COMPLICATIONS

The lethal complications of coarctation are heart failure, aortic rupture, intracranial hemorrhage, and infective endocarditis.[31] In one of the largest series so far reported, congestive failure was present in two-thirds of patients under 1 year and in two-thirds of those over 40 years, whereas it

Table 27–4
The Murmurs of Coarctation

Timing of Murmur	Produced By
Systolic	1. Coarctation itself
	2. Aortic ejection
	a. Dilation of aorta
	b. Bicuspid valve
	c. Associated aortic stenosis
	d. Associated subaortic stenosis
	3. Other associated lesions
	a. Ventricular septal defect
	b. Patent ductus arteriosus
	c. Mitral regurgitation
Diastolic	1. Coarctation itself
	2. Aortic regurgitation due to:
	a. Bicuspid aortic valve
	b. Dilated ring
	c. Infective endocarditis
	3. Diastolic component of PDA murmur
	4. LV inflow murmur
	a. Associated mitral stenosis
	b. Dilated left ventricle
	c. Increased flow (L-to-R shunts)
	d. Austin Flint
	e. Obstruction from LV hypertrophy
	f. Fibroelastotic change in mitral valve
Continuous	1. Coarctation itself
	2. Patent ductus
	3. Collaterals

Profile: Coarctation of the Aorta

M:F = 2 or 3:1, but complicates 30% of webbed-neck syndromes
Note different syndromes: postductal ("adult"); preductal ("fetal")

Postductal

Often symptom-free, chance diagnosis
Minority (with PDA) have heart failure in infancy
Coldness, numbness, "heaviness" of feet, legs
Cramps at rest, intermittent claudication
Headaches, epistaxis, vertigo
Dyspnea, angina, palpitations
Complications: heart failure, infective endocarditis or aortitis, aortic rupture, stroke

Prominent arterial pulsations in neck ("carotid swell")
Thrill in suprasternal notch, sometimes at base and over scapula
Hypertension in arms, lower pressure in legs
Weak and delayed (compared with radial) pulses in legs
Pulsating collateral vessels around thorax
Blanching time increased in toes
LV impulse, aortic ejection click, accentuated A2
Numerous potential murmurs:
  From coarctation itself—systolic or continuous
  From aortic ejection
  From associated lesions
  From collaterals

Preductal

Respiratory distress, heart failure, cyanosis of legs, abdominal pain
Right ventricular impulse

affected only 4% of those between 1 and 40 years.[13] Of 304 autopsied cases,[26,32] the cause of death was unrelated to the coarctation in 29%; in the remainder, the fatal events were:

Heart failure, 26%,
Aortic rupture, 21%,
Infective endocarditis, 18%, and
Intracranial hemorrhage, 12%.

Bacterial infection involves either the bicuspid aortic valve (endocarditis) or the aorta itself (aortitis) in the ascending arch or just distal to the coarctation. When pregnancy complicates coarctation, rupture of the ascending aorta is the main hazard, occurring most often in the third trimester, less often during labor.[33,34]

According to Campbell's analysis in 1970, of those who survive the stormy first 2 years of life, one-quarter die before the age of 20 years, one half by 32 years, three-quarters by 46 years, and 90% by 58 years.[31] Obviously today's survival can be improved if earlier recognition is followed by timely surgery.

REFERENCES

1. Tawes RL, et al. Congenital bicuspid aortic valves associated with coarctation of aorta in children. Br Heart J 1969;31:127.
2. Becker AE, et al. Anomalies associated with coarctation of the aorta: particular reference to infancy. Circulation 1970;41:1067.
3. Liberthson RR, et al. Coarctation of the aorta: review of 234 patients and clarification of management problems. Am J Cardiol 1979;43:835.
4. Hesslein PS, et al. Prognosis of symptomatic coarctation in infancy. Am J Cardiol 1983;51:299.
5. Glancy DL, et al. Juxtaductal coarctation. Am J Cardiol 1983;51:537.
6. Haddad HM, Wilkins L. Congenital anomalies associated with gonadal aplasia. Pediatrics 1959;23:885.
7. Campbell M, Poloni PE. The aetiology of coarctation of the aorta. Lancet 1961;1:463.
8. Simon AB, et al. Familial aspects of coarctation of the aorta. Chest 1974;66:687.
9. Sehested J. Coarctation of the aorta in monozygotic twins. Br Heart J 1982;47:619.
10. Jarcho S. Coarctation of the aorta (Reynaud 1828). Am J Cardiol 1962;9:591.
11. Gasul BM, et al. Heart disease in children: diagnosis and treatment. Philadelphia: JB Lippincott, 1966:898, 904.
12. Subramanian AR. Coarctation or interruption or aorta proximal to origin of both subclavian arteries: report of three cases presenting in infancy. Br Heart J 1972;34:1225.
13. Glass IH, et al. Coarctation of the aorta in infants: a review of 12 years experience. Pediatrics 1960;26:109.
14. Freundlich E, et al. Coarctation of the aorta in infancy: analysis of a 10-year experience with medical management. Pediatrics 1961;27:427.
15. Edwards JE. The congenital bicuspid valve. Circulation 1961;23:485.
16. Kempton JJ, Waterston DJ. Coarctation of aorta presenting as cardiac failure in early infancy. Br Med J 1957;2:442.
17. Shinebourne EA, et al. Coarctation of the aorta in infancy and childhood. Br Heart J 1976;38:375.
18. Taussig HB: Congenital malformations of the heart. Cambridge: Harvard University Press, 1960:802.
19. Strafford MA, et al. Coarctation of the aorta: a study in delayed detection. Pediatrics 1982;69:159.
20. Braimbridge MV, Yen A. Coarctation in the elderly. Circulation 1965;31:209.
21. Cleland WP, et al. Coarctation of the aorta. Br Med J 1956;2:379.
22. Campbell M, Baylis JH. The course and prognosis of coarctation of the aorta. Br Heart J 1956;18:475.
23. Campbell M, Suzman S. Coarctation of the aorta. Br Heart J 1947;9:185.
24. Levine SA, Kalstone CE. The blanching test for coarctation of the aorta. Am J Med Sci 1963;246:702.
25. Eisalo A, et al. Fluorescence angiography of the fundus vessels in aortic coarctation. Br Heart J 1970;32:71.
26. Abbott ME. Coarctation of the aorta of the adult type. Am Heart J 1928;3:381 and 574.
27. Spencer MP, et al. The origin and interpretation of murmurs in coarctation of the aorta. Am Heart J 1958;56:722.
28. Christensen NA, Hines EA. Clinical features in coarctation of the aorta: a review of 96 cases. Proc Mayo Clin 1948;23:339.
29. Wood P. Diseases of the heart and circulation. Philadelphia: JB Lippincott, 1956:378.
30. Nadas AS. Pediatric cardiology. Philadelphia: WB Saunders, 1963.
31. Campbell M. Natural history of coarctation of the aorta. Br Heart J 1970;32:633.
32. Reifenstein GH, et al. Coarctation of the aorta: a review of 104 autopsied cases of the "adult type," 2 years of age or older. Am Heart J 1947;33:146.
33. Rosenthal L. Coarctation of the aorta and pregnancy: report of five cases. Br Med J 1955;1:16.
34. Deal K, Wooley CF. Coarctation of the aorta and pregnancy. Ann Intern Med 1973;78:706.

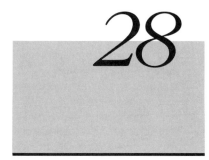

28

Patent Ductus Arteriosus

During fetal life, blood flows from the pulmonary artery (PA) into the aorta (right-to-left) through a functioning ductus, because the unexpanded lungs and fetal state of the pulmonary arterial tree maintain a high pulmonary vascular resistance. After birth, expansion of the lungs lowers their vascular resistance, while tying the umbilical cord raises systemic resistance so that the flow is reversed from aorta to PA (left-to-right). At the same time, lung expansion produces a positional change while increased oxygen tension stimulates the muscular ductus to constrict; both of these influences favor functional closure of the ductus during the first few days of life. In the newborn, you may hear a ductus murmur, maximal in the 3rd and 4th left interspaces: A crescendo systolic murmur leading up to the second sound and fading quickly in early diastole.[1] Apparently asphyxia and high body temperature favor temporary persistence of patency. Rubella affecting the mother during her first trimester may cause permanent patency of the ductus, and this is sometimes associated with bilateral cataracts, deaf-mutism, and pulmonary stenosis or segmental PA stenoses.

The ductus remains patent two or three times more often in females than in males, and the defect shows a definite familial tendency[2]; patency is more likely to afflict the premature than the full-term baby[3]—in one series of 111 premature infants, 17 had patent ductuses.[4] Spontaneous closure of ductuses that remain patent occurs at the rate of 0.6% per annum.[5]

In most series, PDA ranks second or third among congenital defects, and accounts for about 15% of all congenital heart disease (see Table 26-1). Like coarctation, PDA can kill rapidly in infancy, or, at the other extreme, permit symptom-free survival to a ripe old age.[6-9] Of 804 patients, 37 (4.6%) attained an age of 50 years.[10] One remarkable patient lived to the age of 90 years before symptoms developed.[11]

CLINICAL PICTURE

Clinical findings depend on the size of persisting shunt and the state of the pulmonary vasculature. Pulmonary vascular obstruction may be present in infancy or may be acquired in later life as the consequence of increased flow. In many cases the ductus is functionally small, the child is entirely free of symptoms, and the lesion is discovered by chance. In White's long-lived patient,[11] patency of the ductus was first recognized at the age of 48 years. Others, with larger shunts, suffer from varying degrees of fatigability, dyspnea, and underdevelopment. Respiratory infections may be frequent and troublesome.

Pulses

Arterial pulses are vigorous, even waterhammer, with low diastolic and high pulse pressures: the pulse pressure was 50 mm Hg or more in 19 of 20 infants.[12] The diastolic pressure may drop to zero with exercise.[13]

In infants, where blood pressure measurements are not the easiest undertakings, palmar pulsation is a useful sign: You feel the superficial arch pulsating forcibly as it crosses the metacarpal heads. This sign corresponds with a pulse pressure of 40 mm Hg or more, and is only rarely present in controls under the age of 2 years, whereas it was found in eight of nine infants with PDA.[14] Capillary pulsation is common.

The Precordium

The left ventricular impulse may be hyperactive, reflecting its increased diastolic load. A systolic, or diastolic, or continuous thrill is often palpable at the left upper sternal border, in the suprasternal notch, and perhaps higher in the neck. The first sound may be accentuated. The second sound—if audible—may be normal, single, or, when the left ventricular load is excessive, paradoxically split.[15] Be sure to listen for the components of S2 away from the site of maximal murmur intensity, where they are likely to be "drowned in sound." In many cases, because of "eddy sounds" (Fig. 28-1) and the engulfing murmur (Figs. 28-1, 28-2), it is impossible to distinguish and analyze S2[16]; as pulmonary hypertension develops, loudening the pulmonic component and curtailing the murmur, the second sound may become audible (Fig. 28-3).[17] An opening snap and third sound (Fig. 28-3) are heard in some patients.

Murmurs

The typical "machinery" murmur, produced at the PA end of the ductus—where two opposing currents "crash head on" during systole, and the shunted stream continues to pour forth in diastole—is continuous and varies with the size of the shunt; if small, the murmur is high-pitched and occupies more of diastole; if large, it is coarser and ends much earlier.[18] Its intensity is noticeably uneven, because of "eddy sounds," and it envelopes S2. (See Fig. 28-1.) Maximal at the left upper sternal border, it is well heard outward under the left clavicle, and often in the neck. Some have described its intermittent disappearance—probably due to kinking of the ductus,[19] or to a valve situated at its PA end.[20]

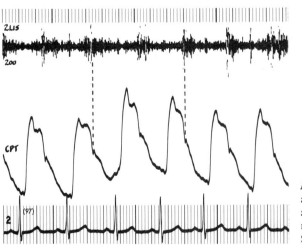

Figure 28–1. From a patient with patent ductus arteriosus, illustrating the unevenness and the waxing and waning of the "continuous," "machinery" murmur, which reaches its maximum at about the time of S2 (dashed lines).

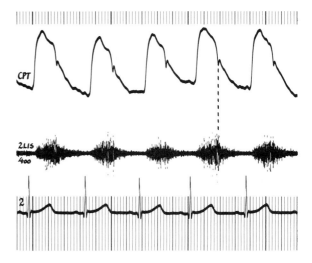

Figure 28–2. From an 18-month-old child with patent ductus arteriosus. Note the murmur reaching its maximum at the time of a submerged S2 and spilling over into diastole (timing of the invisible S2 is indicated by the dashed line).

When the shunt is sizeable, a short apical mid-diastolic murmur (Fig. 28-3) announces the increased mitral flow—which must increase to keep pace with the left sided loss via the aortic run-off. The combination of this murmur with an accentuated first sound (Fig. 28-3), fullness of the left atrium on x-ray, bifid P waves, and raised pulmonary capillary ("wedge") pressure, has led French cardiologists to speak of the "pseudomitral syndrome."

In infants, even without pulmonary vascular obstruction, the typical continuous murmur is often lacking. This can make an important diagnosis difficult, since a large ductus, without the typical murmur, can produce severe symptoms in infancy that require prompt surgery.[21,22] Of 165 cardiac defects causing death or severe distress in the first few weeks of life, PDA accounted for four of them.[23] Echocardiography, or cardiac catheterization and retrograde aortography may be required for diagnosis.

Of 23 patent ductuses studied during the first year of life, only three had continuous murmurs, whereas 16 had apical mid-diastolic murmurs.[12] When you see the following clinical picture in infancy:

Failure to grow and thrive,
Repeated episodes of pneumonia,
Dyspnea with early heart failure,

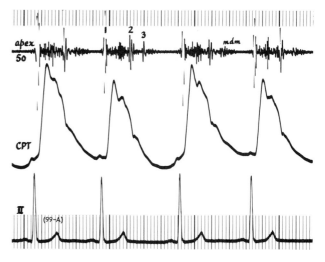

Figure 28–3. From an 8-year-old boy with large ductus—same caliber as his aorta. There is no continuous murmur, but at the apex an audible S3 and mid-diastolic murmur (mdm) attest to the large left-to-right shunt.

Systolic murmur at left sternal border,
Bounding pulse with high pulse pressure,
Accentuation of P2, and
Apical mid-diastolic murmur,

the differential diagnosis is between PDA, aortopulmonary window, and large ventricular septal defect.[24]

When only a systolic murmur is present, but a PDA is suspected, the diastolic aortic/PA gradient can be increased by giving mephentermine (10–30 mg IV or IM), and this may bring a lurking continuous murmur to light.[25]

Pulmonary Hypertension

When severe pulmonary hypertension clouds the picture and eventuates in an Eisenmenger syndrome, in addition to the expected symptoms of dyspnea, fatigue, and palpitations, precordial pain, hemoptysis, and hoarseness may develop.[26] On the other hand, the patient may be less symptomatic than one with a large left-to-right shunt. When PA pressure equals aortic ("balanced ductus") or exceeds it ("reverse ductus"), there is no continuous murmur, and indeed there may be no murmur at all,[27] but there is usually a systolic ejection murmur. The pulse pressure remains wide, P2 is pal-

pable and loud, a pulmonic ejection click usually appears, and an early diastolic murmur of pulmonic regurgitation may develop. In the "reverse" cases, "differential" clubbing (more marked in toes than fingers)[28] and cyanosis (more pronounced in feet than hands) develop.

The murmurs of patent ductus may evolve in orderly fashion (Fig. 28-4) as pulmonary hypertension progresses: to a shorter, but still continuous, machinery murmur with audible mid-diastolic murmur (Fig. 28-4**B**); to pansystolic murmur alone with now audible S2 (Fig. 28-4**C**); to a less than pansystolic murmur (Fig. 28-4**D**); to little or no systolic murmur with early diastolic (Graham Steell) murmur (Fig. 28-4**E**) dominating the auscultatory scenario.[17]

THE COMPLICATED DUCTUS

The congenital lesions found most often in association with PDA are aortic valve disease,[29] coarctation of the aorta, ventricular septal defect, and pulmonic stenosis.[30] With all of these, the ductus adds an extra handicap. But bear in mind that patent ductuses don't always make matters worse; in conjunction with the following congenital lesions, the patent ductus may be beneficial or even life-

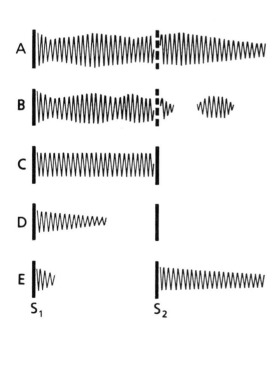

Figure 28–4. Murmurs of patent ductus as modified by development of pulmonary hypertension. (**A**) Continuous murmur obscuring S2. (**B**) Shortening of continuous murmur, still obscuring S2, with apical mid-diastolic murmur. (**C**) Murmur now confined to systole, but pansystolic; S2 audible. (**D**) Murmur abbreviated to less than pansystolic; S2 loud. (**E**) Dominant murmur now early diastolic (Graham Steell) from pulmonic regurgitation secondary to pulmonary hypertension. (After Perloff.[17])

	PDA	*APW*
Symptoms	Majority asymptomatic	Majority symptomatic
Pulse	Usually strong and bounding	Seldom strong and bounding
Continuous murmur	In 95%	In only 15%
Site of maximal murmur intensity and thrill	2nd left interspace	3rd left interspace
Cyanosis	Differential	Diffuse

sparing: Tetralogy of Fallot; tricuspid, pulmonic or aortic atresia; single ventricle with pulmonic stenosis; and transposition of the great arteries with pulmonic stenosis.

Apart from heart failure and pulmonary hypertension, the most important acquired complication of PDA is infective endarteritis, which is said to occur in 0.45% per year.[5] Rarely, aneurysm of the ductus itself or of the PA may develop.

AORTOPULMONARY WINDOW

The aortopulmonary (AP) window (or fenestration) is also sometimes called partial persistent truncus or aortic septal defect. This is a rare defect in which the blood is shunted through a large porthole between the ascending aorta and the main pulmonary trunk, a short distance above the semilunar valves. The picture closely simulates a large PDA. Starting as a large left-to-right shunt, the pulmonary vascular resistance mounts rapidly with the development of pulmonary hypertension and consequent right-to-left shunt. Cyanosis usually appears in adolescence and progresses. A retrograde aortogram may be necessary for final diagnosis. The "average" AP window differs from the "average" patent ductus as shown in display above.

These differences are the result of the generally larger shunt and its location. The cyanosis is evenly distributed, because the shunt is proximal to all the branches of the aortic arch.

In a series of 17 patients,[31] the second sound was accentuated in 14, there were major associated cardiovascular defects in nine (three of them PDAs), cyanosis in seven, an ejection click in five, an early diastolic murmur in four, and a continuous murmur in only two.

REFERENCES

1. Burnard ED. A murmur from the ductus arteriosus in the newborn baby. Br Med J 1958;1:806.
2. Anderson RC. Causative factors underlying congenital heart malformations: 1. patent ductus arteriosus. Pediatrics 1954;14:143.
3. Nadas AS. Patent ductus revisited. N Engl J Med 1976; 295:563.
4. Kitterman JA, et al. Patent ductus arteriosus in premature infants: incidence, relation to pulmonary disease and management. N Engl J Med 1972;287:473.
5. Campbell M. Natural history of persistent ductus arteriosus. Br Heart J 1968;30:4.
6. Fishman L. Patent ductus arteriosus in a patient surviving to seventy-four years. Am J Cardiol 1960;6:685.
7. Fishman L, Silverthorne MC. Persistent patent ductus arteriosus in the aged: including the report of the oldest case on record with diagnosis confirmed post mortem. Am J Cardiol 1951;41:762.
8. Bain CWC. Longevity in patent ductus arteriosus. Br Heart J 1957;19:574.
9. Hornsten TR, et al. Patent ductus arteriosus in a 72 year old woman: successful corrective surgery. 1967;199:580.
10. Marquis RM, et al. Persistence of ductus arteriosus with left to right shunt in the older patient. Br Heart J 1982; 48:469.
11. White PD, et al. Patency of the ductus arteriosus at 90. N Engl J Med 1969;280:146.
12. Rudolph AM, et al. Patent ductus arteriosus: a clinical and hemodynamic study of 23 patients in the first year of life. Pediatrics 1958;22:892.
13. Taussig HB. Congenital malformations of the heart. Cambridge: Harvard University Press, 1960:495.
14. Stuckey D. Palmar pulsation: a physical sign of patent ductus arteriosus in infancy. Med J Aust 1957;44:681.
15. Gray I. Paradoxical splitting of the second sound. Br Heart J 1956;18:21.
16. Neill C, Mounsey P. Auscultation in patent ductus arteriosus: with a description of two fistulae simulating patent ductus. Br Heart J 1958;20:61.
17. Perloff JK. Auscultatory and phonocardiographic manifestations of pulmonary hypertension. Prog Cardiovasc Dis 1967;9:303.
18. Gasul BM, et al. Heart disease in children: diagnosis and treatment. Philadelphia: JB Lippincott, 1966:316.
19. Shapiro W, et al. Intermittent disappearance of the murmur of patent ductus arteriosus. Circulation 1960;22:226.
20. Keith TR, Sagarminaga J. Spontaneously disappearing

murmur of patent ductus arteriosus: a case report. Circulation 1961;24:1235.

21. Ziegler RF. The importance of patent ductus arteriosus in infants. Am Heart J 1952;43:553.

22. Adams P, et al. Diagnosis and treatment of patent ductus arteriosus. Pediatrics 1953;12:664.

23. Lambert EC, et al. Congenital cardiac anomalies in the newborn: a review of conditions causing death or severe distress in the first month of life. Pediatrics 1966;37:343.

24. Dammann JF, Sell CGR. Patent ductus arteriosus in absence of continuous murmur. Circulation 1952;6:110.

25. Crevasse LE, Logue RB. Atypical patent ductus arteriosus: the use of a vasopressor agent as a diagnostic aid. Circulation 1959;19:332.

26. London F, et al. Patent ductus arteriosus with reverse flow. South Med J 1957;50:160.

27. Evans DW, Heath D. Disappearance of the continuous murmur in a case of patent ductus arteriosus. Br Heart J 1961;23:469.

28. Young D, Mark H. Fate of the patient with the Eisenmenger syndrome. Am J Cardiol 1971;28:658.

29. Mark H, et al. Coexistence of patent ductus arteriosus and congenital aortic valvular disease. Circulation 1958;17:359.

30. Heiner DC, Nadas AS. Patent ductus arteriosus in association with pulmonic stenosis: a report of six cases with additional noncardiac congenital anomalies. Circulation 1958;17:232.

31. Blieden LC, Moller JH. Aorticopulmonary septal defect: an experience with 17 patients. Br Heart J 1974;36:630.

29

Ventricular Septal Defects

Defects of the ventricular septum are the most common form of congenital cardiac anomaly, and account for about 20% of all congenital heart disease. There is evidence that the number in the United States is increasing—and not because of improved diagnosis.[1] In Atlanta, between 1970 and 1977, the number of new cases reported each year more than doubled. Acquired septal defects may result from myocardial infarction, stab or bullet wounds, and even blunt trauma.[2,3]

Congenital defects show no prejudice for either sex. Like other simple defects, the ventricular septal defect (VSD) embraces a wide spectrum of syndromes, ranging from symptom-free longevity to neonatal death; and defects range from pinhead size to several centimeters in diameter. Unfortunately, small defects and modest pulmonary-to-systemic flow ratios are not guarantees against an increasing pulmonary vascular resistance (PVR).[4] Defects as small as 2 mm can be rapidly fatal in infancy.[5]

Circumscribed defects occupy any part of the septum, and are distributed as in Figure 29-1; thus, four-fifths of defects are located in a small fraction of the septal expanse, the membranous septum. Note that part of the membranous septum extends above the tricuspid valve so that certain defects provide direct communication between the left ventricle and the right *atrium* (Fig. 29-2).

The clinical picture depends mainly on two things: Size of shunt and degree of PVR. Large shunts stimulate a reaction in the pulmonary bed and the PVR rises; they also overload the right ventricle and may cause secondary outflow tract obstruction through muscular hypertrophy of the crista. Clinical features of the various syndromes are presented in Table 29-1.

CLINICAL CATEGORIES

Despite inevitable overlap, the clinical syndromes can be usefully divided into six general categories[6]:

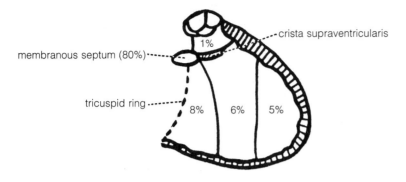

Figure 29–1. Approximate distribution of ventricular septal defects.

I. A few, with *tiny defect and negligible shunt*, have only a short systolic murmur (Fig. 29-3**E**) without a thrill. Some of these may be small muscular defects that close off as systolic contraction proceeds.[7]

II. With *small defect and shunt*, the pulmonary artery pressure remains normal and the patient symptom-free. There is a thrill at the left sternal border maximal in the 4th interspace, and a corresponding pansystolic murmur, which is typically high-pitched and sometimes harsh. It may be "plateau" (Fig. 29-3**A**) or diamond-shaped with early, mid-, or late systolic peaking (Fig. 29-3 **B–D**). It is usually well transmitted to the right of the sternum as well as to the apex, and is often well heard over the whole precordium. In 20% the murmur is maximal at the 2nd rather than the 4th interspace, and then the defect may be indistinguishable

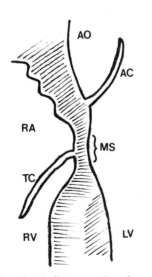

Figure 29–2. Sketch illustrating the relationship of the membranous septum (MS) to both the right ventricle (RV) and the right atrium (RA). AO, aorta; AC, aortic cusp; TC, tricuspid cusp; LV, left ventricle.

from mild pulmonic stenosis. Inhalation of amyl nitrite diminishes the murmur.

To my ear, the epithet that describes the murmur's usual quality most aptly is "squeezing"; if you carefully select and listen at the interspace in which the murmur is loudest, inspiration there diminishes its intensity; but if you then apply your stethoscope one, or more often two, interspaces lower, the murmur grows *louder* with inspiration (Fig. 29-4)—thus simulating a tricuspid event.

III. With a *larger shunt, but still normal pulmonary artery pressure*, patients may still have no symptoms with physical findings similar to those in category II. However, a third sound is always present, and a mid-diastolic murmur is usually heard. The apex beat may be somewhat overactive and displaced leftward. Moderate cardiac enlargement may be detectable.

IV. With a *sizeable shunt and moderately increased pulmonary artery pressure*, symptoms develop: "Feeding" problems in infancy, dyspnea at rest, respiratory infections, stunting of growth, and frank congestive failure.[8,9] There is a precordial bulge, right ventricular lift, and a hyperactive displaced left ventricular impulse. In addition to the usual thrill and murmur, third sound, and mid-diastolic murmur at the apex, there is wide splitting of the second sound with accentuated and palpable P2, and a pulmonary flow murmur.[7]

V. With *large shunts and considerable pulmonary hypertension*, the child is ill, underdeveloped, and subject to pulmonary infections. There is hyperemia of the fingertips, but no true cyanosis except with severe exertion or with pneumonia. Other signs are similar to those in category IV, except that the thrill is less frequent, the defect murmur shorter and softer, and the murmur of pulmonic regurgitation is added. The right ventricular lift is more marked and P2 more easily felt, in keeping with a single loud S2.

Table 29–1
The VSD Spectrum

Minute Defect; Negligible Physiologic Disturbance	PAP Normal, Shunt <40% (Roger's)	PAP Normal, Shunt >40%	PAP Raised, Shunt >40%	PAP = Systemic, Shunt >40%	Bidirectional Shunt (Eisenmenger)
Percentage					
5.5%	34%	15.5%	17%	15%	13%
Symptoms					
None	None	None	At early age	At early age	Cyanosis
Precordial Pulsations					
None	None	Normal or slightly overactive LVI	Overactive, thrusting LVI; RVOT lift	RVOT lift + + + +	RV heave
Thrill					
None	4LIS	4LIS	4LIS	Often none	None
Sounds					
S2					
Normal	Normal or wide split	Normal or wide split	Normal or wide split c̄ palpable P2	Easily felt, single and loud	Palpable shock, single and loud
S3					
0	+	+	+	+	0
EC					
0	0	0	0	(+)	+
Murmurs					
Systolic					
Short at 4LIS, 3/6	Pan at 4LIS (20% 2LIS), 4–5/6	Pan at 4LIS, 4–5/6	Pan (sometimes less) at 4LIS, 4–5/6	Short 2–4/6 at 4LIS	Short 2/6 at 2LIS; or none
Diastolic					
None	Usually none	Apical MDM	Apical MDM easily heard	Apical MDM, ?EDM of PR	No MDM, EDM of PR

PAP, pulmonary artery pressure; RVOT, right ventricular outflow tract; LVI, left ventricular impulse; 4LIS, 4th left interspace; EC, ejection click; MDM, mid-diastolic murmur; EDM, early diastolic murmur; PR, pulmonic regurgitation.

VI. When PVR exceeds systemic vascular resistance and the shunt is reversed (right-to-left) or bidirectional, the Eisenmenger reaction is present—see further on.

SERIAL STUDIES

Serial catheterizations of patients with VSDs have established various trends that the disease may follow, and these are of diagnostic interest and importance:

1. After the first year of life there is a tendency for pulmonary flow and blood pressure to decrease,[10] so that even the seriously sick infant, if he survives, may enjoy marked clinical and hemodynamic improvement. Of 200 consecutive infants with isolated VSDs followed for the first 5 years of life, those with a pulmonary-to-systemic flow ratio less than 2:1 became asymptomatic because the size of the defect decreased; in 20% it closed completely. Of those with flow ratios of more than 2:1, only 6% closed spontaneously, 15% died in infancy, and 10% developed Eisenmenger syndromes.[11]

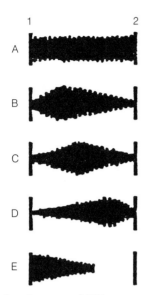

Figure 29–3. Contours of VSD murmurs. (**A**) Pansystolic plateau (the usual form). (**B**) Pansystolic early-peaking. (**C**) Pansystolic mid-peaking. (**D**) Pansystolic late-peaking. (**E**) Less-than-systolic (found in defects of muscular septum, in presence of increased pulmonary vascular resistance, and in a few supracristal defects).

2. The defect closes spontaneously in something like 25% of all patients,[12,13] and 90% of spontaneous closures take place before the age of 8 years.[14] Among *small* defects, the record is encouragingly better: 24% close by the age of 18 months, 50% by the end of 4 years, and 75% by 10 years.[15] The usual mechanism of closure is either adherence of the medial leaflet of the tricuspid valve to the defect, or proliferation of fibrous tissue. Closure may occur even when the defect is relatively large,[14,16] even as late as the 4th or 5th decade,[17] and even in the presence of congestive heart failure and elevated PVR.[14]

3. Even in older patients the relative size of the defect can decrease, and the PVR may decrease progressively despite the continued large left-to-right shunt.[18]

4. As the disease progresses, manifestations of secondary pulmonary infundibular stenosis may result from hypertrophy of the crista supraventricularis.[10]

ADDITIONAL DIAGNOSTIC POINTS

An *ejection click* in the presence of a VSD, if it is best heard in expiration at the lower left sternal border, is questionably related to aneurysm of the septum[19,20] (and may possibly be a harbinger of spontaneous closure); or, if it originates in the pulmonary artery, signals increased PVR and pulmonary hypertension.

Wide splitting of S2 is frequently noted, and is due to a combination of premature aortic closure and delayed pulmonic closure[7]; this wide splitting and the pansystolic murmur indicate absence of serious, irreversible pulmonary vascular disease, and are good guides to operability.[21] In a number of patients, splitting of S2 may be relatively "fixed" (Fig. 29-5), that is, with respiratory variation of only 0.01 second.[22]

Supracristal defects may be recognizable clinically: The pansystolic murmur is harsh and loud, distinctly crescendo-decrescendo with late peaking, and is maximal in the 2nd *and 1st* intercostal spaces on the left with upward radiation to the left

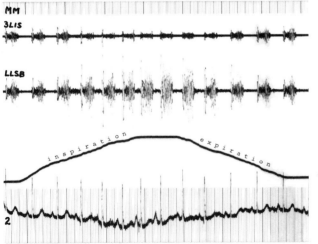

Figure 29–4. Simultaneous phonocardiograms recorded at third left interspace (3LIS) and at the lower left sternal border (LLSB). During inspiration the murmur becomes less intense at the third interspace while it progressively loudens at the lower site.

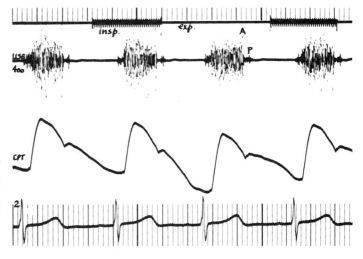

Figure 29–5. From a 5-year old boy with a large ventricular septal defect and pulmonary hypertension (pulmonary artery pressure = 63/21). The phonocardiogram records the pansystolic murmur and fixed splitting of S2 (A-P interval = 0.05 s). The carotid pulse is normal.

clavicle; P2 is soft and S2 widely split in expiration.[23,24] A more recent Japanese study of 37 consecutive supracristal defects demonstrated pansystolic murmurs in 89% of them, with late systolic accentuation in half of these; the remaining 11% had only early systolic murmurs.[25]

Multiple septal defects are sometimes present, but the clinical picture is indistinguishable from that of the single defect.[26] A *left ventricular–right atrial septal defect* cannot be distinguished clinically from an interventricular septal defect.[27]

The VSD is much the most commonly acyanotic lesion to present in infancy with congestive heart failure and a loud systolic murmur maximal at 3rd and/or 4th interspaces; but this combination *can* result from a number of other lesions, including A-V canal, patent ductus, tricuspid atresia, to-

tal anomalous pulmonary return, aortic stenosis, single ventricle, truncus arteriosus without pulmonic stenosis, and mitral regurgitation.[28]

As the VSD murmur is regurgitant, its intensity does not increase at the end of a long cycle, as, for instance, in a postextrasystolic beat (Fig. 29-6).

THE COMPLICATED VSD

VSD with Patent Ductus

VSD with ''silent'' patent ductus[29] is worth recognizing because of required differences in therapy. The usual VSD murmur, with or without a thrill, is present, and there is invariably an apical

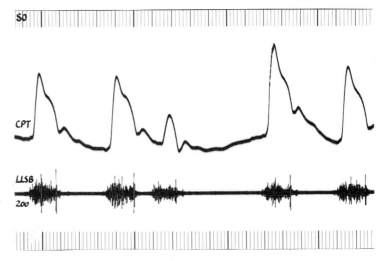

Figure 29–6. From a 28-year-old man with a ventricular septal defect (and repaired coarctation). The phonocardiogram at the lower left sternal border shows the failure of the lengthened postextrasystolic cycle to intensify the regurgitant pansystolic murmur.

mid-diastolic rumble,[30] but it is most unusual to find the typical continuous murmur of the ductus. Points that may suggest the associated ductus are: History of maternal rubella, gross undernourishment, wide pulse pressure,[30] or an early diastolic murmur confined to the left upper sternal border.[21]

VSD with Aortic Regurgitation

In a large French series of 790 patients with VSDs, aortic regurgitation complicated 6.3%.[31] The defect is either immediately under the pulmonic valve (''subpulmonic'') or infracristal, and the acquired lesion assumes the leading clinical role and dwarfs the congenital defect. The aortic cusp (usually right, sometimes noncoronary cusp) is drawn down into the high septal defect, opens the floodgates for free regurgitation, and at the same time partially plugs up the defect and reduces the shunt.

In the Japanese series,[25] there was a correlation between the pattern of the VSD murmur and the development of aortic valve prolapse: They found serious prolapse more often in the group that had pansystolic murmurs *without* late accentuation; and there was no prolapse among the few patients with only early systolic murmurs.

The onset is insidious, but the diagnosis is usually easy: An asymptomatic child, with signs of VSD since infancy, between the age of 2 and 10 years—and most often at about 6 years[32]—begins to notice pulsations in the neck and vigorous precordial pulsations, especially when lying on his left side. Examination reveals the early diastolic murmur and the hemodynamic signs of aortic regurgitation.

The systolic-diastolic (to-and-fro) murmurs of VSD plus aortic regurgitation are easily distinguished from the continuous murmur of a patent ductus, which peaks at the time of and envelopes the second sound. By auscultation alone, the diastolic murmur cannot be distinguished from the Graham Steell murmur of pulmonic regurgitation, but the accompanying signs of pulmonary hypertension versus aortic regurgitation make the distinction clear.

Infundibular pulmonic stenosis sometimes further complicates the picture and adds a systolic thrill and ejection murmur at the left upper sternal border.[33] The regurgitation may progress rapidly to death in congestive heart failure; or infective endocarditis, to which the incompetent and trau-matized aortic valve is susceptible, may close the clinical scene.

Eisenmenger's Syndrome

Severe pulmonary hypertension resulting from increased PVR and producing a reversed or bidirectional shunt through a large VSD is Eisenmenger's syndrome. The essential pathophysiologic feature of the complex is not the VSD but the high PVR with resulting pulmonary hypertension: It matters little whether the shunt is through the ventricular septum or at another level. Therefore the term Eisenmenger syndrome (or reaction) can reasonably apply to any situation that gives rise to the sequence: High PVR—pulmonary hypertension—right-to-left shunt, and this may result from the following lesions[34]:

At aortic level: Patent ductus, aortopulmonary window,
At ventricular level: VSD, single ventricle, common A-V canal, persistent truncus, transposition of the great arteries, corrected transposition, and
At atrial level: atrial septal defect, single atrium, anomalous pulmonary venous drainage.

Of Wood's first 1000 congenital hearts, the Eisenmenger syndrome accounted for 8%.

The Eisenmenger reaction probably requires a pulmonary blood flow four to six times systemic, amounting to 16 to 30 L/minute. But flow is not the whole story, since 70 years of pulmonary plethora is not enough to elicit the reaction in some; and whereas over half those with large patent ductuses or VSDs develop the syndrome, less than 10% of atrial septal defects with comparable pulmonary flow develop it; and again, its development in atrial septal defects occurs at a later age and shows a disproportionate bias for women.[33] About 80% of those with VSD or patent ductus who develop the syndrome acquire it in infancy; in contrast, 90% of those with atrial septal defects wait until adult life.

Clinical Similarities

Regardless of the shunt's level, some features of the reaction are similar. Angina (14%–20%), syncope (10%–15%), congestive heart failure (8%–12%), and polycythemia have a similar incidence. All have a right ventricular lift. Pulmonary artery pulsation and pulmonic ejection clicks occur in

Table 29–2
Differing Incidences in the Eisenmenger Syndromes

	VSD	PDA	ASD
Hemoptysis	33% (100% by age 40)	12%	25%
Cyanosis: Absent	0	60	intermediate
Gross	42	4	intermediate
Clubbing: Absent	3	76	intermediate
Gross	36	5	intermediate
Differential	0	50	0
Squatting	15	3	5
S2: Single	55	6	0
Wide split	12	50 (persistent)	86 (fixed)
P2 loud, palpable	90	90	57

VSD, ventricular septal defect; PDA, patent ductus arteriosus; ASD, atrial septal defect.

about 65%, pulmonic ejection murmurs in about 80%, and murmurs of pulmonic regurgitation in 50% to 65% of all cases. Thrills accompany the pulmonic ejection and regurgitant murmurs in about 10%.

When high PVR complicates the prototypical VSD, the shunt murmur undergoes a series of predictable transformations. As PVR relentlessly advances, the murmur changes from a pansystolic plateau (see Fig. 29-3**A**) into a pansystolic murmur that peaks early (see Fig. 29-3**B**); as time passes and the right ventricular pressure mounts, the murmur is cut off before the second sound (see Fig. 29-3**E**). Finally, with pressures equalized and shunt eliminated, the murmur of the defect disappears and is replaced by a pulmonic ejection murmur.[35] A Graham Steell murmur of pulmonic regurgitation may preempt diastole.

Clinical Differences

Certain other features present with differing frequencies, and may be diagnostically helpful:

1. Cataracts, deafness, or maternal rubella point to a patent ductus,
2. Shortness of breath on effort is much less common and less marked with a patent ductus than with the septal defects, and
3. Giant "a" waves and right atrial gallops are much more common in atrial septal defect (38%) than in ventricular septal defect or patent ductus (2%–3%). Other differences are listed in Table 29-2, with percentages according to Wood.[34]

Profile:　*Ventricular Septal Defect*

M = F

 I. A few: *short* murmur, no thrill, no symptoms

 II. (Roger, 1879) *Pansystolic murmur* and thrill at LSB, diminished by inspiration and amyl nitrite. No symptoms or signs.

 III. Murmur and thrill as in II
 Overactive LV impulse
 S3 and MDM

 IV. Symptoms: feeding problems, retarded growth, dyspnea, respiratory infections, heart failure.
 Murmur and thrill as in II
 RV lift, LV impulse displaced leftward
 Palpable S2, wide splitting of S2
 Pulmonary flow murmur

 V. Cyanosis with pulmonary infections, hyperemic fingertips
 Murmur shorter than pansystolic, may be no thrill
 Pulmonary insufficiency with marked RV lift and S2 easily felt
 Single loud S2

 VI. Eisenmenger complex

Despite their limitations, some patients continue to live fairly active and tolerable lives for a decade or so.[36] The probability of 5-year survival has been calculated at 95% between the ages of 10 and 19 years, but only 56% at 20 years or over.[37] Eisenmenger patients tolerate surgery and pregnancy poorly.[38]

Complications that can cause death are: Hemoptysis (accounts for 30% of deaths), cerebral abscess, infective endocarditis, and heart failure.

REFERENCES

1. Layde PM, et al. Is there an epidemic of ventricular septal defects in the U.S.A.? Lancet 1980;1:407.
2. Rubenstein P, Levinson DC. Acquired intraventricular septal defects due to myocardial infarction and non-penetrating trauma to the chest. Am J Cardiol 1961;7:277.
3. Williams GD, et al. Traumatic ventricular septal defects. Am J Cardiol 1966;18:907.
4. Bisset G, Hirschfeld SS. Severe pulmonary hypertension associated with a small ventricular septal defect. Circulation 1983;67:470.
5. Engle MA. Ventricular septal defect in infancy. Pediatrics 1954;14:16.
6. Schrire V, et al. Ventricular septal defect: the clinical spectrum. Br Heart J 1965;27:813.
7. Leatham A, Segal B. Auscultatory and phonocardiographic signs of ventricular septal defect with left-to-right shunt. Circulation 1962;25:318.
8. Morgan BC, et al. Ventricular septal defect: I. congestive heart failure in infancy. Pediatrics 1960;25:54.
9. Zachariaudakis SC, et al. Ventricular septal defects in the infant age group. Circulation 1957;16:374.
10. Lynfield J, et al. The natural history of ventricular septal defects in infancy and childhood. Am J Med 1961;30:357.
11. Collins G, et al. Ventricular septal defect: clinical and hemodynamic changes in the first five years of life. Am Heart J 1972;84:695.
12. Nadas AS, et al. Spontaneous functional closing of ventricular septal defects. N Engl J Med 1961;264:309.
13. Agustsson MH, et al. Spontaneous functional closure of ventricular septal defects in 14 children. Pediatrics 1963;31:958.
14. Li MD, Keith JD. Spontaneous closure of ventricular septal defect. Am Heart J 1977;80:432.
15. Alpert BS, et al. Spontaneous closure of small ventricular septal defects: ten-year follow-up. Pediatrics 1979;63:204.
16. Evans JR, et al. Spontaneous closure of ventricular septal defects. Circulation 1960;22:1044.
17. Campbell M. Natural history of ventricular septal defect. Br Heart J 1971;33:246.
18. Lucas RV, et al. The natural history of isolated ventricular septal defect. Circulation 1961;24:1372.
19. Pickering D, Keith JD. Systolic clicks with ventricular septal defects: a sign of aneurysm of the ventricular septum? Br Heart J 1971;33:538.
20. Pieroni DR, et al. Auscultatory recognition of aneurysm of the membranous ventricular septum associated with small ventricular septal defect. Circulation 1971;44:733.
21. Hollman A, et al. Auscultatory and phonocardiographic findings in ventricular septal defect. Circulation 1963;28:94.
22. Harris C, et al. "Fixed" splitting of the second heart sound in ventricular septal defect. Br Heart J 1971;33:428.
23. Farru O, et al. Auscultatory and phonocardiographic characteristics of supracristal ventricular septal defect. Br Heart J 1971;33:238.
24. Steinfeld L, et al. Clinical diagnosis of isolated subpulmonic (supracristal) ventricular septal defect. Am J Cardiol 1972;30:19.
25. Mori K, et al. Analysis of patterns of heart murmur in relation to types of supracristal ventricular septal defect. Am J Noninvas Cardiol 1991;5:338.
26. Fox KM, et al. Multiple and single ventricular septal defect: a clinical and hemodynamic comparison. Br Heart J 1978;40:141.
27. Levy M, Lillehei CW. Left ventricular–right atrial canal. Am J Cardiol 1962;10:623.
28. Lambert EC, et al. Differential diagnosis of ventricular septal defect in infancy: a common problem. Am J Cardiol 1963;11:447.
29. Elliott LP, et al. Silent patent ductus arteriosus in association with ventricular septal defect. Am J Cardiol 1962;10:475.
30. Sasahara AA, et al. Ventricular septal defect with patent ductus arteriosus: a clinical and hemodynamic study. Circulation 1960;22:254.
31. Corone P, et al. Natural history of ventricular septal defect: a study involving 790 cases. Circulation 1977;55:908.
32. Nadas AS, et al. Ventricular septal defect with aortic regurgitation. Circulation 1964;29:862.
33. Keck EWO, et al. Ventricular septal defect with aortic insufficiency. Circulation 1963;27:203.
34. Wood P. The Eisenmenger syndrome, or pulmonary hypertension with reversed central shunt. Br Med J 1958;2:701 and 755.
35. Perloff JK. The clinical recognition of congenital heart disease, ed 3. Philadelphia: WB Saunders, 1987:380.
36. Young D, Mark H. Fate of the patient with the Eisenmenger syndrome. Am J Cardiol 1971;28:658.
37. Clarkson PM, et al. Prognosis for patients with ventricular septal defect and severe pulmonary vascular obstructive disease. Circulation 1968;38:129.
38. Pitts JA, et al. Eisenmenger syndrome in pregnancy. Am Heart J 1977;93:321.

Atrial Septal Defect (ASD)

Defects in the atrial septum account for about 12% of all congenital heart disease and constitute the fourth most common congenital lesion. They are more common in women in a ratio of 3:2. They are classified into four types:

Patent foramen ovale: The foramen ovale remains probe-patent in about 20% of adults but does not permit left-to-right shunting; but if pressure in the right atrium exceeds that in the left, a right-to-left shunt develops.

Ostium secundum: This accounts for about 85% of open defects, and of these, two-thirds are centrally located (Fig. 30-1); the sinus venosus type is situated near the orifice of one of the venae cavae—about a quarter are situated near the inferior vena caval opening, and only about 5% are near the superior vena caval opening.

Ostium primum: This defect accounts for 12% of atrial defects, and occupies the most anterior portion of the septum abutting on the A-V rings; it is often part of a more extensive endocardial cushion defect (A-V canal, A-V communis) involving mitral and tricuspid leaflets and the ventricular septum.

Common atrium: This is the virtual absence of the septum (cor triloculare-biventriculare) and accounts for the remaining 4% of defects.

OSTIUM SECUNDUM

General features that characterize the common secundum defect are its preference for women, its rare discovery in infancy, the absence or mildness of symptoms during the first three decades of life, and then in the '30s increasing disability with the late development of heart failure and pulmonary hypertension. By the age of 40 years, half have symptoms, and of those who reach 50, more than three-quarters are more or less disabled.[1] Of 412 patients with proved ASDs reported from Boston,[2] 71% were asymptomatic under the age of 10 years, but only 4% over the age of 40 years remained symptom-free. Some patients, however, live into their seventh decade,[3] and rarely manage to live to a ripe old age, including one who attained the age of 94 years.[4] When deterioration sets in, it is

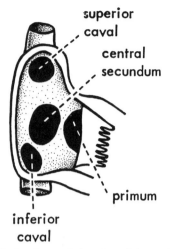

Figure 30–1. Anatomic location of the various types of atrial septal defect.

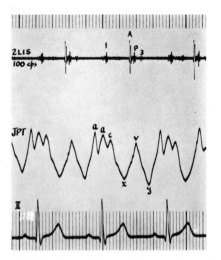

Figure 30–2. From a 5-year-old girl with atrial septal defect. The jugular pulse manifests a bifid "a" wave (a,a), the first peak due to right atrial contraction and the second peak to the impact of left atrial contraction transmitted through the defect.

usually on the basis of one of three complications: Atrial arrhythmias,[5,6] decreased compliance of the left ventricle resulting from ischemic or hypertensive disease and increasing the left-to-right shunt,[7] or increasing pulmonary arterial pressure.[5,8–10]

Of those infants who develop symptoms in their first year of life, the defect spontaneously closes in a significant minority,[11–15] but is unlikely to close after the first year.[12] In Keith's Toronto series of 445 patients with proven ASDs, 15 (3%) closed spontaneously.[14]

Clinical Findings

Some patients may be underdeveloped, but most are normal in development and stature.[16] Deformities perhaps related to secundum defects are high-arched palate, hyperteleorism and arachnodactyly,[17] and the Holt-Oram type of hand and arm deformity.[18] A number of other malformations are sometimes accompanied by ASDs.[19] Limb buds and the primitive heart tube differentiate simultaneously in the embryo's 4th to 6th week, so it is not surprising that congenital abnormalities of the limbs go hand in hand with heart defects. ASDs are sometimes familial.[20–22]

In infants and young children with large defects, a precordial bulge and Harrison's grooves develop. In symptomatic older patients, the earliest complaint is fatigue or dyspnea.[5,8,10,23] Recurrent respiratory infections are sometimes troublesome.[24]

Inspection and Palpation

The jugular pulse is normal, or the "v" wave may be exaggerated and be equal to or larger than the "a" wave,[25] but caution must be exercised in comparing the size of "a" and "v" waves, because in both the normal subject and the patient with an ASD, their relative heights may vary considerably with the cardiac rate.[26] A bifid "a" wave in the jugular pulse has been described (Fig. 30-2). In advanced cases with pulmonary hypertension, the "a" wave becomes prominent and may attain "giant" status.

The peripheral pulse is normal or small, the pulse pressure seldom over 40 mm Hg. Widespread precordial pulsations are characteristic: A tapping apex beat displaced outward, a right ventricular lift in midprecordium and at the left sternal border,[27] and visible and palpable pulmonary artery pulsation. A thrill at the pulmonic area in uncomplicated ASD is rare and immediately suggests associated pulmonic stenosis, though thrills have been reported in as many as 14% of presumably uncomplicated secundum defects.[28] The second sound, and indeed its two splitting components, may sometimes be felt.

Auscultation

At the apex, the first sound is often loud thanks to the accentuation of the tricuspid component.[29] On phonocardiographic analysis, T1 was louder than M1 at the apex in 15 of 19 ASDs, and this apical prominence of T1 may afford a useful clinical clue to the presence of an ASD.[30] Others suspect that the so-called tricuspid component of the first sound in ASD is in reality an opening sound of the pulmonic valve.[31] However, an audible pulmonic ejection click is generally regarded as rare in the absence of pulmonary hypertension.

The second sound is often widely and fixedly split (Fig. 30-3); for the mechanism of fixed splitting, see Chapter 11. But in an appreciable number the splitting is persistent—never closing with expiration—rather than fixed[32,33]; according to Harvey, the splitting is persistent rather than fixed in more than a third of the patients.[34] Splitting is difficult to identify in infants,[1] but it remains a valuable sign in the important diagnosis of large ASDs in infancy, and should be painstakingly sought.[35] P2 is often transmitted to the apex even in the absence of pulmonary hypertension.[28] A fourth sound is often recorded, but is seldom audible unless there is associated pulmonary hypertension. You may hear a tricuspid opening snap.

Pulmonary systolic flow murmurs are audible in virtually all patients[34] except those with severe pulmonary hypertension. When carefully sought, a tricuspid diastolic murmur is found in up to 68% of patients without pulmonary hypertension.[16] It often has a surprisingly high pitch, and of course varies markedly with respiration—sometimes only audible at the height of *inspiration*. It may be difficult to distinguish from the sometimes delayed diastolic murmur of pulmonic regurgitation; and the murmur of pulmonic regurgitation may develop in patients with large defects and copious pulmonary flow even in the absence of pulmonary hypertension.[36]

Early and Late

Atrial septal defect is an uncommon cause of early disaster,[37] and is sometimes compatible with long life.[4,38] But large defects with large flows, without significant pulmonary hypertension, *can* lead to heart failure and death in infancy.[35,39] Early diagnosis is therefore important, and it can be difficult; in fact it is uncommon for ASD to be recognized in infancy. In the unusual case in which ASD causes trouble in early life, one encounters feeding problems, frequent respiratory infections, and stunted growth. The combination of right ventricular thrust, fixed splitting of S2, systolic ejection murmur with or without thrill, and a mid-diastolic murmur best heard between the left lower sternal border and the apex is highly suggestive.

Atrial septal defect in middle age presents a different and often confusing clinical picture.[40] Symptoms include fatigue, dyspnea, palpitation, cough, and recurrent bronchitis. Atrial fibrillation, which develops in about one in five adult patients

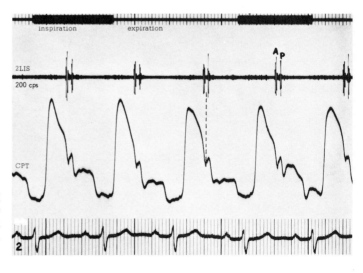

Figure 30–3. From a 37-year-old woman with a large ASD and pulmonary flow four times systemic. The second sound is fixedly split at 0.06 second throughout inspiration and expiration.

with large ASDs,[41] and a variety of murmurs beget the impression of rheumatic heart disease: Pulmonic, mitral, and tricuspid flow and regurgitation supply six murmurs, three systolic and three diastolic, that are not uncommon. Atrial septal defect is the most common form of congenital heart disease among the aged.[42]

Associated Lesions

About 70% of secundum defects are isolated; the rest are complicated by pulmonic stenosis (5%–10%), anomalous pulmonary venous return (10%),[43] or mitral stenosis (Lutembacher's syndrome).[33,44] Many have pulmonic pseudostenosis—a modest pressure difference (less than 20 mm Hg) across the pulmonic valve as a result of the increased blood flow alone.

Lutembacher's Syndrome
(ASD + Mitral Stenosis)

Mitral stenosis is an uncommon complication of ASD, occurring in 2% to 8%.[33,44–46] Do not diagnose it just because there is a diastolic rumble at the apex—remember that half of the patients with ASDs have tricuspid diastolic flow rumbles, and a few primum defects with associated mitral regurgitation have mitral flow rumbles; either of these may trap the unwary into diagnosing a nonexistent mitral stenosis. When true mitral stenosis complicates an ASD, the complex may not be clinically evident: The patient may present signs suggesting only rheumatic heart disease or only ASD.[47]

Some authorities claim that longstanding mitral disease can, by stretching the left atrium, produce incompetency of a foramen ovale defect with resulting left-to-right shunt[40]; undoubtedly, however, most of the Lutembacher duos consist of a congenital atrial defect with subsequent acquired rheumatic mitral stenosis.[46]

OSTIUM PRIMUM

In primum defects, the sex incidence is about equal. Right ventricular hypertrophy and pansystolic murmurs are more common than in secundum defects.[34] Suggestive clinical points are a large heart in childhood with pulmonary hypertension;

retardation or mongolism; and a pansystolic murmur and thrill with mid-diastolic rumble at apex[44] due to the almost invariably associated mitral regurgitation.

The low primum defect is but one segment of the four-part endocardial cushion defect, the other three components being high ventricular septal defect, cleft mitral, and cleft tricuspid leaflet. The presence of all four constitutes a common A-V canal (A-V communis). Small primum defects with cleft mitral valve may simulate and be mistaken for pure mitral regurgitation.

Congestive heart failure tends either to develop before the age of 6 years or to wait until after 30 years.[48] The most common cause of deterioration leading to disability or death is development of persistent arrhythmia, especially atrial fibrillation or complete A-V block.[49] Atrial fibrillation in primum defects develops earlier but less often than in secundum defects. Involvement of the tricuspid valve worsens the prognosis.

Pulmonary Hypertension

Approximately 16% of all ASDs develop pulmonary hypertension—with a reversed (right-to-left) shunt, the Eisenmenger reaction, complicating the situation in 6%.[50] Pulmonary hypertension is rare under the age of 20 years but common over the age of 40. At least in childhood, it is much more common in primum defects than in secundum.[44]

Pulmonary hypertension may result from increased flow alone ("hyperkinetic"); or from increased pulmonary vascular resistance ("obstructive"); or it may be secondary to the Lutembacher combination. Palpitation and dyspnea, right ventricular lift, and a loud, palpable P2 are common to all, but there are clinical differences[50]: Anginal pain, effort syncope, central cyanosis, clubbing, giant "a" wave, atrial gallop, and absence of a systolic murmur are found only in the obstructive type; whereas atrial fibrillation and a tricuspid mid-diastolic rumble occur predominantly in the hyperkinetic and Lutembacher types.

COMMON (SINGLE) ATRIUM

Common, or single, atrium has only a vestigial septum or none at all. It is the most common heart lesion in patients with the Ellis-van Creveld syndrome (ectodermal dysplasia, polydactyly, chondroplasia, and congenital heart defect). Mixing of venous and arterial blood in the common chamber is inevitable, but the respective streams are remarkably channelled, and cyanosis is usually mild and episodic. A cleft mitral leaflet is often present. The clinical picture is naturally similar to that of a large atrial septal defect.

ANOMALOUS PULMONARY VENOUS RETURN (APVR)

To describe the anomalous anatomy that produces APVR, "connection" is the preferred word, whereas "drainage" is used to describe the hemodynamic situation. The anomalous drainage may be total or partial, and there are so many and varied anatomic possibilities that a communication from Leiden contains diagrams of over 40 different anomalous connections.[51] The more common are summarized in Table 30-1.

Total APVR

If all the pulmonary veins drain into the systemic venous system or right atrium, an atrial septal defect (or patent foramen ovale) is obligatory to maintain life—otherwise oxygenated blood would have no access to the systemic circulation and would just recirculate through the lungs. The main factor adversely influencing survival is obstruction to pulmonary venous flow[52-54]; such obstruction is

Table 30-1
The More Common Anomalous Venous Connections

Total Into	Partial Into
Persistent left superior vena cava or innominate vein (almost half the cases)	Right atrium
	Superior vena cava
	Innominate vein
Right atrium	Inferior vena cava
Superior vena cava	
Coronary sinus	
Inferior vena cava	
Portal vein or system	

Table 30-2
Profiles of Total Anomalous Pulmonary Venous Drainage

Without Obstruction (Usually Above Diaphragm)	With Obstruction (Usually Below Diaphragm)
Equal sex incidence	Mostly males
May seem normal at first	Failure to thrive as neonate
Respiratory infections	Tachypnea and dyspnea
Slight or subclinical cyanosis	Definite cyanosis
Continuous murmur with drainage into left SVC or innominate	Continuous murmur at site of obstruction
Loud, palpable S1	Loud, palpable S2
Other signs like ASD	Other signs of pulmonary hypertension
Death before 1 year in 75%–80%	Death in 1 or 2 months

almost invariable in those that drain into abdominal veins (infradiaphragmatic type), and decidedly uncommon in those that drain above the diaphragm.[55] Clinical profiles are summarized in Table 30-2. Although most victims die in infancy, a rare individual may attain adult life and live for a few decades.

With drainage into the inferior vena cava—the so-called "scimitar syndrome" because of the peculiar x-ray—there are characteristic features including repeated respiratory infections; diminished chest expansion, vocal resonance, and breath sounds on the right; and heart sounds loudest on the right side (because the heart is displaced towards the right in the majority). If drainage is into the left innominate, there is a continuous murmur at the left upper sternal border.

Partial APVR

If the anomalous drainage is only partial (ie, one or some, but not all, veins drain anomalously), the situation is hemodynamically equivalent to an ASD with a comparable left-to-right shunt; and clinical signs are indistinguishable from those of ASD, including prominent "v" waves in the jugular pulse, fixed splitting of the second sound, and a pulmonic ejection murmur, as in Figure 30-4.

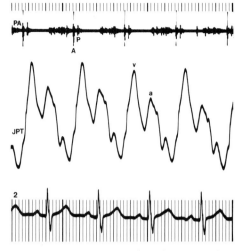

Figure 30–4. From a 5-year-old girl with partial anomalous pulmonary venous return producing a left-to-right shunt with pulmonary flow 2.3 times systemic. Note the flow murmur at the pulmonic area (PA) and fixed splitting of S2 at 0.05–0.06 second; also the dominant "v" wave in the jugular pulse (JVP).

Profile: Atrial Septal Defect

N.B. Suspect ASD in presence of wide S2 splitting and pulmonic ejection murmur

F:M = 3:2

Seldom recognized in infancy

Arachnodactyly, high arched palate, hyperteleorism, Holt–Oram deformity, etc.

Occasionally underdeveloped, frail

Pulse normal, sometimes small

Jugular pulse often normal; may be large "v"

RV lift, PA pulsation

Wide S2 splitting may be palpable

"Split S1" sometimes loud; T1>M1

Wide fixed or persistent splitting of S2

Pulmonic flow murmur; thrill rare

Tricuspid diastolic flow murmur*

Usually no symptoms for three decades; then progressive disability with heart failure; pulmonary hypertension in 12%, including Eisenmenger reaction in 6%

*If no tricuspid middiastolic flow murmur, differential diagnosis rests between ASD, idiopathic dilation of PA, mild PS, or mild PS + ASD

REFERENCES

1. Campbell M, et al. The prognosis of atrial septal defect. Br Heart J 1961;23:587.
2. Hamilton WT, et al. Atrial septal defect secundum: clinical profile with physiologic correlates in children and adults. In: Roberts WC, Brest AN, eds. Congenital heart disease in adults. Philadelphia: FA Davis, 1978:267.
3. Dalen JE, et al. Life expectancy with atrial septal defect. JAMA 1967;200:442.
4. Perloff JK. Ostium secundum atrial septal defect: survival for 87 and 94 years. Am J Cardiol 1984;53:388.
5. Craig RJ, Selzer A. Natural history and prognosis of atrial septal defect. Circulation 1968;37:805.
6. Tikoff G, Kuida H. Pathophysiology of heart failure in congenital heart disease. Modern Concepts of Cardiovascular Disease 1972;41:1.
7. Andersen M, et al. The natural history of small atrial septal defect: long-term follow-up with serial heart catheterizations. Am Heart J 1976;92:302.
8. Gault JH, et al. Atrial septal defect in patients over the age of 40 years. Circulation 1968;37:261.
9. Saksena FB, Aldridge HE. Atrial septal defect in the older patient. Circulation 1970;42:1009.
10. Dave KS, et al. Atrial septal defects in adults. Am J Cardiol 1973;31:7.
11. Cayler GG. Spontaneous functional closure of symptomatic atrial septal defect. N Engl J Med 1967;276:65.
12. Mody MR. Serial hemodynamic observations in secundum atrial septal defect with special reference to spontaneous closure. Am J Cardiol 1973;32:978.
13. Cockerhan JT, et al. Spontaneous closure of secundum atrial septal defect in infants and young children. Am J Cardiol 1983;52:1267.
14. Keith JD, et al. Heart disease in infancy and childhood, ed 3. New York: Macmillan, 1978:400.
15. Ghisla RP, et al. Spontaneous closure of isolated ostium secundum atrial septal defects in infants: an echocardiographic study. Am Heart J 1985;109:1327.
16. Schrire V, et al. Atrial septal defect: I. secundum and sinus venosus defects. S Afr Med J 1963;37:727. II. endocardial cushion defects. S Afr Med J 1963;37:839.
17. Wood P. The Eisenmenger syndrome or pulmonary hypertension with reversed central shunt. Br Med J 1958; 2:701.
18. Holt M, Oram S. Familial heart disease with skeletal malformations. Br Heart J 1960;22:236.
19. Lin AE, Perloff JK. Upper limb malformations associated with congenital heart disease. Am J Cardiol 1985;55:1576.
20. Johansson B, Sievers J. Inheritance of atrial septal defect. Lancet 1967;1:1224.
21. Lynch HT, et al. Hereditary atrial septal defect. Am J Dis Child 1978;132:600.
22. Richer TJ, et al. Familial atrial septal defect in a single generation. Br Heart J 1972;34:198.
23. Nasrallah AT, et al. Surgical repair of atrial septal defect in patients over 60 years of age. Circulation 1976;53:329.
24. Perloff JK. The clinical recognition of congenital heart disease, ed 3. Philadelphia: WB Saunders, 1987:280.
25. Reinhold J. Venous pulse in atrial septal defect: a clinical sign. Br Med J 1955;1:695.
26. Thiron J-M, et al. Variations in height of jugular "a" wave in relation to heart rate in normal subjects and in patients with atrial septal defects. Br Heart J 1980; 44:37.

27. Nagle RE, Tamara FA. Left parasternal impulse in pulmonary stenosis and atrial septal defect. Br Heart J 1967;29:735.

28. DuShane JW, et al. Differentiation of interatrial communications by clinical methods: ostium secundum, ostium primum, common atrium and total anomalous pulmonary venous connection. Circulation 1960;21:363.

29. Leatham A, Gray I. Auscultatory and phonocardiographic signs of atrial septal defect. Br Heart J 1956;18:193.

30. Lopez JF, et al. The apical first heart sound as an aid in the diagnosis of atrial septal defect. Circulation 1962;26:1296.

31. Barritt DW, et al. Heart sounds and pressures in atrial septal defect. Br Heart J 1965;27:90.

32. Dimond EG, Benchimol A. Phonocardiography in atrial septal defect: correlation between hemodynamics and phonocardiographic findings. Am Heart J 1959;58:343.

33. Evans JR, et al. The clinical diagnosis of atrial septal defect in children. Am J Med 1961;30:345.

34. Harvey WP. Auscultatory findings of congenital heart disease. In: Roberts WC, Brest AN, eds. Congenital heart disease in adults. Philadelphia: FA Davis, 1979:53.

35. Hastreiter AR, et al. Secundum atrial septal defects with congestive heart failure during infancy and early childhood. Am Heart J 1962;64:467.

36. Liberthson RR, et al. Pulmonic regurgitation in large atrial shunts without pulmonary hypertension. Circulation 1976;54:966.

37. Disenhouse RB, et al. Atrial septal defect in infants and children. J Pediatr 1954;44:269.

38. Colmers RA. Atrial septal defect in elderly patients. Am J Cardiol 1958;1:768.

39. Ainger LE, Pate JW. Ostium secundum atrial septal defects and congestive heart failure in infancy. Am J Cardiol 1965;15:380.

40. Kuzman WJ. Atrial septal defects in the older patient. Geriatrics 1967;22:107.

41. Tikoff G, et al. Atrial fibrillation in atrial septal defect. Arch Intern Med 1968;121:402.

42. Kelly JJ, Lyons HA. Atrial septal defect in the aged. Ann Intern Med 1958;48:267.

43. Gotsman MS, et al. Partial anomalous pulmonary venous drainage in association with atrial septal defect. Br Heart J 1965;27:566.

44. Bedford DE. The anatomical types of atrial septal defect: their incidence and clinical diagnosis. Am J Cardiol 1960;6:568.

45. Nadas AS, Alimurung MM. Apical diastolic murmurs in congenital heart disease: the rarity of Lutembacher's syndrome. Am Heart J 1952;43:691.

46. Steinbrunn W, et al. Atrial septal defect associated with mitral stenosis. Am J Med 1970;48:295.

47. Espino-Vela J. Rheumatic heart disease associated with atrial septal defect: clinical and pathologic study of 12 cases of Lutembacher's syndrome. Am Heart J 1959;57:185.

48. Weyn AS, et al. Atrial septal defect: primum type. Circulation 1965;32(Suppl 3):13.

49. Somerville J. Ostium primum defect: factors causing deterioration in the natural history. Br Heart J 1965;27:413.

50. Besterman E. Atrial septal defect with pulmonary hypertension. Br Heart J 1961;23:587.

51. Snellen HA, et al. Patterns of anomalous pulmonary venous drainage. Circulation 1968;38:45.

52. Elliott LP, Edwards JE. The problem of pulmonary venous obstruction in total anomalous pulmonary venous connection to the left innominate vein. Circulation 1962;25:913.

53. Hastreiter AR, et al. Total anomalous pulmonary venous connection with severe pulmonary venous obstruction. Circulation 1962;25:916.

54. Scott LP, Welch CC. Factors influencing survival in total anomalous pulmonary venous drainage in infants. Am J Cardiol 1965;16:286.

55. Kauffman SL, et al. Two cases of total anomalous pulmonary venous return of the supracardiac type with stenosis simulating infradiaphragmatic drainage. Circulation 1962;25:376.

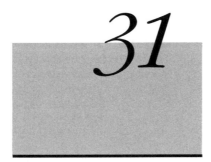

Tetralogy of Fallot

The tetralogy (TET), described by several others before the classic account by Fallot (1888), accounts for approximately 12% of all congenital heart disease. It is the second to fourth most common congenital lesion in most series, and the most common cyanotic lesion in all series. It consists of:

1. *Pulmonic stenosis or atresia*: The critical lesion—severe enough to produce resistance to outflow greater than systemic vascular resistance, so that a right-to-left (or at least bidirectional) shunt results,
2. *Ventricular septal defect (VSD)*: Always confluent with the aortic orifice and always "nonrestrictive," that is, large enough to ensure equality of pressure in the two ventricles at all times,[1]
3. *Dextroposed aorta*: Overriding the septal defect to variable extent, and
4. *Right ventricular hypertrophy*: Secondary to 1 and 2 above.

Pulmonic stenosis, usually infundibular, is the critical lesion, because the degree of outflow obstruction is the main determinant of the severity of the clinical syndrome. If stenosis is mild, the shunt will be predominantly left-to-right, despite the overriding aorta, and there will be no cyanosis. At the other extreme, if there is pulmonic atresia (with resulting "pseudotruncus"), all right ventricular blood must enter the aorta, and the lungs be supplied only through bronchial arteries and an obligate patent ductus. In Keith's series of 329 autopsied cases, atresia was present in 20%, valvar stenosis in 10%, infundibular stenosis in 48%, and combined infundibular and valvar stenosis in 22%.[2]

CLINICAL PICTURE

Subtle variations in the pathologic anatomy of this tetrad can result in major differences in clinical presentation.[3] Some present with no murmur but severe cyanosis during the first month of life, others may have a systolic murmur but cyanosis only when crying; in other cases, the presenting symptom may be episodic unconsciousness, and in still others there may be no cyanosis, but congestive heart failure with dyspnea, hepatomegaly, and a left-to-right shunt. Some authorities have never encountered congestive heart failure in unoperated patients[4]; others claim an incidence of heart failure as high as 33% in adults.[5] When you do find heart failure in a patient with the tetralogy, you should be at pains to exclude an associated condition such as cardiomyopathy,[6] anemia, systemic hypertension, or a complicating infection.

The Classic TET

Symptoms

In the classic form, the infant is not cyanosed, and the picture is that of a large ventricular septal defect. In one series,[7] 40 of 59 patients (68%) had no cyanosis at birth. *Cyanosis* usually develops in 3 to 6 months, and by 6 months at least three-quarters are cyanosed.[2] *Clubbing* of fingers and toes follows in the wake of cyanosis.

Hypoxic spells occur in 35% to 40%,[8] mainly between 6 and 18 months (mean 13.4 months),[7] characterized by rapidly increasing dyspnea and cyanosis, *decrease or disappearance of murmur*, tachycardia, syncope with or without convulsions, and occasional death.[1,9,10] Three mechanisms seem to be operative: A fragile respiratory control center (especially vulnerable to effort—feeding, crying, etc.—after prolonged sleep), muscular spasm of the infundibulum,[9] and atrial tachycardia.[11] All of these increase the right-to-left shunt and intensify hypoxia.

More than three-quarters of patients with a TET squat for relief of dyspnea and faintness, but *squatting* is not specific—some patients with transposition of the great arteries, Eisenmenger's complex, or tricuspid atresia also squat. Squatting increases systemic vascular resistance and so deflects more blood into the pulmonary circulation; this in turn increases the amount of oxygenated blood available for left ventricular output. At the same time, squatting traps venous blood in the legs and so reduces the return of unsaturated blood to the heart,[12] which in turn improves the oxygen saturation of right ventricular blood that is then expelled into the aorta. Although squatting is the favored maneuver, alternative postures that patients sometimes adopt include the knee-chest position, standing with the legs crossed, and lying down.[11]

Of 147 adult patients with TET reported from India and who had not been subjected to surgery, 95% had dyspnea and cyanosis, well over half squatted, and nearly 15% had *hemoptysis*.[13]

Some patients who were in trouble in childhood spontaneously improve as teenagers, perhaps because of increasing arterial collaterals to the lungs.[5] *Chest pain*, which may be due to right ventricular ischemia, is a fairly common complaint in adult patients.[5] Important complications include *brain abscess* (which occurs in 2% of patients with cyanotic congenital heart disease, but seldom before the age of 2 years),[14] and *cerebrovascular accidents* producing hemiplegia, which affect 1% to 2% of cyanotic patients (usually babies under 2 years), due to venous or arterial thrombosis.[15]

Signs

On examination, a few have prominent "a" waves in the jugular pulse (Fig. 31-1).[16,17] There is little evidence of cardiomegaly except for a modest right ventricular lift in some cases, which, like the large jugular "a" wave, is much less striking than in pure pulmonic stenosis. The second sound is loud and single, P2 being inaudible in almost all,[16,18] but phenylephrine may bring out P2 and reveal the latent wide splitting.[19]

Thrill and murmur at the left sternal border may be maximal in 2nd, 3rd, or 4th interspace. In contrast with pure pulmonic stenosis, in which the length of the murmur is directly proportional to the severity of the stenosis, in TET the more severe the stenosis, the shorter the murmur (Fig. 31-2; compare with Fig. 26-4) Therefore, in TET, after effective surgery on the stenotic valve itself, the murmur lengthens and P2 becomes audible; whereas after a successful Blalock procedure, P2 becomes audible but the murmur's length remains unchanged.[20] The length of murmur and other physical signs may be more accurate in assessing the severity of a TET than more sophisticated techniques.[21]

Systemic hypertension is not uncommon,[22] and an occasional TET case presents with systemic hypertension, cardiomegaly, and congestive heart failure; five of 22 patients with hypertension had diastolic pressures over 110 mm Hg.[17]

Life Expectancy

Of patients not subjected to surgery, two-thirds reach the age of 1 year, half attain 3 years, and one-quarter 10 years.[23] Approximately 10% live to the age of 20 years or more.[5]

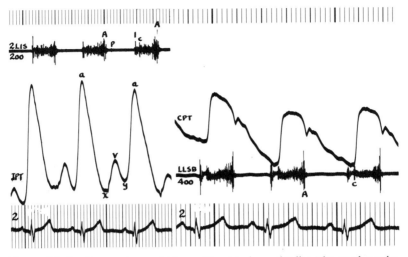

Figure 31–1. From a 4-year-old boy with a tetralogy of Fallot. The jugular pulse (JPT) contains a giant "a" wave, secondary to right atrial hypertension, and a barely recordable P2. Both phonocardiograms show the pansystolic murmur—typical of a mild tetralogy—peaking in late systole. The carotid pulse (CPT) is normal.

Before the open heart surgery era, a rare patient would survive to the fourth or fifth decade—the longest survivor attained 69 years. But with surgical "total correction" most patients will attain adult life. Certainly the average patient who enjoys surgical repair has a life expectancy many times longer than one who lived before the first palliative Blalock–Taussig procedure was undertaken in 1944. It is estimated that there is now a 75% probability that a "totally corrected" TET patient will live for 40 years or more.

Of patients with total repair, 81% have unlimited exercise tolerance, but they all have a crescendo-decrescendo murmur at the 3rd left interspace, and 55% have a low-pitched decrescendo diastolic murmur of pulmonic regurgitation.[4] A

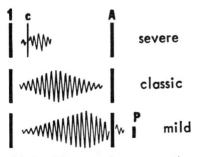

Figure 31–2. Diagrammatic representation of the usual auscultatory findings in severe, "classic," and mild tetralogy. c, ejection click; 1, first heart sound; A and P, aortic and pulmonic components of second sound.

few patients have a separate, pansystolic, plateau murmur from a residual VSD.

The Severe TET

In the extreme form with tight pulmonic stenosis or atresia, the infant is deeply cyanotic at birth and life is precarious—dependent on the ductus remaining patent. An aortic ejection click is audible (Fig. 31-2) in most cases, S2 is single, and the ejection murmur is absent, or soft with no thrill. You may hear a continuous murmur from an associated patent ductus or a softer one from dilated bronchial arteries. The combination of cyanosis, a continuous murmur heard over the entire chest, a separate systolic murmur audible at the left sternal border, a single second sound, and an aortic ejection click suggests the diagnosis of pseudo-truncus.[24]

The "Pink" TET

About one in ten patients have mild enough pulmonic stenosis to comprise the acyanotic form ("pink tetrads"), in which the large ventricular septal defect dominates the clinical picture and the lungs show increased vascularity despite the pulmonic stenosis.[25–27] The heart is large with active apex beat and right ventricular lift. A parasternal

Table 31–1
*Differentiation Between Mild Tetralogy
and Pure Pulmonic Stenosis*

	Tetralogy	Pure Pulmonic Stenosis
A2	Not obscured by murmur	Partially obscured
S2	Single; or wide split with soft P2	Wide split with soft P2
AN: S2	P2 disappears	P2 remains
SM	softer and shorter	Louder and longer
PE: S2	P2 louder	Delays A2, narrows
SM	Increases	Little change

AN, amyl nitrite; PE, phenylephrine; SM, systolic murmur.

thrill accompanies the pansystolic murmur reaching to or beyond a widely split S2 with normal P2. A third sound and occasionally an apical mid-diastolic murmur are heard.

The important distinction between mild TET and moderately severe pure pulmonic stenosis can be difficult. The main points of difference are contrasted in Table 31-1. The diagnosis may be clinched at the bedside with the help of amyl nitrite: In valvar or infundibular obstruction with intact septum, amyl nitrite causes a striking increase in the loudness of the ejection murmur; in TET, the inhalation causes a reduction in the murmur's duration and intensity.[28]

Atypical Syndromes

Atypical, tetrad-like syndromes include congenital absence of the pulmonic valve,[29] which is suspected when a cyanotic patient presents harsh to-and-fro murmurs and thrills at the left sternal border with marked dilation and pulsation of the pulmonary artery[30]; some may show evidence of respiratory obstruction from compression of the left main bronchus by the dilated pulmonary artery, or may manifest a more marked right ventricular lift than the usual tetrad.

Pulmonic stenosis with an atrial septal defect can create a syndrome that needs to be differentiated from TET. Several points of modest differential value are listed in Table 31-2. The systolic

Profile: *Tetralogy of Fallot*
M:F = 2:1

I. *Classic form*
  a. Precyanotic phase
     Infants
     Simulates large VSD
  b. Cyanotic phase
     Begins usually 3–6 months, sometimes later
     Cyanosis → clubbing
     Anoxic spells in up to 50%: sudden restlessness, gasping respirations, tachycardia, deepening cyanosis, decrease in murmur, convulsions, syncope, occasional death
     Squatting (80%)
     No respiratory distress at rest
     Large "a" wave in jugulars (occasional)
     No cardiomegaly (RV lift)
     S2 loud and single: phenylephrine may bring out P2 revealing wide split
     Thrill and murmur at LSB
     Polycythemia (after 1–3 years)

II. *Extreme form* (tight PS or atresia)
     Cyanosis at birth
     Aortic EC
     Soft short basal systolic or no murmur (in atresia)
     Sometimes continuous murmur (PDA or bronchials)

III. Acyanotic form (10%—"pink" tetralogy)
     Child remains acyanotic or cyanotic on exertion only
     Enlarged heart with hyperactive apex beat
     Thrill and **pansystolic murmur** at LSB
     RV lift
     S2 widely split, P2 normal
     S3 at apex
     Amyl nitrite distinguishes from pure PS (see Table 31-1)

murmur behaves quite differently in the two conditions: If you listen where the murmur is loudest, in TET the murmur reaches maximal intensity by midsystole and then fades rapidly, ending before

Table 31–2
Differentiation Between Cyanotic Tetralogy and Pulmonic Stenosis with Atrial Septal Defect

	Tetralogy	PS + ASD
Hypoxic spells	Common	Rare
Squatting	Common	Rare
Cyanosis	Severe	Mild
Heart failure	Uncommon	Common
"a" Waves	In some	In most
Second sound	Loud, single	Wide split, faint P2
Systolic murmur	Shorter	Longer
Associated anomaly	Polydactyly	Turner's, hyperteleorism

the loud, single, and often palpable A2. In pulmonic stenosis with right-to-left atrial shunt the murmur is prolonged and drowns the normal A2 of the widely split S2; the faint, delayed P2 may or may not be audible.

REFERENCES

1. Harley HRS. What is Fallot's tetralogy? Am Heart J 1961;62:729.
2. Keith J, et al. Heart disease in infancy and childhood. New York: Macmillan, 1958.
3. Shinebourne E, et al. Variations in clinical presentation of Fallot's tetralogy in infancy. Br Heart J 1975;37:946.
4. Garson A, et al. Tetralogy of Fallot in adults. In: WC Roberts, ed. Congenital heart disease in adults. Philadelphia: FA Davis, 1979:341.
5. Higgins CB, Mulder DG. Tetralogy of Fallot in the adult. Am J Cardiol 1972;29:837.
6. Chesler E, et al. Tetralogy of Fallot and heart failure. Am Heart J 1971;81:321.
7. Bonchek LI, et al. Natural history of tetralogy of Fallot in infancy: clinical classification and therapeutic implications. Circulation 1973;48:392.
8. Morgan BC, et al. A clinical profile of paroxysmal hyperpnea in cyanotic congenital heart disease. Circulation 1965;31:66.
9. Wood P. Attacks of deeper cyanosis and loss of consciousness (syncope) in Fallot's tetralogy. Br Heart J 1958;20:286.
10. Braudo JL, Zion MM. Cyanotic spells and loss of consciousness induced by cardiac catheterization in patients with Fallot's tetralogy. Am Heart J 1960;59:10.
11. Perloff JK. The clinical recognition of congenital heart disease, ed 3. Philadelphia: WB Saunders, 1987:404.
12. Guntheroth WG, et al. Venous return with knee-chest position and squatting in tetralogy of Fallot. Am Heart J 1968;75:313.
13. Abraham KA, et al. Tetralogy of Fallot in adults: a report on 147 patients. Am J Med 1979;66:811.
14. Fischbein CA, et al. Risk factors for brain abscess in patients with congenital heart disease. Am J Cardiol 1974;34:97.
15. Phornphutkul C. Cerebrovascular accidents in infants and children with cyanotic congenital heart disease. Am J Cardiol 1973;32:329.
16. Leatham A, Weitzman D: Auscultatory and phonocardiographic signs of pulmonic stenosis. Br Heart J 1957;19:303.
17. Holladay WE, Witham AC. The tetralogy of Fallot: the variability of its clinical manifestations. Arch Intern Med 1957;100:400
18. Vogelpoel L, Schrire V. The role of auscultation in the differentiation of Fallot's tetralogy from severe pulmonary stenosis with intact ventricular septum and right-to-left interatrial shunt. Circulation 1955;11:714.
19. Vogelpoel L, et al. The use of phenylephrine in the differentiation of Fallot's tetralogy from pulmonic stenosis with intact ventricular septum. Am Heart J 1960;59:489.
20. Vogelpoel L, Schrire V. Pulmonary stenosis with intact ventricular septum and Fallot's tetralogy: assessment of postoperative results by auscultation and phonocardiography. Am Heart J 1960;59:645.
21. Vogelpoel L, Schrire V. Auscultatory and phonocardiographic assessment of Fallot's tetralogy. Circulation 1960;22:73.
22. Taussig H. Congenital malformations of the heart. Cambridge: Harvard University Press, 1960:25.
23. Bertranou EG, et al. Life expectancy without surgery in tetralogy of Fallot. Am J Cardiol 1978;42:458.
24. Lafargue RT, et al. Pseudotruncus arteriosus: a review of 21 cases with observations on oldest reported case. Am J Cardiol 1967;19:239.
25. Rowe RD, et al. Atypical tetralogy of Fallot: a noncyanotic form with increased lung vascularity. Circulation 1955;12:230.
26. Hubbard TF, Koszewski BJ. Pulmonary stenosis with increased pulmonary blood flow. Arch Intern Med 1956;97:327
27. McCord MC, et al. Tetralogy of Fallot: clinical and hemodynamic spectrum of combined pulmonary stenosis and ventricular septal defect. Circulation 1957;16:736.
28. Vogelpoel L. The use of amyl nitrite in the differentiation of Fallot's tetralogy and pulmonary stenosis with intact ventricular septum. Am Heart J 1959;57:803.
29. Lakier JB, et al. Tetralogy of Fallot with absent pulmonic valve: natural history and hemodynamic considerations. Circulation 1974;50:167.
30. Miller RA, et al. Congenital absence of the pulmonary valve: the clinical syndrome of tetralogy of Fallot with pulmonary regurgitation. Circulation 1962;26:266.

SOME CLINICAL CYANOTIC BURRS

In cyanotic congenital heart disease after the age of 1 year, the diagnostic odds are 4:1 in favor of *Tetralogy*

Cyanosis with right sternoclavicular pulsation: *Tetralogy*

Cyanosis at birth in a second (or later) born, overweight male with a diabetic family history: *Transposition*

Cyanosis with both right and left ventricular impulses: *Transposition*

Cyanosis with large jugular ''a'' wave but no right ventricular enlargement: *Tricuspid Atresia*

Cyanosis in infancy, disappearing, then reappearing: *Ebstein's Anomaly*

Cyanosis with Wolff-Parkinson-White syndrome and/or paroxysmal supraventricular tachyarrhythmia: *Ebstein's Anomaly*

Cyanosis with telangiectasias: *Pulmonary Arteriovenous Fistula*

Cyanosis of toes with pink nailbeds of right hand: *Patent Ductus with Reversed Shunt*

Cyanosis of the right hand with pink toes: *Transposition with Reversed Ductus*

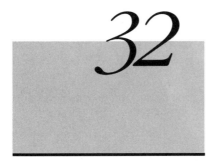

The Other Transpositions

TRANSPOSITION OF THE GREAT ARTERIES

In transposition of the great arteries (TGA), the aorta and pulmonary artery (PA) are transposed in two respects: In relation to the ventricle of origin, and in relation to each other. Thus, the aorta arises from the morphologic right ventricle while the PA arises from the morphologic left ventricle; and instead of the PA arising anterior to the aorta, the aorta occupies the more anterior site with the PA posterior to it.

Whereas Fallot's tetralogy is by far the most common cause of cyanotic congenital heart disease encountered after the age of 1 year, about 90% of patients seen with TGA are infants in their first year. Without surgical intervention the prognosis is miserable. Analysis of 742 cases[1] revealed the following life expectancies: At birth 0.65 year, at 1 week 0.87 year, at 1 month 1.12 years, and at 1 year 3.92 years. More than a quarter of the infants die during the first week, over half before the end of the first month, and almost 90% by the end of the first year.[1] With aggressive surgical management, about half of them survive and function well for 5 years.[2] TGA is found in about 12% of autopsied cases of congenital heart disease.[3]

Although slightly more than half the cases have no additional developmental defects,[4] to maintain life at all, some communication between the two circuits is obligatory: It may be a persistent fetal pathway—patent ductus or foramen ovale—or it may be an additional developmental defect—ventricular septal defect (46%), atrial septal defect (21%), or absent ventricular septum (6%). Pulmonic stenosis complicates a small minority—5% in one series of 85 patients.[5]

For purposes of definition only, and without pretending to depict the relationship of the great arteries to each other, Figure 32-1 indicates their ventricular origin in the various transposition syndromes and compares them with the situation in a tetralogy, itself a form of partial transposition. Table 32-1 lists the features that may help to differentiate the two most common cyanotic syndromes. Transposition of the great arteries affects three times as many males as females. The infant may have an enlarged, "square" head,[6] and cyanosis

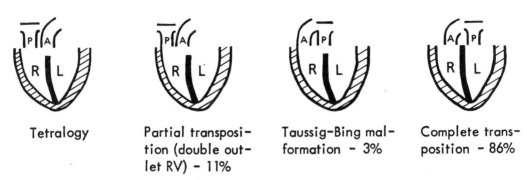

Tetralogy	Partial transposition (double outlet RV) – 11%	Taussig–Bing malformation – 3%	Complete transposition – 86%

Figure 32–1. Diagrammatic relationships of great arteries to ventricles and to the ventricular septum in transposition complexes. In the tetralogy, the aorta overrides the defective septum; in double outlet right ventricle (RV), both great arteries open out of the RV and the ventricular septal defect alone affords egress from the left ventricle (LV); in the Taussig-Bing malformation, the pulmonary artery (PA) overrides the defective septum; and in complete transposition, the aorta arises from the RV and the PA from the LV. R, RV; L, LV; P, PA; A, aorta.

is present at birth or soon appears. If it is intense at birth, one suspects pulmonic stenosis, whereas mild cyanosis suggests a ventricular septal defect without pulmonic stenosis.[7] Differential cyanosis (cyanosis deeper in legs than arms) indicates the presence of a patent ductus. On the other hand, 12 of 18 patients with patent ductus manifested only slight cyanosis, and ten of them failed to show a differential pattern of cyanosis.[8] Patients with patent ductus are predisposed to the early development of pulmonary vascular disease.[9] Cardiomegaly, affecting both left and right ventricles, is detectable by the age of 1 month.

Abnormalities were noted on their first day of life in 89% of infants with TGA.[10] In this series of 66 patients, cyanosis was eventually observed in 98%, tachypnea in 42%, respiratory distress in 34%, murmurs in 29%, and tachycardia in 20%.

If the ventricular septum is intact, heart failure sets in early; on the other hand, absence of early failure points to the presence of a ventricular septal defect together with pulmonic stenosis.[7] Clubbing and polycythemia regularly develop.

The second sound is either split with a normal pulmonic component, or is single (because P2 is inaudible). If the pulmonic component is audible, one may be able to detect paradoxical splitting.[11]

If no murmur is audible, a ventricular septal defect is most unlikely. If a murmur is present, it is usually maximal at the 4th left interspace and peaks at or before midsystole. A presystolic murmur may be heard at the apex.

The *double-outlet right ventricle*—a partial transposition in which pulmonary artery and aorta both open out of the right ventricle, and a ventricular septal defect provides the only outlet from the left ventricle—is indistinguishable, if pulmonic stenosis is present, from the cyanotic tetralogy.[12,13] If there is no pulmonic stenosis, a ventricular septal defect with pulmonary hypertension is simulated; there is minimal cyanosis but gross cardiomegaly.

The *Taussig–Bing malformation*[14]—consisting of a transposed aorta, large overriding pulmonary trunk, and a ventricular septal defect—is characterized by progressive cyanosis from birth and a right ventricular lift. The second sound is loud and palpable, single or closely split. At the left upper

Table 32–1

Differentiating Features of the Two Most Common Cyanotic Syndromes

	Tetralogy	Transposition
Familial tendency	Occasional	Rare
Birth weight	Below average	Above average
Sex ratio	Equal	Mostly males
Age influence	75% of all cyanotic cases over age 4	85% mortality in first 6 months
Heart failure	Rare	Common
Onset of cyanosis	Delayed months	Soon after birth
Anoxic spells	Common	Rare
Murmur	Harsh	Faint or absent unless PS or VSD
Extracardiac congenital defects	Common	Rare

sternal border, one hears an ejection click and soft ejection systolic murmur; an early diastolic murmur of pulmonic regurgitation may be heard.

"CORRECTED" TRANSPOSITION OR VENTRICULAR INVERSION

In complete TGA, atria and ventricles are appropriately aligned: The LEFT atrium leads into the LEFT ventricle, and the RIGHT atrium into the RIGHT ventricle. But then the great arteries mar the anatomy: The aorta opens out of the RIGHT ventricle while the pulmonary artery opens out of the LEFT (Fig. 32-2).

In "corrected" transposition (von Rokitansky, 1875), the LEFT atrium leads into the RIGHT ventricle (through a tricuspid valve), and the RIGHT atrium into the LEFT ventricle (through a bicuspid, mitral valve); but then the circulation straightens itself out as the aorta leaves the RIGHT ventricle and the pulmonary artery leaves the LEFT (Fig. 32-2). In corrected transposition, therefore, the circulation is normal, since RIGHT atrial (venous) blood enters the pulmonary artery (after passing through a "left" ventricle), and LEFT atrial (oxygenated) blood enters the aorta (after passing through a "right" ventricle). A better name, therefore, for corrected transposition is "ventricular inversion"since this site-swapping of the ventricles is *the* defect; and, in the uncomplicated cases, the sole handicap is the strain imposed on the (anatomic) right ventricle in coping with the

Table 32–2
Percent Incidence of Complicating Congenital Defects

	Author		
	Allwork[17]	Friedberg[18]	Huhta[19]
Total no.	32	60	107
% With TA	91	—	34
% With VSD	78	52	77
% With PS	44	45	53

TA, tricuspid anomalies; VSD, ventricular septal defect; PS, pulmonic stenosis.

systemic circulation, which indeed may prove too much for it.[15,16]

Unfortunately, other anomalies (Table 32-2) usually accompany corrected transposition[17–19]: the most common are left A-V valve ("mitral") incompetence, ventricular septal defect, pulmonic stenosis, and conduction disturbances; less common associations are single ventricle, pulmonary regurgitation, and an Ebstein-like deformity of the left-sided ("tricuspid") valve. In these complicated cases, it is the additional defects that mainly determine the prognosis.

Since corrective surgery became feasible, many authors[17,18,20–23] attach "congenitally" to "corrected transposition"—to distinguish the naturally occurring type from transpositions that have been surgically corrected.

Clinical Findings

Sex distribution is about equal, with males perhaps preponderant.[20,21]

Symptoms depend exclusively, and signs mainly, on the associated defects.[24] The symptom-free patient may present because of a detected murmur, mild cyanosis, or bradycardia. In the uncomplicated case, the patient may remain asymptomatic for many years, only to succumb to heart failure in his fifth or sixth decade, thanks to the overloaded "right" ventricular myocardium.[16] The complicated case may present with congestive heart failure, marked cyanosis, or Adams–Stokes attacks. Cyanosis and clubbing develop only when pulmonic stenosis or pulmonary hypertension engineer a right-to-left shunt.[25]

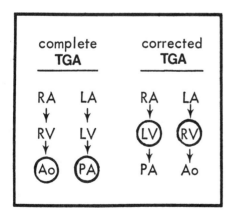

Figure 32–2. The atrium-ventricle-artery line-up in complete and in "corrected" transpositions of the great arteries. The vessels/chambers actually transposed in each are circled.

Physical signs in the uncomplicated case may include[22] a palpable, loud S2 at the left upper sternal border (because of the proximity of the aortic valve to the chest wall); the pulmonic component of S2 is often inaudible at the conventional "pulmonic" area, but may be heard to the right of the sternum. There may be an unimpressive ejection systolic murmur at the left upper sternal border.

In the complicated cases, the signs are those of the associated lesions: Left-sided A-V valve regurgitation,[22,26] pulmonic stenosis, ventricular septal defect, or A-V block. The murmur of "mitral" regurgitation may be heard better medially than at the apex, and is then readily mistaken for that of a ventricular septal defect.[27] A Graham Steell murmur may signal the presence of pulmonary hypertension.

The murmur of pulmonic stenosis is typical except that it is often heard better at the right than the left,[21] and on the left often better at the lower than upper sternal border. An apical mid-diastolic murmur is common in cases with ventricular septal defect or "mitral" regurgitation. With single ventricle, the most striking clinical finding is an early diastolic murmur of pulmonic regurgitation; it was present in eight of nine cases.[23]

In a series of 60 patients, congestive heart failure was present in 28%, and complete heart block in 12%.[18] The risk of developing A-V block apparently persists throughout life.[19]

Because the ventricular conduction system is inverted along with the ventricles,[20] the "left" bundle branch supplies the morphologic left ventricle (now the more rightward ventricle), and this ventricle is activated slightly earlier than the morphologic right ventricle (now the more leftward ventricle). With the help of an electrocardiogram and precordial displacement tracings (measuring the interval from onset of QRS to onset of right-sided and left-sided precordial pulsations), one may be able to demonstrate that parasternal precordial displacement precedes apical.[28]

The following paired findings should alert you to the possibility of corrected transposition:

1. Bradycardia (because of 2:1 or complete A-V block) in the presence of congenital heart disease,
2. Apparent pulmonary hypertension (loud S2 at left upper sternal border) without right ventricular hypertrophy, and
3. Splitting of the second sound at the "aortic" but not at the "pulmonic" area.

Death may result from congestive heart failure, secondary to ventricular diastolic overloading from A-V valve regurgitation or from a large left-to-right shunt through a ventricular septal defect; or failure may result from the systemic overburdening of "right" ventricular myocardium. Rarely, the development of A-V block may precipitate sudden death. Although most patients with corrected transposition fail to live beyond the fifth decade, a rare victim may survive into the eighth.[29]

PERSISTENT TRUNCUS ARTERIOSUS

In this lethal anomaly, which affects males and females equally,[30] one great vessel guarded by a single semilunar valve containing anywhere from two to six (usually three or four) cusps, supplies the entire circulation—coronary, pulmonary and systemic. Clinical features depend on the size of the pulmonary vessels given off and the consequent pulmonary blood flow (PBF). There is always a ventricular septal defect, and the situation may be complicated with a right aortic arch[31] or incompetence of the single semilunar valve with truncal regurgitation.[32] Up to 75% die in the first year, but an occasional patient survives into the fourth decade.[33] Most die from congestive heart failure secondary to the increased PBF, with or without the truncal regurgitation that complicates about 20% of cases.[30]

With large pulmonary arteries and excessive PBF, cyanosis is minimal or absent; there is a precordial bulge with evident cardiomegaly. An ejection click is audible in at least 40% of victims[30] at the apex and at the left sternal border (Fig. 32-3). In about the same proportion[30] there is a loud, single second sound, though it is not always as singly "pure" as one might expect.[34,35] A loud third sound is often audible at the apex.

Murmurs may be audible at birth or soon thereafter, are heard in about 60% in the first week of life,[30] and are certainly detectable by the third month in all who survive.[36] At the left sternal border there is a harsh systolic murmur ending before S2,[35] accompanied by a thrill.

If the afflicted infant survives, pulmonary vascular resistance increases, cyanosis deepens, the heart becomes greatly enlarged, and the early diastolic murmur of truncal regurgitation may appear. The older child may complain of chest pain and hemoptysis.

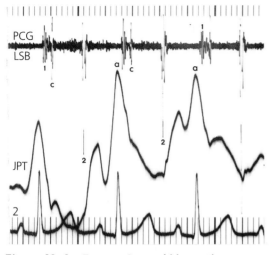

Figure 32–3. From an 8-year-old boy with persistent truncus arteriosus. Note ejection click (c) and loud, single second sound (2) at the left sternal border (LSB), with giant "a" wave in the jugular pulse tracing.

If the pulmonary arteries are small, with consequently only moderately increased PBF, symptoms are less severe and failure less common. Auscultatory findings are similar, however, except that a high-pitched, continuous murmur is often heard best in the back.

If pulmonary arteries are nonexistent, with consequent diminished PBF, cyanosis is present at birth or soon after, and polycythemia and clubbing of the fingers and toes develop. Cardiomegaly is more modest, there is a right ventricular lift, and sometimes a continuous murmur.

One should think of a persistent truncus when one encounters a cyanotic baby with an ejection click, a single loud S2, and a continuous murmur. But clearly the definitive diagnosis requires additional studies, of which the most helpful noninvasive investigation is two-dimensional echocardiography.[37]

REFERENCES

1. Liebman J, et al. Natural history of transposition of great arteries: anatomy and birth and death characteristics. Circulation 1969;40:237.
2. Gutgesell HP, et al. Prognosis for the newborn with transposition of the great arteries. Am J Cardiol 1979;44:97.
3. Keith JD, et al. Transposition of the great vessels. Circulation 1953;7:830.
4. Van Mierop LHS. Transposition of the great arteries:
clarification or further confusion? Am J Cardiol 1971; 28:735.
5. Gasul BM, et al. Heart disease in children: diagnosis and treatment. Philadelphia: JB Lippincott, 1966:519.
6. Miller RA, et al. Transposition of the great vessels. Pediatr Clin North Am 1958;5:1109.
7. Noonan JA, et al. Transposition of the great arteries: a correlation of clinical, physiologic and autopsy data. N Engl J Med 1960;263:592, 684 and 739.
8. Waldman JD, et al. Transposition of the great arteries with intact ventricular septum and patent ductus arteriosus. Am J Cardiol 1977;39:232.
9. Newfeld EA, et al. Pulmonary vascular disease in complete transposition of the great arteries: a study of 200 patients. Am J Cardiol 1974;34:75.
10. Levin DL, et al. d-Transposition of the great vessels in the neonate: a clinical diagnosis. Arch Intern Med 1977; 137:1421.
11. Zuberbuhler JR. Paradoxical splitting of the second sound with transposition of the great vessels. Am Heart J 1967; 74:816.
12. Neufeld HN, et al. Origin of both great vessels from the right ventricle: I. without pulmonic stenosis. Circulation 1961;23:399.
13. Neufeld HN, et al. Origin of both great vessels from the right ventricle: II. with pulmonic stenosis. Circulation 1961;23:603.
14. Taussig HB, Bing RJ. Complete transposition of the aorta and a levoposition of the pulmonary artery. Am Heart J 1949;37:551.
15. Schaefer JA, Rudolph LA. Corrected transposition of the great vessels. Am Heart J 1957;54:610.
16. Nagle JP, et al. Corrected transposition of the great vessels without associated anomalies: report of a case with congestive failure at age 45. Chest 1971;60:367.
17. Allwork SP, et al. Congenitally corrected transposition of the great arteries: morphologic study of 32 cases. Am J Cardiol 1976;38:910.
18. Friedberg DZ, Nadas AS. Clinical profile of patients with congenitally corrected transposition of the great arteries. N Engl J Med 1970;282:1054.
19. Huhta JC, et al. Complete atrioventricular block in patients with atrioventricular discordance. Circulation 1983; 67:1374.
20. Anderson RC, et al. Corrected transposition of the great vessels of the heart: a review of 17 cases. Pediatrics 1957;20:626.
21. Schiebler GL, et al. Congenital corrected transposition of the great vessels: a study of 33 cases. Pediatrics 1961; 27:851.
22. Cumming GR. Congenital corrected transposition of the great vessels without associated intracardiac abnormalities. Am J Cardiol 1962;10:605.
23. Morgan AD, et al. Clinical features of single ventricle with congenitally corrected transposition. Am J Cardiol 1966;17:379.
24. Honey M. The diagnosis of corrected transposition of the great vessels. Br Heart J 1963;25:313.
25. Perloff JK. The clinical recognition of congenital heart disease, ed 3. Philadelphia: WB Saunders, 1987:69.
26. Malers E, et al. Transposition functionally corrected associated with "mitral" insufficiency. Am Heart J 1960; 59:816.
27. Gasul BM, et al. Corrected transposition of the great vessels: demonstration of a new phonocardiographic sign of this malformation. J Pediatr 1959;55:180.
28. Kraus Y, et al. Precordial pulsations in corrected trans-

position of the great vessels: diagnostic value of the electromechanical intervals. Am J Cardiol 1969;23:684.

29. Lieberson AD, et al. Corrected transposition of the great vessels in a 73-year-old man. Circulation 1969;39:96.

30. Calder L, et al. Truncus arteriosus communis: clinical, angiocardiographic and pathologic findings in 100 patients. Am Heart J 1976;92:23.

31. Rowe R, Vlad P. Persistent truncus arteriosus: report of two cases with right aortic arch. Am Heart J 1953;46:296.

32. Deely WJ, et al. Truncus insufficiency: common truncus arteriosus with regurgitant truncus valve: report of four cases. Am Heart J 1963;65:542.

33. MacGilpin HH. Truncus arteriosus communis persistens. Am Heart J 1950;39:615.

34. Gasul BM, et al. Heart disease in children: diagnosis and treatment. Philadelphia: JB Lippincott, 1966:621.

35. Victorica B, et al. Phonocardiographic findings in persistent truncus arteriosus. Br Heart J 1968;30:812.

36. Tandon R, et al. Persistent truncus arteriosus: a clinical, hemodynamic, and autopsy study of 19 cases. Circulation 1963;28:1050.

37. Huhta JC, et al. Two-dimensional echocardiographic assessment of the aorta in infants and children with congenital heart disease. Circulation 1984;70:417.

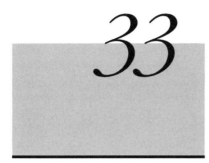

Ischemic Heart Disease

The bulk of ischemic heart disease (IHD) is due to atheromatous coronary artery obstruction. But other lesions can impair coronary flow and so produce ischemic symptoms; included in these are aortic valve disease, syphilitic aortitis, and embolization of a coronary artery. Other rare forms of coronary arterial disease are polyarteritis, rheumatic arteritis, thromboangiitis, medial calcification, aneurysm, and congenital lesions. Cheitlin[1] was able to list over 40 uncommon or rare causes of "nonatheromatous" coronary obstruction.

The balance of coronary supply and demand can also be upset by increased requirements (myocardial hypertrophy, hyperthyroidism) or decreased oxygen delivery (right ventricular hypertension, severe anemia, lung disease).

DEFINITIONS

Angina (Latin, "strangling") may be applied to any discomfort or pain resulting from myocardial ischemia. Coronary insufficiency is an inclusive term applicable to all manifestations of inadequate coronary blood supply, short of myocardial infarction. Clear-cut angina of effort and myocardial infarction represent black and white poles in the ischemic field; although the gray zone between them has attracted a number of descriptive titles, most of them have fallen into disuse (see under *Unstable Angina*). Nowadays, ischemic behavior is generally considered under the headings in Table 33-1.

The division of angina into several types or syndromes is somewhat artificial because there is considerable clinical overlap between them, and both fixed obstruction and intermittent spasm appear to play roles in varying proportions across the anginal spectrum: All the way from pure fixed obstruction in some patients with classical angina, to pure spasm in otherwise normal arteries in some with variant angina; and varying combinations of spasm and fixed obstruction in between (Fig. 33-1). Note that this diagram is deliberately simplistic and takes no account of the roles of plaque disruption, thrombus formation, etc., that no doubt contribute to the capricious behavior of "unstable" angina. No classification in medicine is ever completely satisfactory: The most that can be asked of one is that it provide a framework on which to construct a reasonable system of diagnosis and therapy.

Table 33–1
Syndromes of Myocardial Ischemia

Stable angina of effort
Unstable angina
Variant angina
Mixed angina
Syndrome X
Silent ischemia

CLINICAL FINDINGS

Symptoms

Regardless of the "syndrome," in all of them the discomfort of myocardial ischemia may range from minor distress to agonizing and incapacitating pain; and in all it has many of the same characteristics. The pain is described as crushing, constricting, like a vise, burning, searing, bursting; or it may be passed off as "indigestion." When the symptom does not amount to pain, it is variously described as pressure, tightness, constriction, fullness, heaviness, or "an elephant sitting on my chest." At times dyspnea is the anginal equivalent.

The discomfort or pain is behind the sternum and often radiates to the left arm; less often it travels to shoulder, jaw, teeth, throat, back, or right arm. It is said to radiate to both arms in 17% of patients.[2] Rarely, it is exclusively epigastric, and is then particularly likely to be taken for indigestion.

In a large series of 1200 patients with coronary insufficiency, 974 of whom went on to myocardial infarction, the pain was of no help in diagnosis in a significant minority; it was completely absent in 4.4%, mild and insignificant in 2.9%, and situated elsewhere than in the anterior chest in 8.3%.[3]

In taking the history, refer back to the schema in Chapter 1; three particularly important questions that are too often overlooked are:

1. Does the pain begin with maximal intensity or is there a **build-up**?	→ There must be at least a brief period of mounting anoxia, and in parallel with this there must be a crescendo of the pain, if only for a few seconds.
2. Can you point to the pain with **one finger**?	→ Angina is almost never so sharply localized that the victim can indicate its territory with a single fingertip. The corollary of this is the "clenched fist" sign of Levine.
3. Is the pain **superficial** or deep?	→ Angina is a sensation deep inside the chest; although it may spread to involve the surface, it almost never seems exclusively superficial.

Physical Signs

The physical signs of myocardial ischemia without infarction are sparse but worth seeking. Though in no way diagnostic, the presence of xanthomata, myxedema, or premature aging may indicate that the stage is set. Arcus senilis (or corneal arcus, as considerate writers sometimes style it) in white men under 40 suggests an increased susceptibility to IHD.[4]

The jugular veins may be distended if the right ventricle is infarcted—as it is in about 30% of inferior wall infarcts; or if there is a background of congestive heart failure; and there may be a giant "a" wave,[5] especially if there is pulmonary hypertension secondary to left ventricular failure.

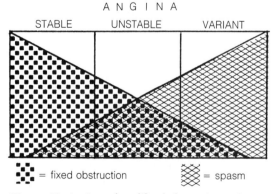

Figure 33–1. Interplay of fixed obstruction and arteriospasm in anginal syndromes.

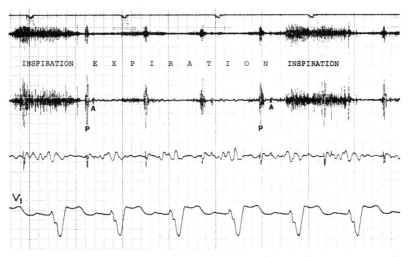

INSPIRATION E X P I R A T I O N INSPIRATION

A

P

A

P

V₁

Figure 33–2. Phonocardiograms documenting paradoxical splitting of the second sound in left bundle-branch block. Pulmonic (P) and aortic (A) components of S2 are closer together at the end of inspiration than at the end of expiration.

You should examine the heart with the patient in both supine and left lateral positions.[6,7] The apex impulse may have an exaggerated presystolic "A" wave that becomes more prominent with the development of angina.[8,9] This abnormal "A" wave is correlatable with an abnormal elevation of left ventricular end-diastolic pressure,[10] and may be reduced by venous tourniquets, an abdominal binder, or nitroglycerin. There may be also an abnormally sustained systolic impulse ("mid-systolic bulge"), exaggerated by exertion or the development of pain, and reduced by nitroglycerin.[11,12]

On auscultation there may be a correspondingly audible S4. The paradoxical splitting of left bundle-branch block (LBBB) may alert you to the possibility of IHD (Fig. 33-2), and such splitting may also be present in the absence of LBBB.[7,13] The systolic murmur of papillary muscle dysfunction may be audible, but perhaps only during attacks of pain.

Carotid sinus massage may assist in diagnosis[14]: With the patient sitting and holding your stethoscope to his chest, you massage one carotid sinus for 3 to 5 seconds. *If significant cardiac slowing results*, stop massaging and ask the misleading question, "Is the pain worse?" Levine claimed that true angina is relieved in a matter of seconds *if slowing occurs*. Others have not found the test so reliable. A Valsalva maneuver may also terminate an attack of angina before the bradycrotic phase.[15] One should never forget that both these maneuvers have inherent dangers.

THE ANGINAL SYNDROMES

Stable Angina Pectoris
(Aliases: Angina of Effort, Heberden's Angina)

In stable angina, the chest discomfort, usually pain, is predictably induced by exercise, emotion (especially anger), exposure to cold (or heat), meals, sexual intercourse, or micturition. Obviously, combinations of these precipitants (eg, exercise in the cold or after a meal) are potent pain purveyors. The attacks of pain are short-lived, usually lasting for only a few minutes, subsiding rapidly with rest or with sublingual nitroglycerin. In most cases, nitroglycerin abolishes the pain in less than a minute.

Angina can present as "breathlessness" rather than pain, it can be respiration-dependent (being felt at only one phase of the respiratory cycle), and it can be precipitated by micturition.[16,17] Sometimes the pain of angina paradoxically relents as the patient perseveres with the precipitating exertion,[18] a phenomenon variously known as "first effort" (or "first hole" if golf is the precipitant), or "second wind" angina.

Unstable Angina

"Unstable" angina has taken the place of numerous terms like coronary failure,[19] intermediate coronary syndrome,[20,21] acute coronary insufficiency,[22] subacute coronary insufficiency,[23] and preinfarction angina[24]—to name a few. It is generally applied to one of three situations: (1) when angina develops at rest, (2) when previously stable angina changes and becomes more troublesome, and (3) when angina of recent onset is frequent and severe.[25]

Angina at Rest

Chest discomfort develops without apparent provocation, and attacks may be prolonged. Response to nitroglycerin is disappointing. These patients have the highest incidence of eventual myocardial infarction.

Crescendo Angina

Changing from a well established pattern of predictable effort angina, the pain becomes more frequent, more intense, or lasts longer; or it may be provoked by significantly less effort. Previously effective nitroglycerin may cease to confer relief.

Angina of New Onset

Chest pain of troublesome intensity begins abruptly. At least at first, it may respond well to nitroglycerin.

Variant Angina
(Aliases: Prinzmetal's Angina, Vasospastic Angina)

Originally described by Prinzmetal in 1959,[26,27] this variant differs from classic angina pectoris in three important respects: (1) It develops at rest and is not provoked by incitants such as exertion or emotion; (2) it tends to recur at about the same time of day or night, sometimes waking the patient after only a short period of sleep, sometimes later at the time of REM sleep,[28] or sometimes occurring repeatedly at about the time of arising; each attack tends to last longer—for 5 to 30 minutes instead of the 2 to 5 minutes of classical angina; and (3) an electrocardiogram (ECG) taken during an episode of pain manifests striking *ST elevation* (instead of the expected depression). The syndrome is attributed to spasm of a coronary artery—usually left anterior descending or right coronary—often associated with fixed obstruction in that artery as well (see Fig. 33-1).

The pain of variant angina does not differ from that of classic angina in quality, location, radiation, or associated symptoms. Dyspnea may accompany the chest discomfort. Syncope during angina occurred in 27% of 59 patients with pure spasm, and significant disturbances of rhythm and conduction in 24%.[29] Victims of variant angina tend to be younger and lack the risk factors commonly found in subjects of classic effort angina; they also are more likely to have additional vasospastic disorders, such as Raynaud's disease or migraine. Attacks tend to occur in clusters, but between attacks the cardiovascular examination is characteristically entirely normal. Spontaneous remissions are common and may be prolonged.[30]

Mixed Angina

This is a purely clinical term applicable to patients who are hapless enough to suffer from angina both on effort and at rest. Clearly there is no fine line between this and some instances of unstable angina.

Syndrome X

This unfortunate term has been given to the combination of typical anginal pain and coronary arteries normal by angiography. It may be due to disease or spasm of smaller, myocardial arteries beyond the purview of arteriography. In many cases it may be esophageal in origin (see further on). In any case, from the point of view of future myocardial infarction and mortality, it has a favorable prognosis, though the symptoms may materially interfere with the patient's life.[31–33]

Silent Ischemia

Since the patient has no pain or discomfort, silent ischemia cannot be classified as a form of "angina." It is, however, a mode of coronary insufficiency. By definition, it is myocardial ischemia recognized objectively (by electrocardiography, Holter monitoring, or stress test) in the absence of subjective awareness.[34] Obviously, if it is truly

Table 33–2
The Chest Pain "Haystack"

Cardiovascular	**Neuromuscular/Skeletal**
Pericarditis	Anterior chest wall syndrome[41,42]
Aortitis, aortic aneurysm	Costochondral (Tietze's) syndrome[43]
Aortic valve disease	Precordial catch[44]
Dissecting aneurysm	**Nerve root pain** from spondylitis,[45] osteoarthritis, cervical disc, etc.
RV hypertension[35]	Costochondral chondrodynia[46]
Cardiomyopathy	Xiphoidalgia
Mitral valve prolapse	Intercostal neuritis
	Pectoral fibrositis
Pleuro-Pulmonary	Herpes zoster
Pulmonary embolism	Epidemic myalgia
Pleurisy, pleurodynia	Diaphragmatic flutter
Pneumonia	Gout
Pneumothorax	
Mediastinal emphysema	**Psychogenic**
Lung tumors	Conversion reactions, malingering, etc.
Gastrointestinal	
Esophageal[36–38]	
Reflux esophagitis	
Diffuse spasm	
Achalasia	
Hiatal hernia[39]	
Splenic flexure syndrome[40]	
Pancreatitis	
Cholecystitis	
Peptic ulcer	

RV, right ventricular.

silent, there is no history of ischemic symptoms to glean, but of course the presence of such risk factors as hypertension, diabetes, nicotine addiction, hypothyroidism, and a family history of coronary disease may alert one to the patient's predisposition; and then the physical examination may reveal some of the physical signs outlined earlier. At this point, one may shrewdly suspect (silent) ischemic disease.

DIFFERENTIAL DIAGNOSIS

Many of the mimics of angina are listed in Table 33-2. Two of the causes of retrosternal pain deserve special mention.

The pain of *right ventricular hypertension* is probably due to ischemia of the right ventricular myocardium,[35] but several clinical differences help to distinguish it from the pain of classic angina pectoris[47,48]: There is often evidence of right ventricular hypertrophy; the patient may have cyanosis or the history of a long-standing cough; the pain is likely to increase with inspiration and is protracted, lasting days or weeks rather than minutes or hours; and there is striking relief from oxygen inhalation, but disappointing response to sublingual nitroglycerin.

Esophageal pain is also retrosternal, may radiate to the jaw and other typical anginal sites, and may be relieved by nitroglycerin. Gastroesophageal reflux is a known, common cause of chest pain, and it can be induced by exertion.[49] But it is often initiated or aggravated by lying down, is more likely than angina to radiate to the back, and it is diagnostically helpful if it is associated with dysphagia, pain on swallowing, or the ingestion of spicy foods.

Table 33-3
Special Mimics with Differential Pointers

Neurocirculatory Asthenia

Symptoms when tired *after* exertion

Left mammary pain

Tenderness at cardiac apex, sensitive to *light* touch

Sighing respiration

Associated with hyperventilation syndrome

Cervical Nerve Root Pain

Aggravated by movement rather than exertion

Worse after sleep or lying down

Aggravated by coughing, straining, etc.

Traction may relieve or worsen

Pain in *outer* aspect of arm

Paresthesias in arms, hands

Hiatal Hernia

Stooping, after meals and lying down

Dysphagia, acid regurgitation, GI bleeding

Respiratory borborygmi

Relief by standing, raised head of bed

Splenic Flexure Syndrome

Air swallower, constipation

Tympanic resonance over LUQ

Relief by passage of flatus

GI, gastrointestinal; LUQ, left upper quadrant.

In all cases of atypical chest pain, both cardiac and esophageal causes should be painstakingly excluded. In a Toronto series, of 105 patients who had atypical chest pain, 43 turned out to have esophageal disease, 21 had both esophageal and cardiac disease, 12 had heart disease, and 29 had neither.[50]

The differentiation of other selected mimics is summarized in Table 33-3.

MYOCARDIAL INFARCTION

Symptoms

The classic, clinical presentation of myocardial infarction is unmistakable: Crushing chest pain, sweating, ''ashen'' pallor. But many presentations are far from typical.

The patient may seem remarkably normal and undistressed, and indeed may have no pain at all, but the usual chest discomfort/pain is described as a heaviness or pressure, or a bursting, crushing, vise-like, constricting pain. Probably only a minority of patients employ one of these classic descriptors. The patient may swallow air to provoke belching in an effort to get rid of the discomfort.[51] He may experience a sense of impending doom.

The location of the discomfort/pain is typically midline, behind the sternum, and is often signalled by the patient with a clenched fist against the midchest (Levine's sign). The pain may radiate to neck, jaw, teeth, left shoulder, and down the left arm, usually down the inside of the arm. Radiation down the right arm is generally associated with inferior wall infarction. The fingers, especially fourth and fifth, may be affected. Less common sites include the occiput, back of neck, interscapular area, and epigastrium.

Reflex gastric dilation, especially in inferior infarction, may lead to nausea and vomiting, and is much more common in transmural than in subendocardial infarction.[52] Intense sweating and syncope are not uncommon. Syncope may result from ventricular tachyarrhythmias, administration of nitrates, vasovagal response to pain, or a bradyarrhythmia.[52]

Almost half the patients have angina for at least a month before experiencing their first infarction.[53] Other prodromal symptoms suffered during the preceding weeks include unusual fatigue, dyspnea, malaise, anorexia, nausea, arm pain, emotional changes, dizziness, and syncope.[54]

On the other hand, a significant minority have no pain even at the time of the infarct. Some of these present with symptoms other than pain: pulmonary edema, shock, syncope, prolonged unconsciousness, arrhythmia, arterial embolism, or obscure pyrexia. Of 500 patients monitored in England within the first hour, pulmonary edema developed in 26%, ventricular fibrillation in 20%, and shock in 12%.[55]

Example　A man of 34 years was admitted to the hospital unconscious. He remained so for 36 hours. Vital signs were entirely normal. An ECG taken during his coma contained the classic changes of acute inferior myocardial infarction.

Angina Plays the Harlot

Although angina is often conventional and behaves as expected, it sometimes shows no respect for orthodox pain paths. In the individual case, the dominant pain of myocardial ischemia may be felt in the tongue, hard palate, mastoid, previous thoracotomy scar, radial side of one wrist, abdomen, kidney region, groin, left testis, rectum, legs, or any "weak" spot, such as the scar of a nephrectomy.

Example An athletic executive of 47 years, while playing tennis on a warm afternoon, was seized with severe pain in the tip of his right shoulder and in the left groin simultaneously—and nowhere else. He broke out into an unathletic sweat, walked to his car and drove himself to the hospital. On admission, he was in frank shock and complaining of pain in the same two regions. His ECG showed the typical pattern of acute inferior infarction. The pain—in these two areas alone--persisted for several hours and then gradually abated. At no time during his illness did he have any sign of chest pain.

Atypical presentations are more common in the elderly, and all of the following are occasionally seen: Sudden dyspnea, acute confusion, cerebrovascular symptoms, peripheral vascular events, and renal failure.[52] Painless infarction is more common in patients with atrial fibrillation or tachycardia, and in those with hypertension[56] or diabetes.

Other heart attacks are not only painless, but totally "silent." In the widely publicized Framingham study, more than a quarter of the infarctions uncovered by electrocardiography were found in patients who could give no history of the antecedent infarction.[57] In populations followed with periodic examinations, apparently 11% to 21% of the myocardial infarctions that develop are silent.[58,59] Of 588 myocardial infarctions found at autopsy, 30% were undiagnosed during life.[60] In another series, 40% of 63 acute and 50% of 113 healed infarctions at autopsy had gone unrecognized before death.[61] And, of course, the initial pain of infarction can be entirely masked by contemporary anesthesia or a concomitant cerebral thrombosis.

Physical Signs

The patient with a heart attack often appears remarkably normal; a few are moribund and look it. In between these extremes, there are numerous compromises. After the first 6 hours,[62] the temperature is slightly elevated, seldom above 101°F.

The pulse may be normal, or, if there has been a significant drop in blood pressure, it may be weak and "thready." The rate may be normal, rapid, or slow. Bradycardia is a good sign if it is associated with evidence of adequate perfusion (warm, dry skin, etc.). In a study from New Zealand,[63] among 735 patients with myocardial infarction, the mortality was only 6% in those who developed sinus bradycardia, compared with 26% in those with sinus tachycardia, and 15% in those who developed neither bradycardia nor tachycardia.

In patients with severe pain or anxiety, the blood pressure may actually be elevated; more often it is at least mildly depressed, often falling during the first day or two to a systolic pressure of 90 to 100 mm Hg.

Depending on the severity of the attack, the patient's breathing pattern may range from complete normality to intense dyspnea. If the heart is "failing," the neck veins are distended; there may be giant "a" wave in the jugular pulse (Fig. 33-3).

"In many patients, perhaps even the majority, the myocardial infarction is palpable."[64] You can sometimes make the diagnosis of infarction standing at the foot of the patient's bed and inspecting the precordium for visible impulses. In the infarct suspect, the presence of an anterior pulsation *in the V3 line* (Fig. 33-4) is excellent corroborative evidence. And if it is visible, it is usually well felt.

Most of the other physical signs of infarction are auscultatory; of these, the most diagnostic is a pericardial rub, which develops in approximately

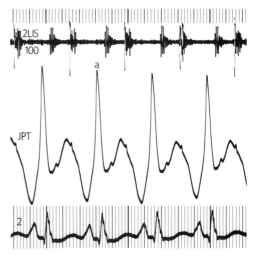

Figure 33–3. Giant "a" waves in the jugular pulse of a patient with severe right ventricular failure secondary to ischemic heart disease.

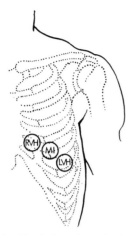

Figure 33–4. Usual sites of maximal pulsation in left ventricular hypertrophy (LVH), right ventricular hypertrophy (RVH), and anterior myocardial infarction (MI).

15% of infarcts (Fig. 33-5). Other audible findings are less specific, including third and fourth heart sounds; the S4 (Fig. 33-6) is so common that its absence makes the diagnosis of infarction unlikely.[65,66] Reversed splitting of the second sound is sometimes present, with or without LBBB (Fig. 33-2). Important murmurs that may develop in the course of an acute infarction are contrasted in Table 33-4.

Complications

Right Ventricular Infarction

The neck veins reveal venous congestion and perhaps become more distended during inspiration (Kussmaul's sign) as the damaged ventricle struggles (and fails) to cope with the augmented influx of blood. Giant "a" waves (see Fig. 33-3) and right-sided atrial (S4) and ventricular (S3) gallops may develop; these, and the pansystolic murmur of tricuspid regurgitation, are best heard at the left lower sternal border, and all become louder with inspiration. A pericardial rub is said to be present in 90% of cases and pulsus paradoxus in 40%.[67] The lung fields are generally clear.

Rupture of the Free Wall

About 2% of infarcts are complicated by rupture of the free wall. There is sudden hemodynamic collapse with electromechanical dissociation (ECG evidence of persisting cardiac rhythm without corresponding pulse or blood pressure.) Tamponade is sometimes recognizable, and a pseudoaneurysm[5,68]—"a pulsating hematoma contained only by the pericardium or adjacent structures"—may develop associated with a loud pericardial rub. A pansystolic murmur may appear at the apex. One-

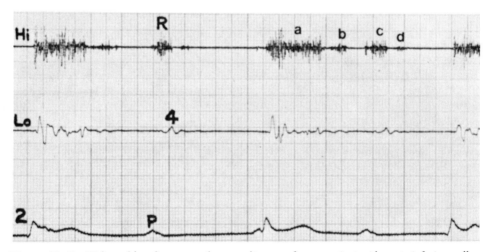

Figure 33–5. High- and low-frequency phonocardiograms from a patient with acute inferior wall myocardial infarction who has developed complete A-V block. In the high-frequency tracing, pericardial friction is recorded in four phases: Ventricular systole (a), ventricular diastole (b), atrial systole (c), and atrial diastole (d). "R" is the rub accompanying a dissociated atrial contraction. (Reproduced with permission from Marriott HJL. Bedside recognition of cardiac arrhythmias. Geriatrics 1975; 30:55.)

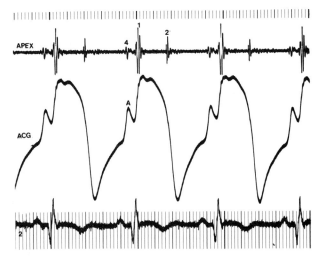

Figure 33–6. Apexcardiogram and phonocardiogram from a patient with recent inferior myocardial infarction. Note the prominent "A" wave coincident with the fourth heart sound (4).

third of all ruptures occur on the first day, half within 4 days.[68]

Rupture of the Ventricular Septum

About 2% of infarctions are complicated by rupture of the ventricular septum. It is characterized by sudden hypotension and biventricular failure, the right ventricle failing before the left.[62] A pansystolic murmur is heard at the left sternal border and somewhat laterally associated with a thrill in about half the patients. As with other ventricular septal defects, the murmur may get louder with

inspiration if you listen one or two interspaces below its maximal point. Amazingly and rarely, a ruptured septum may produce no symptoms.[69]

Mitral Regurgitation

This may result from papillary muscle dysfunction or rupture, rupture of a chorda, or left ventricular dilation or aneurysm. You may suspect chordal rupture if you hear mid or late systolic clicks.[70]

Rupture of a papillary muscle usually happens in the first week, and affects patients with small infarcts and single-vessel disease. The develop-

Table 33–4

The Murmurs of Myocardial Infarction

	Ruptured Ventricular Septum	*Ruptured Papillary Muscle*	*Papillary Muscle Dysfunction*	*Left Ventricular Dilation*
The murmur	Usually *pan*systolic, but may end before S2	*Pan*systolic, but *none* in 40%	*Delayed* systolic or may be pansystolic	May be pansystolic, midsystolic or late systolic
	Maximal at 4th LIS	Maximal at apex (or base)	Maximal at apex	Maximal at apex
Thrill	Common	Rare	No	No
Failure	Rapid, RV before LV	Rapid, with pulmonary edema before RV	Not striking	Not striking
Gallop	RV with TR	LV	No	No

RV, right ventricular; LV, left ventricular; TR, tricuspid regurgitation; LIS, left interspace.

ment of pulmonary edema followed by right ventricular failure in a patient with his first infarct, usually of the inferior wall, should alert one to the possibility of acute mitral regurgitation. The resulting murmur is not always harsh and loud, and not always pansystolic. Papillary muscle dysfunction without rupture produces a systolic murmur that begins after S1 and ends before S2.

The important systolic murmurs that may appear during an infarct are contrasted in Table 33-4.

Cardiogenic Shock

The earliest indication of circulatory failure may be a mental change: Apathy, confusion, or agitation. There is pallor together with a drop in skin temperature (in particular, feel toes, fingers, and forehead). Mild sweating develops, often earliest on the forehead or lower lip. Along with an increase in the cardiac rate, there is a declining blood pressure and urinary output. It is important not to diagnose shock from the blood pressure alone; a systolic pressure below 80 mm Hg usually signals circulatory collapse, but in the absence of other signs a pressure in the 85 to 100 mm Hg range may be well tolerated and may indeed be beneficial.

Heart Failure

Heart failure may develop with the usual symptoms and signs (Chapter 38).

Emboli

Emboli, from the dislodgement of mural thrombi, may occlude cerebral, splenic, mesenteric, renal, or femoral arteries.

Arrhythmias

Arrhythmias develop in almost all patients. Their bedside recognition is dealt with in Chapter 40.

Postmyocardial Infarction Syndrome
(Alias: Dressler's Syndrome)[71]

This complicates 3% or 4% of infarctions.[72] Pain of variable intensity, deceptively similar to that of the antecedent infarction, recurs and lasts anywhere from hours to weeks. The pain may have a more pericardial flavor than the prior infarction pain (ie, it is aggravated by inspiration, yawning,

turning, or swallowing). You suspect the syndrome if the initial fever lasts longer than a week or returns; or if the initial pericardial rub lasts longer than 3 days or recurs. Pericardial effusion is common, and pleurisy, pneumonitis, and even periostitis may complicate the picture.[73] Recurrences are common, and the syndrome may repeat itself several times in the course of 2 years.[74]

Differential Diagnosis

In the differential diagnosis of acute myocardial infarction, one must consider all of the many causes of chest pain. Conditions that require special mention include acute pericarditis, dissecting aneurysm, and pulmonary embolism.

Acute Pericarditis

The pain is sharp and piercing and is definitely influenced by breathing. It is usually aggravated by deep inspiration, swallowing, and turning, and may be somewhat relieved by holding the breath and leaning forward. Pericardial friction and fever are present early on, in contrast with their delayed appearance in acute myocardial infarction.

Dissecting Aneurysm

The pain of dissecting aneurysm (Laennec, 1819), unlike that of myocardial infarction, reaches maximal intensity instantaneously and is described as unbearable, tearing, ripping. It may be focused anteriorly or posteriorly, but it migrates downward as the dissection proceeds. Chest pain accompanied by any of the following should suggest the diagnosis of dissecting aneurysm: Aortic regurgitation, pulsation of the right sternoclavicular joint, unequal carotid pulsation, unequal pulses or blood pressure in the arms, and weakness or paralysis of the legs.

Despite the agonizing standard, about 10% of dissecting aneurysms are said to be painless. The paradoxical combination of ''shock'' with hypertension is characteristic. In general, proximal dissections affect a younger group because they are more likely secondary to a hereditary defect (eg, Marfan's syndrome), whereas distal dissection is the rule in older patients, in whom it is usually initiated by atherosclerosis combined with hypertension. Mysteriously, pregnancy accounts for almost half the dissections that occur before the age

Table 33–5
*Clues that May Help to Differentiate
Special Mimics*

Pericarditis

Sharp, lancinating pain aggravated by respiration, twisting, swallowing

Early fever and rub

Some relief from holding breath, leaning forward

Dissecting Aneurysm

Peak intensity of pain at onset—no build-up

Unequal carotid or arm pulses or BP; or absent pulses

Hypertension + "shock"

Aortic regurgitation

Symptoms in legs

Sternoclavicular pulsation

Wide radiation of pain to back, flanks, etc.

Pulmonary Embolism

The clinical setting: heart failure, postoperative, postpartum, long plane or car trip, etc.

Dyspnea and cyanosis just before or simultaneous with pain onset

Cough, hemoptysis

Acute tricuspid regurgitation

Cardiac signs: fixed splitting of S2, pulmonic ejection murmur, friction over PA, atrial arrhythmias

BP, blood pressure; PA, pulmonary artery.

of 40 years.[75] In the huge series of 925 dissections treated at the Texas Heart Institute, 87% were over 40 years of age and men outnumbered women by 3:1.[75]

Pulmonary Embolism

The clinical context is important: Pulmonary embolism complicates congestive heart failure or thrombophlebitis; or it develops after surgery, delivery, trauma, or prolonged immobilization. Enforced sitting for hours on end, as in a long car ride or plane trip, predisposes to phlebothrombosis in the legs with consequent embolization.

Dyspnea and cyanosis develop simultaneously with, or even anticipate, the chest pain, and there may be cough and hemoptysis. Acute tricuspid regurgitation develops with its characteristic physical signs (see Chapter 25); on auscultation there is fixed splitting of the second sound, a pulmonic

ejection murmur, and friction over the pulmonary artery. Sinus tachycardia or an atrial tachyarrhythmia is almost invariable.

Helpful differential diagnostic pointers are summarized in Table 33-5.

REFERENCES

Myocardial Ischemia

1. Cheitlin MD, et al. Myocardial infarction without atherosclerosis. JAMA 1975;231:951.
2. Harris K. Clinical aspects of atypical coronary disease. Br Med J 1955;2:874.
3. Sigler LH. Subjective manifestations of acute coronary occlusion or insufficiency. Arch Intern Med 1954;94:341.
4. McAndrew GM, Ogston D. Arcus senilis and coronary artery disease. Am Heart J 1965;70:838.
5. Chizner MA. Bedside diagnosis of the acute myocardial infarction and its complications. Curr Probl Cardiol 1982;7:7.
6. Bethell HJN, Nixon PGH. Examination of the heart in supine and left lateral positions. Br Heart J 1973;35:902.
7. Shub C. Stable angina pectoris: 2. Cardiac evaluation. Mayo Clin Proc 1990;64:243.
8. Benchimol A, Dimond EG. The apexcardiogram in ischemic heart disease. Br Heart J 1962;24:581.
9. Dimond EG. Precordial vibrations: clinical clues from palpation. Circulation 1964;30:284.
10. Dimond EG, Benchimol A. Correlation of intracardiac pressure and precordial movement in ischemic heart disease. Br Heart J 1963;25:389.
11. Skinner NS, et al. Angina pectoris: effect of exertion and nitrites on precordial movements. Am Heart J 1961;61:250.
12. Eddleman EE. Kinetocardiographic changes in ischemic heart disease. Circulation 1965;32:650.
13. Crawford MH. Noninvasive assessment of patients with ischemic heart disease. Curr Probl Cardiol 1981;6:7.
14. Levine SA. Carotid sinus massage: a new diagnostic test for angina pectoris. JAMA 1962;182:1332.
15. Levine HJ, et al. Relief of angina pectoris by Valsalva maneuver. N Engl J Med 1966;275:487.
16. Morris JJ, McIntosh HD. Angina of micturition. Circulation 1963;27:85.
17. Marriott HJL, Vogt PA. Micturition angina: a case report. Heart Lung 1977;6:510.
18. MacAlpin RN, Kattus AA. Adaptation to exercise in angina pectoris. Circulation 1966;33:183.
19. Freedberg AS, et al. Coronary failure: the clinical syndrome of cardiac pain intermediate between angina pectoris and acute myocardial infarction. JAMA 1948;138:107.
20. Graybiel A. The intermediate coronary syndrome. United States Armed Forces Medical Journal 1955;6:1.
21. Vakil RJ. Intermediate coronary syndrome. Circulation 1961;24:557.
22. Master AM, et al. Acute coronary insufficiency: its differential diagnosis and treatment. Ann Intern Med 1956;45:561.
23. Wood P. Acute and subacute coronary insufficiency. Br Med J 1961;1:1780.

24. Resnik WH. The significance of prolonged anginal pain (preinfarction angina). Am Heart J 1962;63:290.

25. Munger TM. Unstable angina. Mayo Clin Proc 1990; 65:384.

26. Prinzmetal M, et al. Angina pectoris: I. A variant form of angina pectoris. Am J Med 1959;27:375.

27. Prinzmetal M, et al. Variant form of angina pectoris. JAMA 1960;174:1794.

28. Shub C. Stable angina pectoris: 1. Clinical patterns. Mayo Clin Proc 1990;64:233.

29. Bott-Silverman C, Heupler FA. Natural history of pure coronary artery spasm in patients treated medically. J Am Coll Cardiol 1983;2:200.

30. Waters DD, et al. Spontaneous remission is a frequent outcome of variant angina. J Am Coll Cardiol 1983;2: 195.

31. Kemp HG, et al. The anginal syndrome associated with normal coronary arteriograms: report of a six year experience. Am J Med 1973;54:735.

32. Pasternak RC, et al. Chest pain with angiographically insignificant coronary arterial obstruction. Am J Med 1980;68:813.

33. Ockene LS, et al. Unexplained chest pain in patients with normal coronary arteriograms: a follow-up study of functional status. N Engl J Med 1980;303:1249.

34. Hammill SC, Khanderia BK. Silent myocardial ischemia. Mayo Clin Proc 1990;65:374.

35. Ross RS. Right ventricular hypertension as a cause of precordial pain. Am Heart J 1961;61:134.

36. Bernstein LM, et al. Differentiation of esophageal pain from angina pectoris: role of the esophageal acid perfusion test. Medicine 1962;41:143.

37. Richter JE, et al. Esophageal chest pain: current controversies in pathogenesis, diagnosis, and therapy. Ann Intern Med 1989;110:66.

38. Mellow MH. A gastroenterologist's view of chest pain. Curr Probl Cardiol 1983;7:7.

39. Morris JC, et al. Coronary disease and hiatal hernia. JAMA 1963;183:788.

40. Machella TE, et al. Observations on the splenic flexure syndrome. Ann Intern Med 1952;37:543.

41. Prinzmetal M, Massumi RA. The anterior chest wall syndrome—chest pain resembling pain of cardiac origin. JAMA 1955;159:177.

42. McElroy JB. Angina pectoris with coexisting skeletal chest pain. Am Heart J 1963;66:296.

43. Benson EH, Zavola DC. Importance of the costochondral syndrome in evaluation of chest pain. JAMA 1954;156: 1244.

44. Miller AJ, Texidor TA. The "precordial catch," a syndrome of anterior chest pain. Ann Intern Med 1959;51: 461.

45. Good AE. The chest pain of ankylosing spondylitis. Ann Intern Med 1963;53:926.

46. Carabasi RJ, et al. Costosternal chondrodynia: a variant of Tietze's syndrome. Dis Chest 1962;41:559.

47. Viar WN, Harrison TF. Chest pain in association with pulmonary hypertension. Circulation 1952;5:1.

48. Lassere RP, Genkins G. Chest pain in patients with isolated pulmonic stenosis. Circulation 1957;15:258.

49. Schofield PM, et al. Exertional gastro-oesophageal reflux: a mechanism for symptoms in patients with angina pectoris and normal coronary angiograms. Br Med J 1987; 294:1459.

50. Henderson RD, et al. Atypical chest pain of cardiac and esophageal origin. Chest 1978;73:24.

Myocardial Infarction

51. Fowler NO. Physical signs in acute myocardial infarction and its complications. Prog Cardiovasc Dis 1968;10:287.

52. Lavie CJ, Gersh BJ. Acute myocardial infarction: initial manifestations, management, and prognosis. Mayo Clin Proc 1990;65:531.

53. Francis RL, et al. Angina pectoris preceding initial myocardial infarction. Arch Intern Med 1963;112:226.

54. Simon AB, et al. Components of delay in the pre-hospital phase of acute myocardial infarction. Am J Cardiol 1972;30:476.

55. O'Doherty M, et al. Five hundred patients with myocardial infarction monitored within one hour of symptoms. Br Med J 1983;286:1405.

56. Evans WB, Sutton GC. Painless cardiac infarction. Br Heart J 1956;18:259.

57. Kannel WB, Abbott RD. Incidence and prognosis of unrecognized myocardial infarction. N Engl J Med 1984; 311:1144.

58. Stokes J, Dawber TR. The "silent coronary": the frequency and clinical characteristics of unrecognized myocardial infarction in the Framingham study. Ann Intern Med 1959;50:1359.

59. Lindberg HA, et al. Totally asymptomatic myocardial infarction: an estimate of its incidence in the living population. Arch Intern Med 1960;106:628.

60. Gould SE, Cawley LP. Unsuspected healed myocardial infarction in patients dying in a general hospital. Arch Intern Med 1958;101:524.

61. Johnson WJ, et al. Unrecognized myocardial infarction. Arch Intern Med 1959;97:253.

62. Nellen M, et al. Value of physical examination in acute myocardial infarction. Br Heart J 1973;35:777.

63. Norris RM, et al. Sinus rate in acute myocardial infarction. Br Heart J 1972;34:901.

64. Silverman ME, Hurst JW. Abnormal physical findings associated with myocardial infarction. Modern Concepts of Cardiovascular Disease 1969;38:69.

65. Hill JC, et al. The diagnostic value of the atrial gallop in acute myocardial infarction. Am Heart J 1969;78:194.

66. Turner PP, Hunter J. The atrial sound in ischemic heart disease. Br Heart J 1973;35:657.

67. Lorell B, et al. Right ventricular infarction: clinical diagnosis and differentiation from cardiac tamponade and pericardial constriction. Am J Cardiol 1979;43:465.

68. Lavie CJ, Gersh BJ. Mechanical and electrical complications of acute myocardial infarction. Mayo Clin Proc 1990;65:709.

69. Davies AH, Westaby S. Silent myocardial infarction complicated by asymptomatic ventricular septal defect. Texas Heart Institute Journal 1990;17:139.

70. Steelman RB, et al. Midsystolic clicks in arteriosclerotic heart disease: a new facet in the clinical syndrome of papillary muscle dysfunction. Circulation 1971;44:503.

71. Dressler W. The post-myocardial infarction syndrome: a report on 44 cases. Arch Intern Med 1959;103:28.

72. Weiser NJ, et al. The postmyocardial infarction syndrome: the nonspecificity of the pulmonary manifestations. Circulation 1962;25:643.

73. Roesler H. Periosteal chest wall pain as part of the post-myocardial-infarction syndrome. Am J Med 1960;240: 407.

74. Dressler W, Leavitt SS. Pericarditis after acute myocardial infarction. JAMA 1960;173:1225.

75. Massumi A, Mathur VS. Clinical recognition of aortic dissection. Texas Heart Institute Journal 1990;17:254.

Cardiomyopathy

The word "cardiomyopathy" means "heart-muscle disease," no more, no less. Some authorities[1,2] restrict the term to myocardial disease *of unknown origin*—a usage that is, for both semantic and practical reasons, probably too restricted—and assemble other myocardial diseases under the banner of "specific heart-muscle disease."[1,3] Others would have cardiomyopathy embrace all forms of myocardial mischief, including involvement by infections, the ravages of ischemic disease,[4] etc.; but this usage is too broad and a happier medium is needed.

Logic dictates that the distinction between known and unknown origins should be conveyed by appropriate epithets, and not by arbitrarily assigning one meaning to the English "heart-muscle disease" and another to "cardio-myopathy," the Greek equivalent. The value of the term, cardiomyopathy (CMP), lies in the fact that it segregates a group of diseases that, as far as cardiac involvement goes, begin in and are for practical purposes confined to the myocardium. It is not applied to muscle disease that is secondary to prior involvement of other components of the heart (eg, valves

or coronary arteries). Therefore, the CMPs are best divided into those whose cause is unknown ("idiopathic") and those with known causes ("secondary" or "specific"), and a short classification is presented in Table 34-1.

Approximately 75% of CMP syndromes are idiopathic, the remainder being due to recognizable processes. Exhaustive lists of specific causes are readily available.[1,3,5]

The first step in diagnosis is to recognize, mainly by exclusion, that the disease in question belongs to the "cardiomyopathic" group; the second step is to identify, so far as possible, the individual within the group.

CMP can affect cardiac function in three general ways:[6,7]

1. By producing congestive failure,
2. By obstructing ventricular outflow or inflow, and
3. By restricting cardiac expansion.

In a given case, these effects often overlap and combine.

The congestive picture requires separation from the many causes of heart failure; the obstructive

Table 34–1
Limited Classification of the Cardiomyopathies

Idiopathic	Specific
Dilated (congestive)	Alcoholic
Restrictive/obliterative	Amyloid
Hypertrophic (obstructive)	Hemochromatosis
	Peripartum
	Sarcoid

picture simulates stenosis of one of the heart valves; and the restrictive picture simulates pericardial constriction. Some clinical clues that should make you think of CMP are summarized in Table 34-2. Obviously, myocardial involvement by differing processes will have features in common, and their separation may be clinically impossible; nevertheless, there are some subtle clues that may help to differentiate them.

IDIOPATHIC CARDIOMYOPATHY

Dilated

The "dilated" group used to be called "congestive" because, before diagnostic methods became more sophisticated, all diagnosed cases were already in congestive heart failure. But since we now know that all patients do not necessarily develop heart failure, congestive has been abandoned in favor of dilated. Since fibrosis, infiltration, intoxication, and replacement of the myocardium may all produce ventricular dilation and failure, the re-

Table 34–2
Circumstances Suggesting Cardiomyopathy

1. Onset before 50 years
2. History of familial heart disease
3. Excessive alcoholic intake
4. Recent childbirth
5. Chest pain that comes and goes with heart failure
6. Heart failure without obvious cause
7. Systolic murmurs that get softer as heart failure improves
8. Diastolic blood pressure elevated only with heart failure

sulting clinical picture is largely similar in many forms of CMP, and so, to avoid unnecessary and tedious repetition, let me say at the outset that the following findings are common to all dilated CMPs, both idiopathic and specific:

Symptoms of biventricular congestive failure: Shortness of breath, orthopnea, paroxysmal nocturnal dyspnea, cough, swelling of ankles and abdomen.
Signs of biventricular congestive failure: Bibasilar rales, dyspnea, distended jugular veins, hepatomegaly, edema, ascites; cardiomegaly, S3 gallop, summation gallop, mitral and tricuspid regurgitant murmurs.

The peak onset of symptoms, as exemplified by the relatively "pure" Georgetown series of 115 patients,[5] is in the fourth or fifth decades. Initial symptoms are either those of congestive failure or arrhythmias. Occasionally, the first symptom is chest pain, which may resemble angina but fails to respond to nitroglycerin; there may be syncope or evidence of an embolus, systemic or pulmonary.

Victims of dilated CMP may have diastolic hypertension, but only during heart failure. The neck veins are distended, with large, palpable "a" waves (Fig. 34-1) and paradoxical inspiratory fill-

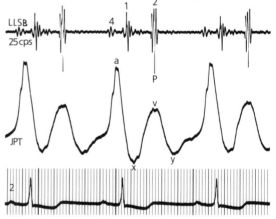

Figure 34–1. From a 34-year-old white man with dilated cardiomyopathy. In the low-frequency (25 cps) phonocardiogram recorded at the lower left sternal border (LLSB), there is an audible fourth sound (4) and an accentuated pulmonic component (P) of the second sound (2); the jugular pulse tracing (JPT) contains a giant "a" wave.

ing (Kussmaul's sign) with steep "x" and "y" descents. A right ventricular lift is sometimes preceded by a presystolic impulse producing a double sternal lift.[8] A palpable and audible triple or quadruple rhythm is common (Fig. 34-1).

Persistent or paradoxical splitting of S2 bespeaks a bundle-branch block, and there is an accentuated P2 (Fig. 34-1). A contiguous S3 and S4 may combine to produce a mid-diastolic rumble, or they may coincide with resulting summation gallop. Systolic murmurs of mitral regurgitation, pulmonary flow, or tricuspid regurgitation are often audible, along with the other typical findings of tricuspid regurgitation. The loudness of the murmur of mitral regurgitation parallels both heart size and degree of congestive failure—the larger the heart and the worse the failure, the louder the murmur.[5] Pulmonary and/or systemic embolism occurs in a significant minority—in the Georgetown series, one in five patients had emboli. At the Mayo Clinic, in a mixed series of idiopathic and specific CMPs, 18% of those not receiving anticoagulant therapy suffered embolization.[9] Many patients develop arrhythmias; in the Georgetown series, a third had atrial fibrillation, and two-thirds had ventricular extrasystoles.

Many of the features of dilated cardiomyopathy are illustrated by the young man whose tracings are shown in Figure 34-1:

Example He presented himself because of shortness of breath at the age of 30 years. He was found to have atrial flutter–fibrillation with a ventricular response rate of about 100/minute. He was digitalized, he improved, and he had no disabling symptoms for the next 4 years, at which time his dyspnea returned and he had a syncopal episode. Over the next 2 months, the dyspnea progressively worsened and he became unable to work. Physical examination revealed distended neck veins, with prominent and palpable "a" wave, Kussmaul's sign, a right ventricular lift, a loud S4 at the lower left sternal border, and an accentuated pulmonic closure sound. At this time his blood pressure was 120/70 mm Hg, the liver edge was not palpable, the lung bases were clear, and there was no pedal edema.

During cardiac catheterization, he developed complete A-V block that spontaneously reverted to normal sinus rhythm with first degree A-V block; from this he temporarily relapsed into atrial flutter. Over the next several months he suffered from intractable arrhythmias with progressive congestive failure, from which he eventually succumbed.

The cause of death is congestive heart failure in about half the patients, whereas another third die suddenly; 10% die from an arrhythmia, and 3% from embolism.[5]

RESTRICTIVE/OBLITERATIVE CARDIOMYOPATHY

From a hemodynamic point of view, it matters little whether restricted ventricular filling is due to external encasement by an unyielding pericardium or by the refusal of a rigid and exuberant endocardium to relax. The presenting symptoms and signs of restrictive CMP, therefore, closely mimic those of constrictive pericarditis. Restrictive CMP is uncommon in the Western world; in the United Kingdom, for example, of a series of 224 patients with CMP, only two were of this genre.[10]

The two time-honored conditions that produce this form of CMP are endomyocardial fibrosis (endemic to and common in the tropics) and Loeffler's syndrome (fibroblastic "endocarditis" with eosinophilia), which is worldwide and rare; in fact, they may each be different expressions of the same disorder.[11] The eosinophil has been characterized as the culpable "rogue" that stimulates the endocardium to proliferate and shrink the ventricular cavity.[2] Restrictive syndromes may also result from such recognizable invasions as amyloidosis, hemochromatosis, glycogen storage, sarcoidosis, scleroderma, and neoplastic infiltration,[12] but these are then regarded as "specific" or "secondary" rather than "idiopathic."

In most cases, both ventricles are affected, but involvement of either may predominate.[3] When right ventricular involvement is predominant, the clinical picture is virtually indistinguishable from constrictive pericarditis.

The affected patient may begin with an apparent febrile illness from which recovery seems complete. After a period of quiescence, during which time the endocardium is presumably fibrosing and proliferating in silence, symptoms may begin with decreased exercise tolerance and cough (from left ventricular involvement) or with abdominal swelling (from ascites and hepatomegaly due to right ventricular involvement). In some series, atypical chest pain has been a prominent feature.[13,14]

On physical examination, you may find evidence of impaired left ventricular output, pulmonary hypertension, and mitral and/or tricuspid regurgitation. Detectable cardiac enlargement is slight. A third heart sound may be mistaken for the pericardial knock of constrictive pericarditis. Embolization of the thrombotic endocardial debris often occurs.

When the right ventricle is mainly affected, you will detect the enlarged liver and ascites; peripheral edema may or may not be evident.[12–14] The venous pressure is much elevated with prominent "v" wave and brisk "y" descent, and Kussmaul's sign is present. There is the usual sinus tachycardia of heart failure, and pericardial effusion and central cyanosis may be present.

A physical sign that may be of some help in differentiating restrictive disease from constrictive pericarditis is a palpably displaced left ventricular impulse—a less likely finding in the constrictive syndrome. Also, the S3 of restrictive CMP is best heard at the apex, whereas in constrictive pericarditis it is best appreciated at the left lower sternal border.[14]

Prognosis is poor, but some symptomatic patients have lived for more than a decade.[12]

HYPERTROPHIC CARDIOMYOPATHY

This form of CMP has been dealt with in Chapter 20.

SPECIFIC CARDIOMYOPATHIES

Although many of the secondary, or specific, CMPs will require endomyocardial biopsy for definitive diagnosis, many present certain clinical clues that may suggest the correct diagnosis.

Alcoholic

Doubt has been expressed that alcoholic CMP is a distinct entity. Some have held the opinion that the cardiac involvement in alcoholics is the result of the malnutrition that often accompanies the excessive intake of alcohol, rather than an effect of alcohol itself. Others have noted the possibility that the commonly associated nicotine addiction is at least a contributing factor.

Complete recovery, however, from the ravages of CMP after a period of total abstinence from alcohol without any other form of therapy[15,16] affords evidence that it is a specific entity; and a report from Moscow—where sudden death is surprisingly common in alcoholics—claims that there is an identifiable complex of microscopic myocardial changes specific for alcoholic CMP.[17] The condition is quite distinct from beri-beri: It is unresponsive to thiamine, and is characterized by low cardiac output with high peripheral resistance. In making the diagnosis in a patient with a history of alcoholism, the exclusion of all other causes of CMP is all-important.

No one knows how much alcohol is needed to damage the myocardium—and if there is a toxic threshold it will obviously vary greatly from individual to individual—but it has been suggested that about a pint of spirit a day for perhaps 10 years will achieve injury to the heart muscle.[18] Far from affecting only "skid row" types, the patient is often an overweight man, successful enough to support his spirituous proclivity; some of the patients are, indeed, well-to-do, martini-sodden executives.

It is crucial to make the diagnosis at an early stage of the disease before extensive, irreversible damage to the myocardium has taken place, because, at the early stage, complete abstention from alcohol can effect a complete cure. The first symptom is likely to be palpitations associated with paroxysmal atrial fibrillation. Fatigability and mild breathlessness are at first attributed to his overweight; but as time passes, the shortness of breath intensifies, and paroxysmal nocturnal dyspnea and the full-blown picture of congestive heart failure may appear. Cough and hemoptysis are occasional complaints. Evans[18] categorically states that chest pain does not result from alcoholic CMP; whereas in patients with dilated, idiopathic CMP, chest pain, indistinguishable from angina, is a presenting symptom in 10%.

Physical findings much depend on the stage at which the disease is seen. There may be no abnormal signs, or the irregular cardiac rhythm of atrial fibrillation or frequent extrasystoles may be present. Both prolonged exposure to and acute intake of excessive alcohol can precipitate atrial fibrillation.[18–20] In the florid stage of CMP, the most common findings are cardiomegaly and an S3 gallop, both of which were present in 100% of a Chicago series of 57 patients.[16] Rales were present in 96%, an S4 gallop in 82%, edema in 70%, and an enlarged liver in 58% of the same series. Murmurs are much less common: pansystolic apical murmurs were heard in only 23%, and ejection murmurs in 19%.[16] And, in fact, the relative inconspicuousness of murmurs in the presence of impressive cardiomegaly is an important tip-off to CMP.

Amyloid

Amyloid affects men more often than women, and is the most common cause of *restrictive* cardiomyopathy encountered in the Western world[21]; most patients are over 50 years. In the Mayo Clinic series of 153 patients with systemic amyloidosis, 41 (27%) had overt CMP.[22] Fatigue is the commonest early symptom, sometimes accompanied by a dramatic loss of weight—one patient in the Mayo series lost 50 lbs in 4 months.[22] Two other usefully suggestive findings are the carpal tunnel syndrome, which is generally bilateral, and purpura, especially of the upper thorax, neck, and face, with a special predilection for the upper eyelid—in which case the petechiae are visible only when the eyes are closed. In a few cases a clue to the presence of amyloid disease may be enlargement of the tongue (macroglossia).

Edema is the most common physical finding in amyloidosis, which may be secondary to a nephrotic syndrome or to the heart failure that insidiously develops. Extensive involvement of the myocardium takes place before there is significant dyspnea or clinically detectable cardiomegaly.[22] As infiltration of the myocardium proceeds, the symptoms and signs of congestive failure progress. Once overt congestive failure develops, survival is brief, usually only a matter of months.[22]

If infiltration affects the ventricular septum disproportionately, hypertrophic CMP may be simulated.

Hemochromatosis

The CMP of hemochromatosis is usually hereditary, affects two or three individuals per 1000 of the general population,[23] and over 90% of them are men. Less often it results from repeated blood transfusions, and rarely from long-term medication with oral iron preparations or from a portal-to-systemic venous shunt.

CMP represents a distressingly late stage of a once curable disease. But even after symptoms of heart failure have developed, some improvement can be expected with appropriate therapy; therefore, early diagnosis is important both to initiate effective treatment and to screen family members, especially siblings, who are most at risk.

The initial symptom is often arthralgia,[24] but the earliest indication may be symptoms or signs of hepatic or cardiac dysfunction, or the discovery of glycosuria. Cardiac arrhythmias are common, especially atrial tachycardia and atrial fibrillation:[3]

It is an often overlooked diagnosis; in the words of the Mayo authors, "it lurks unrecognized among patients with diabetes mellitus, congestive heart failure, idiopathic cardiomyopathy, rheumatoid arthritis, alcoholic cirrhosis, or hypogonadism."[23] Clearly, hemochromatosis should be considered in the differential diagnosis in the presence of any of these diseases.

In its florid stages hemochromatosis is easily recognized by the simultaneous involvement of four organs: skin, liver, pancreas, and heart, with resulting bronze pigmentation, cirrhosis, diabetes, and congestive failure. Hepatocellular carcinoma complicates about one-third of patients with advanced disease.[23]

Peripartum

This form of CMP affects youngish (obviously) black (usually) women; most of them are in their fourth rather than third decade, and are multiparas.[25] The diagnosis is made if congestive heart failure develops during the third trimester or within 3 months of giving birth; if there has been no evidence of heart disease before the pregnancy; and if there is no recognizable cause for the failure.

Symptoms begin within the first 3 months after giving birth in 80% of patients, but in about 10% the onset is even later, and in the remaining 10% symptoms begin during the third trimester of the pregnancy.[26] Although the role of pregnancy and other factors in initiating the disease remains obscure, a report from London suggests that an occult myocarditis may play the underlying pathogenetic role in some cases.[27]

Since this is yet another form of dilated CMP, symptoms and signs are similar to those of other types, and the reported incidence in two series[28,29] is presented in Table 34-3. There appears to be a

Table 34–3
Reported Frequency of Symptoms and Signs in Peripartum Cardiomyopathy

	Burch[28] (34)*	Demakis[29] (27)*
Symptoms		
Dyspnea on exertion	34	20
Orthopnea	30	19
Edema	26	—
Cough	25	19
Paroxysmal nocturnal dyspnea	23	22
Weakness	17	—
Palpitation	13	2
Ascites	8	—
Chest pain	8	13
Hemoptysis	7	7
Abdominal pain	6	13
Signs		
Cardiomegaly	34	27
Mitral regurgitation	20	4
Third sound gallop	19	27
Edema	17	13
Hepatomegaly	17	—
Accentuated P2	14	—
Rales	11	—
Distended jugular veins	9	—
Arrhythmias	9	—

*Number of patients.

higher incidence of pleuritic pain and hemoptysis than in most other forms of CMP. In the Chicago series, half the patients had chest pain.[29]

Sarcoidosis

Most victims of cardiac sarcoidosis develop symptoms between the ages of 15 and 40; in the United States it is at least ten times as common in blacks as in whites, and among blacks it shows a definite predilection for women.[30] Autopsy evidence reveals that the heart is invaded in about one-quarter of sarcoid cases, but most of these are clinically silent, and only about 5% develop symptomatic CMP.[31] Interestingly, when the heart is significantly involved, there is usually little or no involvement of other organs; therefore one cannot depend on visible lesions in the skin, eyes, or lymph nodes to tip one off to the invisible involvement of the heart. A corollary of this is that when a patient with known and obvious sarcoid develops cardiac symptoms, you cannot confidently attribute them to sarcoid involvement of the heart. In fact, Roberts goes so far as to say that when there is evident involvement of other organs, you can predict that there will probably be no clinical CMP.[32]

Ventricular muscle is more often and more heavily invaded than atrial, and ventricular arrhythmias are more common than atrial; in fact, the most common presentation of sarcoid CMP is ventricular tachycardia. The possibility of sarcoid CMP should be entertained in any young person with unexplained cardiac dysfunction, especially heart failure or ventricular tachycardia.[33]

When sarcoid granulomas occupy the myocardium, they appear to have a liking for the upper part of the ventricular septum[32]; they therefore quite often produce A-V block by destroying the A-V node and bundle. Sudden death ends the sarcoid scene in up to two-thirds of patients, and it may be the initial manifestation of cardiac sarcoidosis.[32]

CMP may be of either dilated or restrictive variety. Congestive heart failure may be secondary to the CMP or to associated pulmonary involvement (cor pulmonale). Severe mitral regurgitation may result from invasion of the papillary muscles and their consequent dysfunction. The pericardium is seldom involved, but pericardial syndromes have occasionally been described—bloody effusion, tamponade, and constrictive pericarditis. Ventricular aneurysms complicate about 10% of patients with sarcoid CMP.[34]

REFERENCES

General

1. Report of the WHO/ISFC task force on the definition and classification of cardiomyopathies. Br Heart J 1980;44:672.
2. Goodwin JF. The frontiers of cardiomyopathy. Br Heart J 1982;48:1.
3. Wenger NK, et al. Cardiomyopathy and specific heart muscle disease. In: Hurst JW, ed. The heart, ed 7. New York: McGraw Hill, 1990:1278–1347.
4. Shabetai R. Cardiomyopathy: how far have we come in 25 years, how far yet to go? J Am Coll Cardiol 1983; 1:252.

5. Segal JP, et al. Idiopathic cardiomyopathy: clinical features, prognosis and therapy. Curr Probl Cardiol 1978; 3:9.

Dilated

6. Goodwin JF, et al. Clinical aspects of cardiomyopathy. Br Med J 1961;1:69.
7. Goodwin JF. Cardiac function in primary myocardial disorders. Br Med J 1964;1:1527 and 1595.
8. Massumi RA, et al. Primary myocardial disease: report of 50 cases and review of the subject. Circulation 1965;31:19.
9. Fuster V, et al. The natural history of idiopathic dilated cardiomyopathy. Am J Cardiol 1981;47:525.

Restrictive/Obliterative

10. Goodwin, JF, Oakley CM. The cardiomyopathies. Br Heart J 1972;34:545.
11. Olsen EGJ, Spry CJF. Relation between eosinophilia and endomyocardial disease. Prog Cardiovasc Dis 1985;27:241.
12. Siegel RJ, et al. Idiopathic restrictive cardiomyopathy. Circulation 1984;70:165.
13. Benotti JR, et al. Clinical profile of restrictive cardiomyopathy. Circulation 1980;61:1206.
14. Chew CYC, et al. Primary restrictive cardiomyopathy: non-tropical endomyocardial fibrosis and hypereosinophilic heart disease. Br Heart J 1977;39:399.

Alcoholic

15. Schwartz L, et al. Severe alcoholic cardiomyopathy reversed with abstention from alcohol. Am J Cardiol 1975;36:963.
16. Demakis JG, et al. The natural course of alcoholic cardiomyopathy. Ann Intern Med 1974;80:293.
17. Vikhert AM, et al. Alcoholic cardiomyopathy and sudden cardiac death. The fourth US/USSR symposium on sudden cardiac death. J Am Coll Cardiol 1986;8(supp A):3.
18. Evans W. Alcoholic myocardiopathy. Prog Cardiovasc Dis 1964;7:151.
19. Burch GE, DePasquale NP. Alcoholic cardiomyopathy. Am J Cardiol 1969;23:723.
20. Koskinen P, et al. Alcohol and new onset atrial fibrillation: a case-control study of a current series. Br Heart J 1987;57:468.

Amyloid

21. Swanton RH, et al. Systolic and diastolic ventricular function in cardiac amyloidosis: studies in six cases diagnosed with endomyocardial biopsy. Am J Cardiol 1977; 39:658.
22. Gertz MA, Kyle RA. Primary systemic amyloidosis: a diagnostic primer. Mayo Clin Proc 1989;64:1505.

Hemochromatosis

23. Fairbanks VF, Baldus WP. Hemochromatosis: the neglected diagnosis. Mayo Clin Proc 1986;61:296.
24. Niederau C, et al. Survival and causes of death in cirrhotic and in noncirrhotic patients with primary hemochromatosis. N Engl J Med 1985;313:1262.

Peripartum

25. Walsh JJ, et al. Idiopathic myocardiopathy of the puerperium (postpartal heart disease). Circulation 1965;32:19.
26. Julian DG, Szekely P. Peripartum cardiomyopathy. Prog Cardiovasc Dis 1985;27:223.
27. Melvin KR, et al. Peripartum cardiomyopathy due to myocarditis. N Engl J Med 1982;307:731.
28. Burch GE, et al. The effect of prolonged bed rest on postpartal cardiomyopathy. Am Heart J 1971;81:186.
29. Demakis JG, et al. Natural course of peripartum cardiomyopathy. Circulation 1971;44:1053.

Sarcoidosis

30. Braunstein MS. Sarcoidosis. Compr Ther 1986;12:36.
31. Silverman KJ, et al. Cardiac sarcoid: a clinicopathologic study of 84 unselected patients with systemic sarcoidosis. Circulation 1978;58:1204.
32. Roberts WC, et al. Sarcoidosis of the heart: a clinicopathologic study of 35 necropsy patients (Group I) and review of 78 previously described necropsy patients (Group II). Am J Med 1977;63:86.
33. Lemery R, et al. Cardiac sarcoidosis: a potentially treatable form of myocarditis. Mayo Clin Proc 1985;60: 549.
34. Wilkins CE, et al. Cardiac sarcoidosis: two cases with ventricular tachycardia and review of cardiac involvement in sarcoid. Texas Heart Institute Journal 1985;12:377.

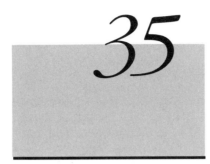

Infective Endocarditis

The clinical picture of infective endocarditis has changed dramatically over the past several decades. Thirty or 40 years ago, most infections were caused by *Streptococcus viridans* engrafted on already diseased rheumatic valves or congenital deformities; but today, as often as not, a more aggressive microbe attacks previously normal valves. And although one may still see the "subacute" form as typified by a smoldering infection hosted by a patient with mitral regurgitation, or the acute form typified by a *Staphylococcus aureus* infection rapidly destroying an incompetent (or previously normal) aortic valve, most infections nowadays mount an intermediate attack.[1] Of course, rheumatic valves and congenital defects are still susceptible to microbial invasion, but they account for a smaller proportion of cases; the most susceptible congenital lesions are patent ductus arteriosus, ventricular septal defect, and tetralogy of Fallot; atrial defects are seldom involved.[2]

Of 145 patients with infective endocarditis reported from Birmingham, England, between 1973 and 1986, only 31 (21%) had previous rheumatic disease, and 81 (55%) had no previous cardiac involvement.[1] The *viridans* streptococcus was the invading organism in 81 (55%) and the *aureus* staphylococcus in 31 (21%). This prevalence appears to hold true on both sides of the Atlantic, as the Mayo experience[3] also finds 75% caused by streptococci and staphylococci. Although *viridans* infections accounted for only 38% of endocarditides in the 1970s, compared with 53% in the 1950s, there is probably no reduction in the total number of such infections; the average number of patients with endocarditis seen at the Mayo clinic increased from 24.5 per year in the 1950s to 39 in the 1970s, and the reduction in the *viridans* percentage is undoubtedly due to the increase in infection by a variety of other organisms—at least in part the result of the burgeoning use of intravascular prostheses and invasive systems, and the proliferation of illicit intravenous drug abuse. The categories into which cases fell in one series[4] are indicated in Table 35-1.

Table 35–1
Hosts of Infective Endocarditis

Native Valve: Drug user	4%
Nondrug user	53%
Prosthetic Valve: Early	6%
Late	37%
	100%

CLINICAL FINDINGS

Because of the former tendency to affect patients with rheumatic or congenital heart disease, most patients were in their first four decades, but nowadays peak incidence is in the sixth decade,[1,3,4] and the disease is quite common in elderly subjects.

In the Texas Heart Institute series of 94 patients seen between 1983 and 1989, there were four times as many men as women.[4] The onset is usually insidious with *viridans* and enterococcal infection, but may be abrupt with an embolic episode; the onset is fulminant if the invaders are staphylococcal.

The first step in diagnosis is a lively suspicion awakened by any febrile patient with a cardiac murmur. Hemiplegia in a young person,[5] or any of the attendant circumstances listed in Table 35-2 should lead you to consider the possibility of infective endocarditis.

Although dental manipulations have long been thought of as the archetype of precipitating causes, in the Hammersmith experience of 544 cases, dental procedures within 3 months of the onset were identifiable in only 13.7%.[6] Poor dental hygiene is probably more dangerous than manipulation, and genitourinary and gastrointestinal procedures are no less important than tooth extraction as a source of infection.[7]

The ways in which infective endocarditis can present are legion (Table 35-2). In the more insidious cases, vague symptoms, such as low-grade fever and malaise, may persist for weeks or months before diagnosis.[8] There may be night sweats, weight loss, and anorexia, with the gradual development of clubbing of fingers and toes, splenomegaly, and peripheral signs including splinter hemorrhages, Roth spots, Osler nodes, and Jane-

Table 35–2
Protean Potential Presentations of Infective Endocarditis

A. General: Malaise, anorexia, weight loss, pallor, fever night sweats

B. Cardiac: Murmur, heart failure, pericardial rub or effusion, myocardial infarction

C. Pulmonary: Pleuritis, hemoptysis, clubbing, pulmonary edema

D. Ophthalmic: Sudden blindness, homonymous hemianopia, eyelid petechiae, Roth spots

E. Neurologic: Hemiplegia, aphasia, headache, ataxia, mental changes

F. Renal: Proteinuria, hematuria, hypertensive crisis

G. Orthopedic: Backache, osteomyelitis, arthritis

H. Peripheral vascular: Splinter hemorrhages, Osler's nodes, Janeway's lesions

I. Immunologic: Arthralgia, myalgia, tenosynovitis

way lesions; but all of these once fashionable signs are now relatively uncommon.[2] In this connection, it is crucial to appreciate the fact that, in the absence of infection, petechiae in the conjunctiva develop in more than half the patients undergoing cardiac surgery with cardiopulmonary bypass.[9] Moreover, splinter hemorrhages are more common in the general hospital population than in patients with infective endocarditis.[2]

Cerebral emboli are not uncommon, and stroke or sudden blindness (from embolus to the central artery of retina) may be the initiating event. Other presentations not especially suggestive of infection include backache, hematuria, congestive heart failure, myocardial infarction (from embolus to a coronary artery), and hypertensive crisis.[10]

Expected findings are sometimes conspicuous by their absence; for example, in the Texas series,[4] 17% had no fever, and 28% had no cardiac murmur, no congestive heart failure, and no embolic episodes. Of an aggregate of 560 cases[11-14] reported from four centers between 1961 and 1966, fever was reported in 98% to 100%, cardiac murmur in 60% to 99%, petechiae in 40% to 70%, splenomegaly in 34% to 53%, and clubbing in 12% to 24%. In a comparable series in the 1990s there is no doubt that the incidence of each of these helpful clinical findings would be significantly less.

Table 35–3
Circumstances Predisposing to Endocarditis

1. Previous infective endocarditis
2. Previous valve surgery
3. Congenital heart disease
4. Rheumatic heart disease
5. Dental procedures; poor oral hygiene
6. Genitourinary manipulations
7. Gastrointestinal procedures
8. Diabetes mellitus
9. Advanced age
10. Intravenous drug abuse
11. Chronic alcoholism
12. Immunosuppressive drugs or steroid

Despite potent and proliferating antibiotics combined with aggressive surgery, mortality remains high at 30% to 40%, and the most common cause is congestive heart failure.[5] The disease is more often fatal when it affects a previously normal valve.[15]

In summary, clinical suspicion is the best, single diagnostic tool. Friedberg is reputed to have commented that any person over 50 years of age who did not feel well should be suspected of having infective endocarditis! One must recognize the patient at risk (ie, the prevalence of any of the circumstances listed in Table 35-3). Eloquent testimony to the difficulty of making the diagnosis — or reluctance to suspect it? — is the fact that of the 18 patients in the Birmingham series who died, 12 were first recognized postmortem. This represents little or no improvement over the diagnostic record of decades past, when, for example, of 96 autopsied patients, the diagnosis was overlooked before death in 70%.[16]

Among intravenous drug abusers, acute endocarditis is especially common. Men are three times as often affected as women, and the average age at presentation is 29 years,[17] compared with an average age in the 50s for all infective endocarditis. The infection most often attacks the previously normal tricuspid valve and leads to pulmonary embolism, abscess, or pneumonia. It is a mistake, however, to think of the valve lesions in addicts as confined to the right side[5]; about half the patients with tricuspid involvement develop infection of left-sided valves as well.[15]

In 60% to 70% of patients with tricuspid valve involvement, there may be no murmur; and in the absence of pulmonary hypertension, the regurgitant murmur is usually not pansystolic.[18] In the absence of a tricuspid murmur, an atrial gallop that intensifies with inspiration may afford a valuable clue.[10]

PROSTHETIC VALVE ENDOCARDITIS

Infections involving prosthetic valves develop in about 2% to 4% of implants[19,20] and are classified into early and late, but the dividing line is unsettled. The "early" cases (usually staphylococcal[19,21] and fulminating) develop symptoms within 2,[5,22] 3,[4] or 4 months[21] of valve surgery and are presumed to represent infection implanted at the time of surgery. A frequent nidus has been staphylococcal infection of the transected sternum[21]; in many cases the culprit may be a postoperative indwelling catheter rather than contamination at the time of operation. The "late" cases (usually streptococcal[19,21] and less severe) develop symptoms after 2 to 4 months, and are assumed to be due to "seeding" by dental extractions or some other source of bacteremia. If native valve endocarditis has previously affected the implantation site, the risk of developing prosthetic valve endocarditis is increased five-fold; other risk factors, in descending order of importance, are being black, having a mechanical rather than homograft valve, and being male.[20]

As in other forms of endocarditis, the most important first step in diagnosis is a towering suspicion of anyone with a prosthetic valve and a fever. Fever, as one would expect, is present in almost all cases, but when coagulase-negative staphylococci are the invaders, absence of pyrexia is not unusual.[4] A diminution in the intensity of opening or closing prosthetic sounds may be an early clue to the presence of an infected valve.[10]

New or changing regurgitant murmurs are present in only about half the cases, and petechiae, splenomegaly, and emboli — of which cerebral are most common — in about one-third. Roth spots, Janeway lesions, and Osler's nodes are uncommon. Septic shock is not unknown.[22] About three-quarters of the early cases and almost half of the late cases are fatal.[19]

REFERENCES

1. Bain RJI, et al. The clinical and echocardiographic diagnosis of infective endocarditis. J Antimicrob Chemother 1987;20(Suppl A):17.
2. Weinstein L, Rubin RH. Infective endocarditis: 1973. Prog Cardiovasc Dis 1973;16:239.
3. Brandenburg RO, et al. Infective endocarditis: a 25 year overview of diagnosis and therapy. J Am Coll Cardiol 1983;1:280.
4. Gentry LO, Khoshdel A. New approach to the diagnosis and treatment of infective endocarditis. Texas Heart Institute Journal 1989;16:250.
5. Reid CL, et al. Infective endocarditis: improved diagnosis and treatment. Curr Probl Cardiol 1985;10:6.
6. Bayliss R, et al. The teeth and infective endocarditis. Br Heart J 1983;50:506.
7. Bayliss R, et al. The microbiology and pathogenesis of infective endocarditis. Br Heart J 1983;50:513.
8. MacGregor JS, Cheitlin MD. Diagnosis and management of infective endocarditis. Texas Heart Institute Journal 1989;16:240.
9. Willerson JT, et al. Conjunctival petechiae after open-heart surgery. N Engl J Med 1971;284:539.
10. Applefeld MM, Woodward TE. Infective endocarditis: a clinical overview. Curr Probl Cardiol 1977;2:7.
11. Pankey GA. Subacute bacterial endocarditis at the University of Minnesota Hospital, 1939 through 1959. Ann Intern Med 1961;55: 550.
12. Vogler WR, et al. Bacterial endocarditis: a review of 148 cases. Am J Med 1962;32:910.
13. Guze LB, Pearce ML. Hospital acquired bacterial endocarditis. Arch Intern Med 1963;112:102.
14. Rabinovich S, et al. A long-term view of bacterial endocarditis: 337 cases 1924 to 1963. Ann Intern Med 1965; 63:185.
15. Roberts WC: Editorial comment. Curr Probl Cardiol 1977; 2:11.
16. Cooper ES, et al. Pitfalls in the diagnosis of bacterial endocarditis. Arch Intern Med 1966;118:55.
17. Reisberg BE. Infective endocarditis in the narcotic addict. Prog Cardiovasc Dis 1979;22:193.
18. O'Rourke RA. Editorial comment. Curr Probl Cardiol 1977;2:16.
19. Wilson WR, et al. Prosthetic valve endocarditis. Proc Mayo Clin 1982;57:155.
20. Ivert TSA, et al. Prosthetic valve endocarditis. Circulation 1984;69:223.
21. Moore-Gillon J, et al. Prosthetic valve endocarditis. Br Med J 1983;287:739.
22. Cogwill LD, et al. Prosthetic valve endocarditis. Curr Probl Cardiol 1986;11:623.

Pericardial Disease

PERICARDITIS

Pericardial disease is often overlooked, yet accurate diagnosis is important since "treatment for pericarditis of one cause may be useless or dangerous in another."[1] Once again, the most important step in diagnosis is to think of it in the appropriate clinical setting. The causes of pericarditis and/or effusion are legion; for an exhaustive listing, see Spodick's review.[2] Some of the important causes are presented in Table 36-1.

Of 403 Mayo patients with pericarditis, the etiologic breakdown was as follows[11]:

Acute nonspecific, 67%
  Without effusion, 44%
  With effusion, 23%
Chronic, 23%
  Constrictive, 20%
  Calcific, 3%
Chronic effusive, 3%
Postmyocardial infarction, 2%
Radiation, 2%
Rheumatoid, 2%
Tuberculous, 1%

This distribution compares with a Spanish series of 231 consecutive patients admitted to a cardiology service in Barcelona: 199 (86%) were acute idiopathic, 13 (6%) were neoplastic, and nine (4%) tuberculous; in addition, purulent, toxoplasmosis, viral, rheumatic fever, and collagen vascular disease accounted for two (1%) each.[12]

The incidence in children differs: Purulent, rheumatic, and rheumatoid disease together accounted for more than half of 32 children with acute pericarditis.[13]

In acute myocardial infarction, a pericardial rub develops in about 10% of cases, usually on the second or third day.[14,15] Patients with rubs have a higher incidence of complications, such as congestive failure and arrhythmias, but apparently no higher mortality. It is important to recognize the development of pericardial friction, because the administration of anticoagulants in the presence of a rub may invite the development of hemopericardium and contribute to a fatal outcome.[14,15]

The close similarity between the clinical features and steroid response of acute "idiopathic"

Table 36–1
Causes of Pericarditis and/or Effusion

Idiopathic
Still the largest group, though many are probably due to unidentified viruses,[3] lupus[4], etc.

Infective
Bacterial: pyogenic; tuberculous (note that onset of symptoms is often acute); etc.
Viral: Cocksackie A & B[5]; influenza A & B[6]; herpes[7]; infectious mononucleosis[8]; etc.
Fungal: histoplasmosis[9]; toxoplasmosis; etc.
Protozoal: amebiasis[10]

Connective Tissue
Rheumatic fever; lupus erythematosus; rheumatoid arthritis; etc.

Hypersensitivity
Serum sickness; drug reactions; postpericardiotomy; postmyocardial infarction; etc.

Metabolic
Uremia; cholesterol pericarditis; myxedema; etc.

Malignant
Metastatic; mesothelioma

Traumatic
Including surgery, catheterization, etc.

pericarditis, the postpericardiotomy syndrome,[16] the postmyocardial infarction syndrome, and the syndrome that may follow traumatic hemopericardium[17] is striking, and suggests that they all represent autoimmune reactions to products of pericardial injury.

Acute Pericarditis

Symptoms may be attributed to either the inflammatory process or to the effects of the effusion. Fever is accompanied by retrosternal pain, which can range from trivial to severe. It may be constant or intermittent, and it may radiate to the neck, the jaw, shoulders, or arms, and sometimes to the back or abdomen. The pain is aggravated by movement, swallowing, and deep inspiration, which may result in splinted breathing; it is often relieved by leaning forward. On occasion, it may imitate the pain of myocardial infarction to perfection.[18] Cough may be troublesome, and the patient may complain of difficulty in swallowing.

The effusion may result in distention of veins in the neck, face, and arms, and the patient may complain of dyspnea and orthopnea with associated fatigue, weakness, and even fainting spells.

Preeminent among the *signs* attributable to the inflammatory process is, of course, the characteristic pericardial rub, supposedly caused by friction between the two layers of inflamed pericardium—though it may persist in the presence of significant effusion. In fact, at least one study has shown no correlation between the size of the effusion and the presence or absence of an associated rub[19]: Audible friction was present in four of 13 patients with small effusions, 23 of 40 with moderate-sized effusions, and in ten of 23 with large.

The rub is characteristically scratchy, creaking, scraping, or grating and superficial; and increasing pressure with the listening diaphragm may make it louder. It is usually triphasic,[20] producing an unmistakable triple cadence, correlating with atrial systole and ventricular systole and diastole (Fig. 36-1). Less often it is diphasic, producing a to-and-fro cadence, when it is usually due to atrial and then ventricular systole; less often the diphasic rub coincides with ventricular systole and diastole. Occasionally it is only monophasic, and then is almost always associated with ventricular systole, rarely with atrial systole. Some of the to-and-fro rubs are potentially triphasic, but acoustically diphasic, because atrial systole and early ventricular diastole have overlapped, thanks to either tachycardia or a prolonged A-V conduction time (P–R interval). An atrial diastolic rub[21] is audible only in the presence of A-V block (Fig. 36-1). The rub often can be felt, especially in uremic pericarditis, as a superficial to-and-fro thrill; it was palpable in 23% of 100 consecutive patients with pericardial friction.[20]

In the same series of 100 patients, the rub was triphasic in more than half, diphasic in a third, and monophasic in 15%. Altogether, a rub was heard in ventricular systole in 99 of the 100 patients, in atrial systole in 69, and in ventricular diastole in 59. You will see that this reported audibility accords well with the relative intensity of the rub in each phase if you look at Figure 36-1: Of the three commonly heard rubs, the loudest and longest is ventricular systolic,[1] next loudest is atrial systolic,[3] and softest is ventricular diastolic.[2]

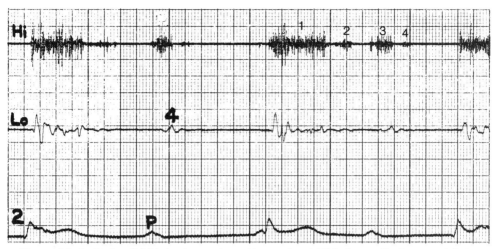

Figure 36–1. Pericardial friction in a patient with complete A-V block complicating acute inferior infarction. In the high-frequency tracing (Hi), the four phases of the rub are labeled as follows: 1, ventricular systolic; 2, ventricular diastolic; 3, atrial systolic; and 4, atrial diastolic. In the low-frequency tracing, 4 represents the atrial sound (S4). Note that the rubs in order of decreasing loudness are 1, 3, 2, and 4. (Reproduced with permission from Marriott HJL. Bedside recognition of cardiac arrhythmias. Geriatrics 1975;30:55.)

Pericardial friction is usually heard best with the diaphragm pressed firmly at the left sternal border as the patient leans forward. Sometimes inspiration makes it louder: In nine of 16 cases, the rub was louder or audible only during inspiration.[22] In the presence of effusion, the rub may be heard only with the patient lying supine in full inspiration. Occasionally the rub may be loudest at the apex or at the right sternal border.

When the rub is typically triphasic, the diagnosis is unequivocal, but when it is diphasic it may be mistaken for to-and-fro aortic murmurs. When it is monophasic, it has to be differentiated from various systolic murmurs, and from a mediastinal "crunch"—Hamman's sign of mediastinal emphysema. A very real trap is the artifact of moist skin, rhythmically with each heart beat, peeling off the diaphragm of the stethoscope to produce a creaking sound; this deception can be rapidly excluded, however, by substituting the bell.

When pleural effusion complicates pericarditis, it tends to be left-sided in contrast with the right-sided tendency in congestive heart failure (see Chapter 38); among 35 patients, it was exclusively left-sided in 21, and in four others it was larger on the left than the right.[23]

Many observers have claimed that pericarditis spawns arrhythmias, but a study by Holter monitoring of 49 consecutive patients with acute pericarditis failed to establish a causal relationship.[24] A significant arrhythmia complicating acute pericarditis, therefore, suggests the presence of underlying heart disease.

Pericardial Effusion and Cardiac Tamponade

The accumulating effusion leads to signs of cardiac embarrassment and compression—"tamponade." If the fluid accumulates gradually, the elastic pericardium can accommodate a liter or two without serious embarrassment of cardiac function; but if it accumulates rapidly—as with rupture of a dissecting aneurysm and consequent hemopericardium—as little as 150 mL can produce fatal compression in a few minutes.[25]

The classic quartet of tamponade consists of tachycardia, hypotension, pulsus paradoxus, and jugular vein distention. The paradoxical pulse can be most helpful in diagnosis; it was present in 55 of 56 patients with tamponade.[26] But it may be absent in various circumstances: With left ventricular hypertrophy, severe left ventricular failure, or severe aortic regurgitation[27]; or in the presence of a large atrial septal defect[28]; and in the presence of severe hypovolemia, neither pulsus paradoxus nor jugular distention may appear.[29] On the other hand, pulsus paradoxus is found in conditions other than pericardial effusion, including pulmonary embolism,[30] and any restrictive myocardial disease.

The patient may squat, or lean forward on a hugged pillow ("pillow sign"—Blechmann, 1922), or emulate the Mohamedan in prayer (Hirtz, 1911). Venous engorgement without inspiratory collapse results, sometimes with paradoxical inspiratory filling (Kussmaul's sign); and this may be accompanied by pulsus paradoxus (Chapter 4). The apical impulse is often impalpable and the heart sounds faint; but a strong impulse and/or loud sounds do not exclude effusion. You may suspect effusion if the heart sounds are louder with the patient on his back (supine) than when he lies face down (prone).[31]

Dressler[32] described a flat percussion note over the lower half of the sternum, sometimes extending into the 3rd left interspace and/or into the right 5th, 4th, and even 3rd interspaces. Dullness in the 5th right interspace is Rotch's sign (1878). A patch of dullness, bronchial breathing and bronchophony below the angle of the left scapula (Ewart's sign, 1896) is due to posterior displacement of the heart compressing the lung and bronchi.[33] The pericardial knock (Chapter 13), characteristic of constrictive pericarditis, is sometimes heard with effusion, resulting from the abrupt check to cardiac relaxation by the enveloping fluid.

Chronic pericardial effusion can persist for years without classic signs. The tip-off is a huge heart with relatively mild cardiac embarrassment[34]: "When the heart is too big for the symptoms, suspect chronic pericardial effusion or Ebstein's disease."

Constrictive Pericarditis

The diagnosis of constrictive pericarditis (CP), frequently referred to as Pick's disease (1896), is important for three reasons: (1) it is potentially curable in many cases by surgical stripping; (2) it is easily mistaken for a number of more common clinical entities, including congestive heart failure and cirrhosis of the liver; and (3) careful attention to the physical examination may be as diagnostic as sophisticated imaging studies.[35]

The causes of CP are listed in Table 36-2. Vir-

Table 36–2
Causes of Constrictive Pericarditis

Infective
  a. Nonspecific (?viral)
  b. Tuberculosis[36]
  c. Purulent
  d. Histoplasmosis[37]
Traumatic
  a. Postcardiac surgery[38]
  b. Postpacemaker implantation[39,40]
Connective tissue
  a. Lupus erythematosus[41]
  b. Rheumatoid[42]
Postirradiation[43]
Neoplastic
Uremic[44]
Methysergide therapy[45]
Mulibrey nanism
Idiopathic

tually any acute involvement of the pericardium may eventuate in CP. In the 1940s and 1950s, undoubtedly the most common cause was tuberculosis,[36] but in the succeeding decades tuberculosis has yielded first place; nowadays, nonspecific (probably viral) pericarditis, rheumatoid, and traumatic pericarditis are more common precursors than tuberculous. Constrictive pericarditis following cardiac surgery is uncommon; it complicated only 11 of over 5000 consecutive operations, developing between 2 weeks and 6 months after surgery.[38] Less common are lupus erythematosus, irradiation, idiopathic pericarditis, and histoplasmosis. An exotic cause is mulibrey* nanism, a dwarfism that seems mainly to affect patients of Finnish origin.

The patient may appear relatively healthy, though virtually all suffer from some degree of dyspnea. A few may present with chest pain, fever, and night sweats.[42] There is usually a distended abdomen, and distended neck veins with abnormal venous pulse showing a sharp "y" descent with deep trough (Friedreich's sign, 1864), and paradoxical venous filling with inspiration

---

*An acronym composed of the first two letters of the tissues mainly affected: MUscle LIver BRain EYe.

Table 36–3
Differentiation Between Constrictive Pericarditis and Cardiomyopathy (CMP)

	CP	CMP
Pulsus paradoxus	+	0
Giant "a" wave	0	+
Dominant "x" descent	+	0
Atrial fibrillation	+	(+)
LV impulse	0	+
MR or TR	0	+
Third sound	Earlier	Later
Hydrothorax	+	0

LV, left ventricular; MR, mitral regurgitation; TR, tricuspid regurgitation.

(Kussmaul's sign). There is a convincing arterial pulsus paradoxus in about one-third of the patients, though some find it rarely,[46] and a tendency to low blood pressure and pulse pressure, though most readings are within normal range.[36] Atrial arrhythmias are common, and the combination of two distinct negative troughs ("x" and "y") in the jugular pulse in the presence of atrial fibrillation at once suggests the diagnosis.

A definable cardiac impulse is almost always absent. The second sound may show a peculiar pattern of splitting[47]: An abrupt, momentary, wide splitting at the onset of inspiration due to precocious aortic valve closure because of the decreased left ventricular ejection—a finding that may suggest the diagnosis even in the absence of a pericardial knock. The early diastolic sound—the pericardial "knock"—is presumably caused by the abrupt cessation to rapid ventricular filling imposed by the constricting encasement,[46,48] and occurs 0.09 to 0.12 second after A2. Nitroglycerin eliminates the knock, whereas squatting and phenylephrine bring it out.[49] With severe constriction there may be no knock and marked venous distention with abrupt systolic "x" descent.[50] Some patients may develop diastolic murmurs, and tricuspid stenosis may be imitated.[51] An enlarged liver and spleen, ascites, and edema complete the picture.

Clues for differentiation from restrictive cardiomyopathy are listed in Table 36-3; keep in mind, however, that the physical signs of chronic constrictive pericarditis do not always separate it from other forms of heart disease causing congestive failure.[52]

REFERENCES

Acute Pericarditis

1. Souders CR. Pericarditis: a problem in diagnosis. Med Clin North Am 1963;47:295.
2. Spodick DH. Differential diagnosis of acute pericarditis. Prog Cardiovasc Dis 1971;14:192.
3. Bradley EC. Acute benign pericarditis. Am Heart J 1964; 67:121.
4. McCuiston CF, Moser KM. Studies in pericarditis: I. differentiation of the acute idiopathic form from that occurring in disseminated lupus. Am J Cardiol 1959;4:42.
5. Desaneto A, et al. Cocksackie B5 heart disease: demonstration of inferolateral wall myocardial necrosis. Am J Med 1980;68:295.
6. Adams C. Postviral myopericarditis associated with the influenza virus. Am J Cardiol 1959;4:56.
7. Winfield CR, Joseph SP. Herpes zoster pericarditis. Br Heart J 1980;43:597.
8. Shugoll GI. Pericarditis associated with infectious mononucleosis. Arch Intern Med 1957;100:630.
9. Picardi JL, et al. Pericarditis caused by *Histoplasma capsulatum*. Am J Cardiol 1976;37:82.
10. Segal I, et al. Amebic pericardial effusion. Heart Lung 1977;6:339.
11. Connolly DC, Burchell HB. Pericarditis: a ten year survey. Am J Cardiol 1961;7:7.
12. Permanyer-Miralda G, et al. Primary acute pericardial disease: a prospective series of 231 consecutive patients. Am J Cardiol 1985;56:623.
13. Nadas AS, Levy JM. Pericarditis in children. Am J Cardiol 1961;7:109.
14. Niarchos AP, McKendrick CS. Prognosis of pericarditis after acute myocardial infarction. Br Heart J 1973;35:49.
15. Yan V. Pericarditis in acute myocardial infarction. Heart Lung 1974;3:247.
16. Engle MA, Ito T. The postpericardiotomy syndrome. Am J Cardiol 1961;7:73.
17. Tabatznik B, Isaacs JP. Postpericardiotomy syndrome following traumatic hemopericardium. Am J Cardiol 1961;7:83.
18. Roman GT, et al. Fatal case of acute idiopathic pericarditis: discussion of the character and origin of thoracic pain in acute pericarditis. Am J Cardiol 1959;4:68.
19. Markiwicz W, et al. Pericardial rub in pericardial effusion: lack of correlation with amount of fluid. Chest 1980;77:643.
20. Spodick DH. Pericardial rub: prospective, multiple observer investigation of pericardial friction in 100 patients. Am J Cardiol 1975;35:357.
21. Spodick DH, Marriott HJL. Atrial diastolic friction. Chest 1975;68:122.
22. Dressler W. Effect of respiration on the pericardial friction rub. Am J Cardiol 1961;7:130.
23. Weiss JM, Spodick DH. Association of left pleural effusion with pericardial disease. N Engl J Med 1983;308:696.
24. Spodick DH. Frequency of arrhythmias in acute pericarditis determined by Holter monitoring. Am J Cardiol 1984;53:842.

Pericardial Effusion and
Cardiac Tamponade

25. Spodick DH. Acute cardiac tamponade: pathologic physiology, diagnosis and management. Prog Cardiovasc Dis 1967;10:64.
26. Guberman BA, et al. Cardiac tamponade in medical patients. Circulation 1981;64:633.
27. Spodick DH. The normal and diseased pericardium: current concepts of pericardial physiology, diagnosis and treatment. J Am Coll Cardiol 1983;1:240.
28. Winer HE, Kronzon I. Absence of pulsus paradoxus in patients with cardiac tamponade and atrial septal defects. Am J Cardiol 1979;44:378.
29. Antmann EM, et al. Low-pressure cardiac tamponade. Ann Intern Med 1979;91:403.
30. Cohen SI, et al. Pulsus paradoxus and Kussmaul's sign in acute pulmonary embolism. Am J Cardiol 1973;32:271.
31. Harvey WP. Auscultatory findings in disease of the pericardium. Am J Cardiol 1961;7:15.
32. Dressler W. Percussion of the sternum: I. aid to differentiation of pericardial effusion and cardiac dilation. JAMA 1960;173:761.
33. Steinberg I. Roentgenography of pericardial disease. Am J Cardiol 1961;7:33.
34. Bedford DE. Chronic effusive pericarditis. Br Heart J 1964;26:499.

Chronic Constrictive Pericarditis

35. D'Cruz I. The noninvasive diagnosis of constrictive pericarditis. Am J Noninvas Cardiol 1990;4:65.
36. Wood P. Chronic constrictive pericarditis. Am J Cardiol 1961;7:48.

37. Shabetai R, et al. Restrictive cardiac disease: pericarditis and the myocardiopathies. Am Heart J 1965;69:271.
38. Kutcher MA, et al. Constrictive pericarditis as a complication of cardiac surgery: recognition of an entity. Am J Cardiol 1982;50:742.
39. Foster CJ. Constrictive pericarditis complicating an endocardial pacemaker. Br Heart J 1982;47:497.
40. Schwartz DJ, et al. Epicardial pacemaker complicated by cardiac tamponade and constrictive pericarditis. Chest 1979;76:226.
41. Yurchak PM, et al. Constrictive pericarditis complicating disseminated lupus erythematosus. Circulation 1965;31:113.
42. John JT, et al. Pericardial disease in rheumatoid arthritis. Am J Med 1979;66:385.
43. Applefeld MM, et al. The late appearance of chronic pericardial disease in patients treated by radiotherapy for Hodgkin's disease. Ann Intern Med 1981;94:338.
44. Lindsay J, et al. Chronic constrictive pericarditis following uremic hemopericardium. Am Heart J 1970;79:390.
45. Orlando RC, et al. Methysergide therapy and constrictive pericarditis. Ann Intern Med 1978;88:213.
46. Fowler NO. Constrictive pericarditis: new aspects. Am J Cardiol 1982;50:1014.
47. Beck W, et al. Splitting of the second sound in constrictive pericarditis, with observation of the mechanism of pulsus paradoxus. Am Heart J 1962;64:765.
48. Tyberg TI, et al. Genesis of pericardial knock in constrictive pericarditis. Am J Cardiol 1980;46:570.
49. Nicholson WJ, et al. Early diastolic sound of constrictive pericarditis. Am J Cardiol 1980;45:378.
50. Gibson R. Atypical constrictive pericarditis. Br Heart J 1959;21:583.
51. Schrire V, et al. Unusual diastolic murmurs in constrictive pericarditis and constrictive endocarditis. Am Heart J 1968;76:4.
52. Lange RL, et al. Diagnostic signs in compressive cardiac disorders. Circulation 1966;33:763.

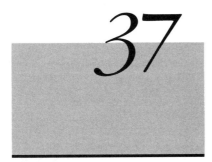

Cor Pulmonale

ACUTE COR PULMONALE

Looking at a woman's legs has often saved her life.

Osler

Although overwhelming pneumonia may produce acute cor pulmonale, much the most common cause is pulmonary embolism. And although much the most common embolus is the blood clot emanating from the leg, numerous other embolic missiles are occasionally encountered (Table 37-1)

Pulmonary Embolism

Pulmonary embolism is both underdiagnosed in the sick[1] and overdiagnosed in the otherwise well.[2] It is of great clinical importance to the cardiologist because it is common in cardiac patients; because we are not very good at diagnosing it; because it simulates, complicates, aggravates, and even initiates heart failure; and because lifesaving interventions are available.

Pulmonary embolism is one of the commonest lung diseases encountered in general hospitals.[3] Careful postmortem examination of the pulmonary tree may uncover old or recent thromboemboli in as many as 64% of *all* autopsies.[4] In one series, lung emboli were found in 57% of all atrial fibrillators, 25% of all patients with any demonstrable heart disease, and in 9% of those who had no evidence of heart disease.[5] But then, autopsies are done on dead people, and may therefore give an exaggerated impression of actual frequency.[2]

Most authors report accurate *ante*mortem diagnosis between 20% and 50%, but the diagnosed percentage in some series has been as low as 7%.[6] In more than three-quarters of those who die, postmortem evidence of previously undiagnosed recent emboli is found.[7]

Every pulmonary embolization does not produce pulmonary infarction, let alone cor pulmonale; in fact, the clinical effects of a single embolus may range from complete silence to almost instantaneous death—75% of those who die, die within the first hour.[8] Only about 10% of emboli produce a demonstrable infarct of the lung (because of its

Table 37–1
Potential Embolic Missiles

Thrombus
Tumor, eg, chorioepithelioma, right atrial myxoma
Amniotic fluid
Fat
Air

double blood supply). Infarction is more likely to develop with occlusion of distal vessels and in those with preexisting cardiac disease, and less likely with proximal pulmonary artery obstruction and in those with normal cardiovascular systems.[9] The main clinical syndromes produced by pulmonary embolism are summarized in Table 37-2.

The Syndromes

If the embolus is small enough, it may produce no recognizable disturbance. Repeated, silent emboli, however, may produce the following insidious train of events: dyspnea and cough → right ventricular hypertrophy with gallop rhythm and harsh pulmonic ejection murmur → intractable heart failure.[10]

Pulmonary embolism and infarction are not synonymous. Sizeable emboli can produce acute cor pulmonale without infarction of the lung because of its dual blood supply. To diagnose pulmonary embolism, one must THINK OF IT in the appropriate clinical context, and one should therefore be well versed in the conditions that predispose to venous thrombosis (Table 37-3). The great majority of pulmonary emboli start life as thrombi in the leg veins[11]; clots forming in the calves are most common, but those in the thigh may be more dangerous.[12] A significant minority arise in pelvic veins and in the right heart (especially in failure

Table 37–2
The Syndromes of Pulmonary Embolism

1. Complete silence
2. "Primary" pulmonary hypertension
3. Pulmonary infarction
4. Acute cor pulmonale
5. Cardiovascular collapse

Table 37–3
Factors Predisposing to Pulmonary Embolization

1. **Heart failure**
2. **Atrial fibrillation**
3. Debilitating diseases, esp. cancer
4. Surgery, fractures, trauma
5. Advancing age
6. Bedrest, immobilization
7. Venous hypertension, prolonged sitting (eg, long flights)
8. Dehydration
9. Obesity
10. Pregnancy; ??contraceptive pills

and fibrillators), and a few originate in axillary or brachial veins. In one series, 17% came from sources other than the calf veins[13]; and in another study no less than 39% were thought to originate in the heart, with a further 27% from abdomino-pelvic veins.[14]

Although it is important to look for local signs of venous thrombosis, it is equally important to remember that venous thrombosis does not always produce detectable signs. In some series of pulmonary embolism, evidence of venous thrombosis has been detected in less than 10%. Indeed, embolism may emulate a "bolt from the blue," and prostrate an active young person who has neither apparent cause for nor clinical evidence of venous thrombosis.[15–17] Absence of signs of venous thrombosis does not militate against, much less exclude, pulmonary embolism. Subtle increase in the girth of calf or thigh may be the only indication of the lurking thrombotic mischief.

Contrary to a popular impression, pulmonary embolism is much more common in medical than in surgical patients[18,19]; it is somewhat more common in women, and it affects the lower lobes in about 75%, the right more than the left.[1]

Clues, Pitfalls, and Symptoms

"Pneumonia" without purulent sputum equals pulmonary embolism.

One should always be especially prepared for pulmonary embolism and/or infarction in patients with mitral stenosis, history of previous embolism, or obscure right ventricular failure. One should

Table 37–4
Incidence of Classic Symptoms

Author	No. Patients	Hemoptysis	Pleural Pain	Anginal Pain	Pleural Friction	Evidence of Venous Thrombosis
Dexter[11]	70	41%	73%		44%	
Gorham[23]	100	12%	26%	19%	9%	19%
Coon[5]	606	11%				19%

never fail to think of it in the presence of acute dyspnea or chest pain. The two diseases for which pulmonary embolism or infarction is most often mistaken are myocardial infarction and pneumonia. Also keep in mind the numerous deceptive ways in which pulmonary embolization may present:

1. Unexplained or unresponsive fever,
2. Recurrent "pleurisy,"
3. Acute abdomen,
4. Unexplained, bloody, pleural effusion,
5. Paroxysmal supraventricular tachyarrhythmia,
6. Unexplained, or increasing congestive heart failure, and
7. Convulsions or syncope—especially orthostatic.

Syncope was the initial or dominant feature of pulmonary embolism in 13% of 132 consecutive cases.[20] Short of frank syncope, tiredness or faintness may be warning symptoms; or a sense of anxiety or apprehension may afford an important "premonitory" indication of a frank embolus in the offing: In 60% of one series, the patients were described as restless, nervous, excited, twitching, concerned, confused, or despondent just before the major episode.[21] Another premonitory circumstance may be an urge to defecate.

The supposedly classical features of pulmonary embolus are variable and sometimes remarkably infrequent (see Table 37-4). For example, the classic triad—dyspnea, chest pain, hemoptysis—was present in but 3% of one series,[6] and in 15% of another.[22] The symptoms actually experienced, in their order of frequency, are listed in Table 37-5; and some clinical triads of occasional diagnostic value are presented in Table 37-6.

There are two distinct pain types: One substernal or precordial that is virtually indistinguishable from anginal pain, and the other pleuritic and usually axillary. In the course of an attack, the pain may shift from "anginal" to "pleuritic," presumably as infarction supervenes.[23]

Physical Signs

The physical examination is of prime importance in reaching a diagnosis. *Dyspnea* is immediate and severe in massive embolism and *precedes* the onset of *pain* (contrast with myocardial infarction); it is OUT OF PROPORTION to cardiac and pulmonary

Table 37–5
Symptoms Experienced in Order of Frequency

Initial Symptoms[14]	Overall Symptoms[11]
Dyspnea	Tachypnea
Sudden death	Tachycardia
Chest pain	Fever
Cyanosis	Pleurisy
Restlessness	Cough
Shock	Hemoptysis
Tachycardia	Icterus
Hemoptysis	Chill

Table 37–6
A Trio of Triads

Rising temperature Rising heart rate Rising respiratory rate	A common presenting triad[11]
Dyspnea Chest pain Hemoptysis	Classic triad, but seen only in minority[6,22]
Tachycardia Digitalis toxicity Intractable edema	May offer clue that PE complicates CHF[29]

PE, pulmonary embolism, CHF, congestive heart failure.

findings. Although there is secondary bronchiolar constriction from liberation of serotonin, histamine, and other substances from the platelet-containing clot,[1] the use of accessory muscles of respiration is not striking since airway obstruction is not the main feature, and breath sounds are loud and clear.[24]

When the embolus is less overwhelming, the most common presenting clue is a *rise in temperature, pulse rate and respiratory rate*[11]; this rising trio may be the *only* sign, usually lasting 2 to 3 days. Although tachypnea obviously occurs in many syndromes apart from pulmonary embolization, absence of tachypnea reliably excludes it.[1] *Cyanosis* is common, appears rapidly, may be minimal or intense, and lasts from a few minutes to days. *Scleral icterus* may be detected after a day or two if pulmonary infarction has occurred. *Distended neck veins* may show Kussmaul's paradoxical filling.[25] The *"red blood wave"*—sudden, momentary passing of a pink flush across the pallid, cyanotic face—is thought to be due to temporary dislodgement of the clot. *Chest expansion* may be diminished on one side. *Pulmonary artery pulsation* may be seen and felt, and may be associated with palpable *friction* at the left upper sternal border—due to a dilated pulmonary artery rubbing its sleeve of pericardium.

The second sound is abnormally split, and the splitting may be fixed.[26] P2 is accentuated—unless the proximal end of the clot is close to the valve.[27] An S4 gallop develops at the left sternal border. *Murmurs* may include:

1. *Systolic ejection* at the left upper sternal border—due to partial obstruction of the pulmonary artery,
2. *Early diastolic* at the left sternal border—due to secondary pulmonic regurgitation,
3. *Interscapular systolic*—due to embolus riding at bifurcation of the pulmonary artery,
4. *Systolic* over lung fields, in particular one that increases with inspiration and spills into diastole—due to partial obstruction of smaller branches of the pulmonary artery, and
5. *Pansystolic* of acute tricuspid regurgitation

Left ventricular failure, with pulmonary edema, can complicate pulmonary embolism, presumably as the combined result of tachycardia, decreased coronary flow, and arterial oxygen unsaturation.[11]

Although it is clear that one cannot depend on the clinical picture to make the diagnosis of pulmonary embolism, bedside examination is of crucial importance in alerting the clinician to the possibility in the predisposed (see Table 37-3), and therefore instigating further investigation.[28]

CHRONIC COR PULMONALE

Chronic heart failure secondary to pulmonary disease can often be diagnosed at a glance. The emphysematous "barrel" chest with evident dyspnea and cyanosis— the "blue bloater"—is easy to spot. With uncomplicated emphysema, the neck veins may be engorged in expiration but are emptied by inspiration; if they are distended even during inspiration, venous congestion is confirmed. The other classic signs of right ventricular failure—enlarged liver and pedal edema—are also present.

The onset of congestive failure in the patient with chronic obstructive pulmonary disease (COPD) is insidious. As failure supervenes, it is likely to be mistaken for a worsening of previous pulmonary symptoms (cough, shortness of breath). Unusual daytime somnolence may suggest the diagnosis.

Physical signs are damped by the voluminous lungs, but accentuation of S2 and a right ventricular lift may be detectable. Hypercapnia produces peripheral vasodilation, and the extremities are consequently warm though cyanosed.

Heart sounds are distant, are best heard in the epigastrium in the neighborhood of the xiphoid, and a right ventricular gallop is often well heard there. As the level of pulmonary hypertension increases, the systolic murmur of tricuspid regurgitation and the diastolic murmur of pulmonic regurgitation may appear.

REFERENCES

1. Rosenow EC, et al. Pulmonary embolism. Mayo Clin Proc 1981;56:161.
2. Robin ED. Overdiagnosis and overtreatment of pulmonary embolism: the emperor may have no clothes. Ann Intern Med 1977;87:775.
3. Israel HL, Goldstein F. The varied clinical manifestations of pulmonary embolism. Ann Intern Med 1957;47:202.
4. Freiman DG, et al. Frequency of pulmonary thromboembolism in man. N Engl J Med 1965;272:1278.
5. Coon WW, Coller FA. Clinicopathologic correlation in thromboembolism. Surg Gynecol Obstet 1959;109:259.
6. Coon WW, Coller FA. Some epidemiological considerations of thromboembolism. Surg Gynecol Obstet 1959; 109:487.

7. Genton E. Therapeutic aspects of pulmonary embolism. Heart Lung 1974;3:233.

8. Donaldson GA, et al. Reappraisal of application of Trendelenburg operation to massive fatal embolism: report of successful pulmonary-artery thrombectomy using cardiopulmonary bypass. N Engl J Med 1963;268:171.

9. Dalen JE, et al. Pulmonary embolism, pulmonary hemorrhage and pulmonary infarction. N Engl J Med 1977; 296:1431.

10. Owen WR, et al. Unrecognized emboli to the lungs with subsequent cor pulmonale. N Engl J Med 1953;249:919.

11. Dexter L, et al. Pulmonary embolism. Med Clin North Am 1960;44:1251.

12. Moser KM, LeMoine JR. Is embolic risk conditioned by location of deep vein thrombosis? Ann Intern Med 1981; 94:439.

13. Marks J, et al. Treatment of venous thrombosis with anticoagulants: review of 1135 cases. Lancet 1954;2:787.

14. Fowler EF, et al. Pulmonary embolism: a clinical study of 97 fatal cases. Surgery 1954;36:650.

15. Cohen H, Daly JJ. Unheralded pulmonary embolism. Br Med J 1957;2:1209.

16. Fleming HA, Bailey SM. Massive pulmonary embolism in healthy people. Br Med J 1966;1:1322.

17. Barraclough MA, Braimbridge MV. Massive pulmonary embolism. Br Med J 1967;1:217.

18. Towbin A. Pulmonary embolism: incidence and significance. JAMA 1954;156:209.

19. Parker BM, Smith JR. Pulmonary embolism and infarction: a review of the physiologic consequences of pulmonary arterial obstruction. Am J Med 1958;24:402.

20. Thames MD, et al. Syncope in patients with pulmonary embolism. JAMA 1977;238:2509.

21. Krause S, Silverblatt M. Pulmonary embolism. Arch Intern Med 1955;96:19.

22. Miller R, Berry JB. Pulmonary infarction: a frequently missed diagnosis. Am J Med Sci 1951;222:197.

23. Gorham LW. A study of pulmonary embolism. Arch Intern Med 1961;108:8 and 418.

24. Bloomfield DA. The recognition and management of massive pulmonary embolism. Heart Lung 1974;3:241.

25. Burdine JA, Wallace JM. Pulsus paradoxus and Kussmaul's sign in massive pulmonary embolism. Am J Cardiol 1965;15:413.

26. Cobbs BS, et al. The second heart sound in pulmonary embolism and pulmonary hypertension. Am Heart J 1966; 71:843.

27. Ball KP. Massive thrombotic occlusion of the large pulmonary arteries. Circulation 1956;14:766.

28. Bettmann MA, Salzman EW. Current concepts in the diagnosis of pulmonary embolism. Modern Concepts of Cardiovascular Disease 1984;53:1.

29. Tench WR. The triad of tachycardia, digitalis toxicity and mercurial-fast edema in congestive heart failure complicated by pulmonary embolism. Am J Med 1955; 19:869.

Heart Failure and Digitalis Intoxication

Heart failure (HF) is the final common path of all forms of heart disease, and there are more than ten million patients with it in this country.[1] When florid, HF is easily recognized; but in its early stages the diagnosis can be difficult.

The diagnosis is almost exclusively made by the history and physical examination; and it is important to establish the diagnosis because most patients can be dramatically helped, and in some the process may actually be reversible.

There are many ways of classifying HF: Acute and chronic (Table 38-1); high output and low output; backward (Hope, 1832) and forward (McKenzie, 1913); left and right ventricular, etc.[2] All of these subdivisions have their merits and uses.

The circulating blood occupies two circuits that form a continuous figure-of-eight (Fig. 38-1). The simplistic way to think of HF is as the inability of the pump to transfer its burden of blood from one circulation (systemic or pulmonary) to the other (pulmonary or systemic). But it is clear that it is

impossible for one ventricle to pump a larger volume than the other for any length of time, without numerous compensatory and complicating mechanisms coming into play; and so it is more realistic to think of HF as the failure of the pump to meet the metabolic demands of the tissues. From the point of view of bedside diagnosis, however, the concept of backward and forward failure is eminently practical, and both mechanisms are operative in most patients with chronic HF.[2]

If the left ventricle fails to adequately transfer its blood from pulmonary circuit to systemic circuit, there are two results (keep an eye on Fig. 38-1): Too much blood stays in the lungs (congestion; backward failure) and too little is propelled into the other organs (forward failure). Congested lungs produce shortness of breath, dyspnea, orthopnea, pulmonary edema, and rales at the lung bases. Inadequate perfusion of other organs results in angina, mental confusion and dizziness, decreased urinary output, impaired muscular capa-

Table 38–1

Some Representative Causes of Congestive Heart Failure

Acute	Chronic
Myocardial infarction	Ischemic heart disease
Rupture of papillary muscle or ventricular septum	Hypertension
	Valvular heart disease
Rupture of chorda tendinea	Congenital heart disease
Pulmonary embolism	Chronic lung disease
Rheumatic fever	Thyrotoxicosis
Myocarditis	Cardiomyopathy
Infective endocarditis	Constrictive pericarditis
Pericardial effusion	Myxedema
Fluid overloading	Beri-beri
Tachycardia or bradycardia	Bradyarrhythmia

bility, etc. The reduction in glomerular filtration activates the renin–angiotensin–aldosterone axis, which leads to the retention of sodium and water in an attempt to maintain a normal left ventricular output. At an early stage of HF, fluid may be retained during daytime activities, only to be excreted during the night's rest; hence nycturia.

If the right ventricle fails to transfer its blood from the systemic into the pulmonary circulation, congestion develops in the systemic circulation, and distended neck veins, enlarged liver (and sometimes spleen), ascites, and edema of the feet and ankles result.

Examples of causes of left ventricular failure are hypertension, aortic stenosis, and ischemic disease. The most common cause of right ventricular failure is left ventricular failure; other causes include mitral stenosis and pulmonary hypertension.

Causes of HF such as rheumatic fever, thyrotoxicosis, myocarditis, and arrhythmias have the potential to affect both sides of the heart equally; and it is important to realize that arrhythmias, especially atrial fibrillation, may both cause HF and be precipitated by it, so that it is sometimes difficult to determine which is cause and which is effect.

In view of the foregoing, when probing for evi-

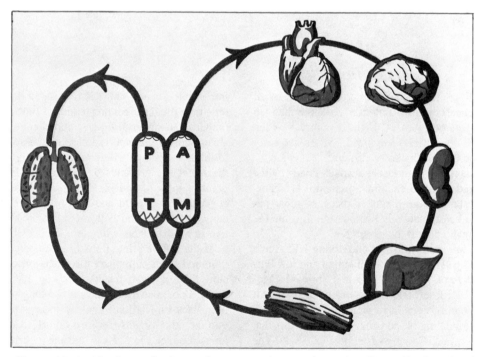

Figure 38–1. The figure-of-eight circulation—an aid to visualizing the effects of backward and forward failure of either ventricle. P, A, T, and M refer to pulmonic, aortic, tricuspid, and mitral valves, respectively.

dence of HF, one should include the following questions in one's interrogation:

How's your breathing?
How many pillows do you sleep on?
Do you ever wake up in the night short of breath?
Do your feet and ankles ever swell up?
Is your weight steady?
Do you have to wake up at night to pass water?

Symptoms

Trouble with breathing is the cardinal indication of left ventricular failure; but never accept "shortness of breath" to mean what *you* mean by it without pressing the patient for a clear description of *his* meaning. Often it turns out to mean "can't-get-enough-air" or the sighing respirations of anxiety. Never take its admission for granted as the equivalent of true dyspnea.

If the patient develops pulmonary edema, sitting upright may be obligatory (Fig. 38-2); the patient with pulmonary edema is frantic, fights for breath, and is cyanosed; paroxysms of coughing extrude pink, frothy sputum. The distraught man depicted in the figure has instinctively assumed an admirable and practical posture for treating this

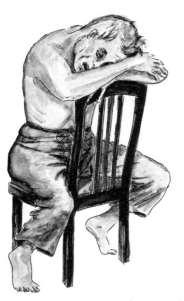

Figure 38–2. Posture instinctively assumed by a patient in acute pulmonary edema—and, incidentally, an excellent arrangement for managing such a patient.

emergency: An upright chair is available in most indoor environments; sitting front-to-back provides a much needed support for the distressed patient; and this position conveniently exposes the back for ready and repeated examination by his attendants.

The chief symptom of right ventricular failure is swelling of the feet, ankles, and other dependent parts. Anorexia and nausea may result from hepatic congestion or from digitalis therapy.

Cardinal Physical Signs

The routine examination for heart failure is directed at four main areas: Neck veins, liver, lung bases, and ankles.

Neck Veins

The jugulars are inspected as outlined in Chapter 3. If they are distended more than 2 or 3 cm above the sternal angle, they are abnormally full, and congestive failure is a likely cause. As a general rule, if the neck veins are easily identifiable and clearly not distended, right ventricular failure is not present; but beware the thick, "bull" neck in which even distended veins may not be readily detectable.

If the level to which the veins fill is obscure, milk the vein empty with the finger and then observe the level to which it *re*fills. With the patient's torso raised to the prescribed critical angle, the normal jugulars fill only from above; but in congestive failure they may fill from below as well.

The hepatojugular reflux—perhaps better renamed the abdominojugular test[3]—may be helpful. Renaming is suggested since it is not necessary to apply pressure over the liver, and since the distention of cervical veins—although the exact mechanism is not known—is probably not due to reflux. Furthermore, the usually recommended 1-minute compression of the abdomen is unnecessary; 10 seconds is enough. Midabdominal compression with the palm of the hand for this period in the normal subject fails to produce jugular distention, but in the presence of a raised pulmonary arterial wedge pressure, the neck veins become engorged.[3]

Liver Enlargement

An enlarged liver is a cardinal sign of congestive failure, but it can be misleading since hepatomegaly has so many noncardiac causes. Doubt may be resolved by applying the abdominojugular test. The liver is tender if its enlargement is due to congestion.

The normal liver is impalpable in most people. Sometimes, however, it can be felt in patients with emphysema but no heart failure; and it is usually palpable in infants and young children.

Lung Bases

Rales at the lung bases also can be misleading— they are probably the least reliable of all the signs of HF. They may be absent in patients with severe dyspnea and dangerous degrees of pulmonary congestion, which may trap the unwary physician into diagnosing psychogenic hyperventilation.[4]

On the other hand, basal rales are sometimes consistently present in chronic cardiacs who can comfortably lie flat in bed and who seem to be little the worse for persistent rales over the years.

Pulmonary edema is usually easy to diagnose except in its early stages, when there may be no adventitious sounds in the chest (in which case, you must exclude hyperventilation); or when rhonchi dominate the picture (exclude bronchial asthma). Patients are often pallid in the early stages with hacking, unproductive cough; in the later stages, there is central cyanosis with pink, frothy sputum.

The following clinical points favor the diagnosis of pulmonary edema: History of hypertension, myocardial infarction, or rheumatic heart disease; history of previous attacks of nocturnal dyspnea or nocturnal coughing relieved by sitting up; the finding of an enlarged heart, gallop rhythm, murmurs of mitral stenosis or aortic disease, or a raised blood pressure; basal rales with or without rhonchi.

Edema of the Ankles

Remember that approximately 10 pounds of excess fluid has already accumulated in the tissues when you can demonstrate pitting. Therefore the insidious retention of water is better recognized by weight gain or nycturia (see above). Early pitting edema is often missed by not prodding long enough. The proper technique to reveal obscure edema was driven home by a distinguished obstetrician with histrionic tendencies wagging a forefinger aloft and declaiming, "ONE finger, for ONE minute, ONE inch above the malleolus!" A full minute is not necessary, but the point is well taken: One should always press firmly for an appreciable time (say, 15 to 30 seconds) before excluding pitting. The quick jab by a hurried examiner is inadequate. In patients not on their feet, the edema may accumulate in dependent parts such as sacrum and scrotum.

Additional Signs

In most cases, regardless of the etiology, cardiac enlargement is evident and tachycardia the rule. A ventricular gallop rhythm is often present, and may in fact be the only auscultatory abnormality[5]; the other "death rattle" of the left ventricle, pulsus alternans, may also be detectable. Left ventricular failure leads to pulmonary hypertension so that P2 becomes loud and may be palpable, and the second sound may be widely split.

There is often a right ventricular lift and audible gallop at the left sternal border. In the presence of emphysema, you may hear the gallop best in the epigastrium.

Depending on the cause of the failure, various findings may surface: For example, an atrial gallop in hypertensive or ischemic heart disease; murmurs of mitral stenosis and/or regurgitation, aortic stenosis and/or regurgitation; signs of hyperthyroidism in thyrotoxic heart failure; a barrel chest in cor pulmonale; etc.

Apart from the murmurs of valvar lesions that cause failure, A-V valve regurgitation may develop secondary to the ventricular dilation of failure; and it may be difficult or impossible to decide whether the regurgitant murmur represents cause or effect.

You may be able to detect a pleural effusion on one or both sides. In most patients the effusion is bilateral,[6–8] but if it is confined to one side it is more often right-sided.[6,8]

In advanced cases, ascites, Cheyne–Stokes respirations, and "cardiac cachexia"[9]—wasting of skeletal muscle—may be present.

Apart from the run-of-the-mill causes of congestive failure, an occasional case is due to a rare disorder; sometimes one is alerted to an unaccustomed etiology by the patient's failure to respond to conventional therapy. This should impel you to search for some unsuspected precipitating factor, for example, an undetected hypocalcemia. Calcium plays a role in myocardial excitation and contraction, and also influences the excretion of sodium; and in patients with hypocalcemia and heart failure, the failure may not respond until a normal level of calcium is restored.[10]

Simple Bedside Tests

If the physical examination is carried out with care and know-how, further tests are seldom needed to make the diagnosis of HF. But there are three simple tests that can be performed at the bedside with minimal fuss, and which may be of considerable value in specific circumstances. The *circulation time* (CT) may be useful in confirming HF. It may also be of value in distinguishing between:

1. Low and high output failure,
2. Bronchial asthma and the cardiac "asthma" of pulmonary edema, and
3. Emphysema alone and emphysema complicated by congestive failure.

The CT is gauged by rapidly injecting Decholin intravenously and having the patient signal a bitter taste as the endpoint; normally, it takes 9 to 16 seconds to reach the sensing tongue. CTs must be assessed at basal conditions with the patient fasting, because exercise, digestion, emotion, hyperventilation, and fever accelerate the circulation and shorten the CT. The CT is shortened in high-output states, such as pregnancy, anemia, hyperthyroidism, arteriovenous fistula, emphysema, and beri-

beri, and in congenital heart disease with right-to-left shunts. In contrast, HF slows the circulation and lengthens the CT—as do myxedema and polycythemia.

The *vital capacity* can be valuable in detecting the earliest sign of HF, especially in situations where symptoms and signs are not easy to assess, as in the pregnant cardiac. In following a cardiac patient through pregnancy, the vital capacity should be measured *at every visit*. If a stable baseline reading has been obtained at return visits, a sudden drop of only 200 mL may be significant of early pulmonary congestion; normally, the vital capacity tends to increase during pregnancy, so that a measurable drop is all the more significant.

The *Valsalva maneuver* is also a useful clinical test for detecting or confirming early HF. It should be standardized by having the patient blow a column of mercury, or the needle of the aneroid, to 40 mm Hg and hold it there for 10 seconds. A Valsalva performed in this way by the normal person produces a triphasic blood pressure response (see Fig. 38-3, which, for simplicity's sake, depicts only the diastolic pressure): The pressure, both systolic and diastolic, (1) rises sharply at the start of straining; (2) returns towards the baseline while the strain continues; (3) dips abruptly below the baseline when the straining ceases; and (4) rebounds above the baseline before settling back to its initial level. Reflex bradycardia follows (Fig. 38-4).

In patients with HF, and in those with pericarditis or large left-to-right shunts, the rebound/overshoot[4] and the bradycardia do not materialize.[11,12]

This sounds like a formidable bedside undertaking, but it can be readily accomplished. The

Figure 38–3. The curve represents the normal fluctuations in diastolic blood pressure during and following a Valsalva maneuver. The dashed line represents the level—a few mm Hg above resting diastolic pressure—at which you set and hold the inflated blood pressure cuff throughout the test. In the normal, Korotkoff sounds are audible before the test begins but disappear as the diastolic pressure rises with straining (A); during the post-straining dip (3) the sounds are again heard (B), only to disappear again (C) during the short-lived rebound (4). In the patient with heart failure, the rebound (4) does not occur, so the sounds do not disappear a second time.

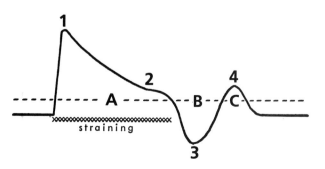

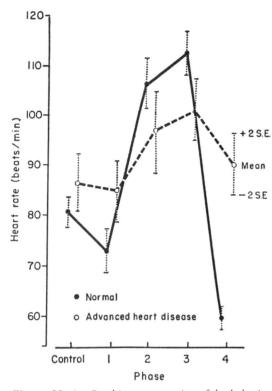

Figure 38–4. Graphic representation of the behavior of the heart rate in the normal subject (solid curve) and in the patient with heart failure (dashed curve) during and after a Valsalva maneuver. In the normal, the straining period is followed by reflex bradycardia, which does not develop in the failing heart. Phases 1 to 4 are the same as in Figure 38-3. (Reproduced with permission from Elisberg EI. Heart rate response to Valsalva maneuver as a test of circulatory integrity. JAMA 1963;186:202.)

intravascular gymnastics can be recognized with the help of a blood pressure cuff, as follows: Obtain stable baseline diastolic pressures; inflate the cuff to a few millimeters above diastolic pressure (dashed line in Fig. 38-3), and have the patient perform the Valsalva maneuver by the standardized technique described above. In the normal person, Korotkoff sounds will first disappear (Fig. 38-3**A**), then return (Fig. 38-3**B**), and then disappear again (Fig. 38-3**C**). In HF, the second disappearance (Fig. 38-3**C**) will not happen. Alternatively, one can simply keep a finger on the pulse (or record the electrocardiogram) during the procedure and observe the presence or absence of the bradycardia.

Heart Failure in Infancy

In the infant, HF may be difficult indeed to recognize: One hears no articulate complaints, edema is less conspicuous, and venous congestion is difficult to appraise. In place of the complaint of breathlessness, one hears that the infant sucks for only short periods, then falls asleep exhausted; the breathing is labored and rapid—by count 50 to 120 per minute instead of the normal 25 to 40. One notices inspiratory indrawing in the suprasternal notch and at the line of attachment of the diaphragm. There may be a hacking, irritable cough. Dependent edema may develop, and, if the baby sleeps face downward, primarily involve the face. The normally palpable liver edge may lose its sharpness and the spleen may become palpably enlarged.

The most common causes of HF at various intervals during the first few months of life are:[13]

1st week: aortic atresia,
2nd–4th week: coarctation of the aorta,
4th–8th week: transposition of the great arteries, and
8 weeks to 6 months: endocardial fibroelastosis.

Other causes of HF in the early months include hypoplastic left ventricle (1st–2nd week); glycogen storage disease (early infancy); A-V fistulas (cerebral, hepatic, etc.); ventricular septal defect; A-V communis; anomalous pulmonary venous drainage; single ventricle; patent ductus arteriosus; and persistent truncus.[13,14] The most common causes of *sudden* failure are paroxysmal tachycardia and myocarditis.

Digitalis Intoxication

A long life is too short to learn enough about this wonderful drug.

                                                        Wenckebach

Although digitalis does not enjoy such frequent use as formerly, it and HF remain as inseparable as Siamese twins, and manifestations of digitalis intoxication still often go unrecognized. The exact frequency of toxicity is impossible to ascertain; it is still common, though less so than a decade or two ago.[15] Most series in the United States—involving predominantly digoxin—have reported an incidence of about 20%, but the prevalence nowadays is more like 10% to 15%. A survey from Norway of 649 patients receiving maintenance digitoxin revealed the surprisingly low incidence of 5.8%.[16]

It is admittedly difficult to diagnose toxicity with certainty—its nonspecific symptoms may be attributable to the underlying cardiac disease for which the drug is being administered.[17]

The common gastrointestinal complaints are well known, as are the more common arrhythmias (such as ventricular bigeminy, and atrial tachycardia with A-V block). Other less popularized rhythm disturbances deserve emphasis; one should especially be on the lookout for accelerated junctional rhythm with resulting A-V dissociation, and for any regular ventricular rhythm in the presence of atrial fibrillation.

Perhaps as important as the arrhythmias—because of its special lure to disastrous overtreatment—is increasing congestive failure.[18] In any patient who is receiving full doses of a digitalis preparation, yet whose heart rate is increasing and failure worsening, one should think of the possibility of digitalis toxicity.

A pharmaceutical blunder in the Netherlands, involving the improper manufacture of digoxin tablets, led to the intoxication of 179 persons, which afforded a rare opportunity to assess the frequency of various symptoms: Fatigue and visual symptoms (usually a disturbance of red/green perception) developed in 95%; weakness, anorexia, and nausea in 80%; psychological complaints and abdominal pain in 65%; dizziness or abnormal dreams in over 50%; headache, diarrhea, or vomiting in 40% or more; and psychosis in 7%.[19]

The abdominal symptom likely to be overlooked is abdominal discomfort or pain without nausea. This has been associated with hemorrhagic necrosis of the intestine,[20] and one should bear this threatening complication in mind whenever abdominal pain follows digitalization.

The neurologic signs are often unrecognized, yet they are not uncommon. In two reported series, they accounted for 41%[21] and 31%[22] of all the toxic symptoms observed. For convenience, they are grouped and listed in Table 38-2—if you remember them, you may well save another life.

"Digitalis delirium" (Duroziez, 1874) is a catchy alliteration embracing a wide variety of mental aberrations resulting from the drug. Always

Table 38–2
Neurologic and Ocular Manifestations of Digitalis Intoxication

Neurologic

Common: headache, drowsiness, dizziness, restlessness and irritability, weakness and fatigue

Less common: paresthesiae; neuralgic pains—in teeth, face, jaw, arms, legs, feet, epigastrium, and generalized in muscles; vertigo; hallucinations, delusions, confusion, delirium

Rare: mood disturbances—euphoria, depression; amnesia, stupor, convulsions, coma

Ocular

Common: flickering, flashes of light, white vision, colored vision, blurring of vision

Rare: photophobia, oscillatory movements of eyeballs, optic neuritis, scotomata; reduced acuity, blindness; paresis of ocular muscles, diplopia

suspect digitalis toxicity in any patient receiving a digitalis preparation who exhibits any mental changes, ranging from calm disorientation to violent psychosis.[23] These dangerous effects of digitalis have not received the attention they deserve, although, as long ago as 1921, "dementia produced by digitalis" was upheld in court in defense of homicide.

A further point worth remembering is that the duration of toxic symptoms is not predictable. They have been known to last for many days after withdrawal of even the "short-acting" preparations.

You are less likely to overlook the toxic signs of digitalis if you are familiar with the circumstances that predispose to their development: Old age, diuresis, hypokalemia, hypernatremia, alkalosis, azotemia, chronic lung disease, and myxedema. And remember that quinidine, verapamil, nifedipine, amiodarone, erythromycin, and tetracycline all increase the plasma concentration of the drug.

REFERENCES

Heart Failure

1. Srebro J, Karliner JS. Congestive heart failure. Curr Probl Cardiol 1986;23:305.
2. Braunwald E. Heart disease, ed 3. Philadelphia: WB Saunders, 1988:471–474.

3. Ewy GA. The abdominojugular test: technique and hemo-dynamic correlates. Ann Intern Med 1988;109:456.

4. Bradlow BA. Cardiac emergencies: diagnosis and treatment. London: Butterworth, 1963:33.

5. Bristow JD, Metcalfe J. Physical signs in congestive heart failure. Prog Cardiovasc Dis 1967;10:236.

6. Race GA, et al. Hydrothorax in congestive heart failure. Am J Med 1957;22:83.

7. Peterman TA, Brothers SK. Letter to editor. N Engl J Med 1983;309:313.

8. Weiss JM, Spodick DH. Laterality of pleural effusions in chronic congestive heart failure. Am J Cardiol 1984; 53:951.

9. Morrison WL, Edwards RHT. Cardiac cachexia. Br Med J 1991;302:301.

10. Connor TB, et al. Hypocalcemia precipitating congestive heart failure. N Engl J Med 1982;307:869.

11. Knowles JH, et al. Clinical test for pulmonary congestion with use of the Valsalva maneuver. JAMA 1956;160:44.

12. Elisberg EI. Heart rate response to Valsalva maneuver as a test of circulatory integrity. JAMA 1963;186:200.

13. Keith JD. Congestive heart failure. Pediatrics 1956;18: 491.

14. Engle MA. Cardiac failure in infancy: recognition and management. Modern Concepts of Cardiovascular Disease 1963;32:825.

Digitalis Intoxication

15. Smith TW. Digitalis: mechanisms of action and clinical use. N Engl J Med 1988;318:358.

16. Storstein O, et al. Studies on digitalis: XIII. a prospective study of 649 patients on maintenance treatment with digitoxin. Am Heart J 1977;93:434.

17. Smith TW, et al. Digitalis glycosides: mechanisms and manifestations of toxicity. Prog Cardiovasc Dis 1984; 27:21.

18. Batterman RC, Gutner LB. Increasing congestive heart failure: a manifestation of digitalis toxicity. Circulation 1950;1:1052.

19. Lely A, van Enter C. Large-scale digitoxin intoxication. Br Med J 1970;3:737.

20. Gazes PC, et al. Acute hemorrhage and necrosis of the intestines associated with digitalization. Circulation 1961; 23:358.

21. Batterman RC, Gutner LB. Hitherto undescribed neurological manifestations of digitalis toxicity. Am Heart J 1948;36:582.

22. Church G, et al. Deliberate digitalis intoxication. Ann Intern Med 1962;57:946.

23. Church G, Marriott HJL. Digitalis delirium. Circulation 1959;20:549.

39

Cardiac Tumors

The right location for a rare diagnostic possibility is the "back" of one's mind—kept available to be marched forward when the clinical situation merits its consideration. Rare though it is, the cardiac neoplasm is to cardiology what syphilis was to medicine: The Great Imitator. And as the Proteus of heart disease, the tumor can assume the guise of valvular or pericardial disease, congestive heart failure or pulmonary hypertension, embolization or arrhythmia, hemolytic anemia or infectious endocarditis; or the patient's presenting symptom may be stroke, syncope, chest pain, fever, or loss of weight.[1] Tumor therefore enters into the differential diagnosis of virtually every cardiovascular syndrome; and we should think of it in the early stages of our physical assessment of the patient because the most common cardiac tumor, atrial myxoma, is "devastating *but curable*."[2] Yet it is gloomily claimed that only 5% to 10% of cardiac tumors are clinically diagnosable.[3]

More than 20 different primary neoplasms, about half of them benign and half malignant, are recognized[4]; but although their categories are numerous, a primary cardiac tumor is found in only a small fraction of 1% of autopsies.

To a considerable extent, the clinical manifestations of each tumor depend on the layer of the heart predominantly involved. When the tumor is endocardial, it mimics and/or causes valve disease and produces constitutional effects; when it invades the myocardium, it produces congestive heart failure, arrhythmias, and blocks; and when it involves the pericardium, chest pain, effusion, and tamponade are likely. Some of the salient features of a few important primary cardiac tumors are summarized in Table 39-1.

MYXOMAS

These many-faceted tumors account for about half of all primary cardiac neoplasms, and they may grow in any of the four cardiac chambers: 75% occupy the left atrium, and 18% the right atrium, while the remainder are equally divided between the two ventricles.[4,5]

261

Table 39–1
Salients of Some Important Cardiac Tumors[3]

"Benign"	*Age Range*	*Site*	*Clinical Manifestations*
Myxoma	3–83 yr	Atria	Obstructive, embolic, and constitutional
Papillary fibroelastoma	25–80 yr	Valve	Paroxysmal angina, SD
Rhabdomyoma	15 yr	RV, LV	Tuberous sclerosis; obstructive
Fibroma	Children	Ventricular myocardium	Heart block, VF, SD
Hemangioma	7 mo–80 yr	Anywhere	Like myxoma if endocardial
Mesothelioma	Newborn to 80 yr	AV node	AV block, SD
Malignant			
Angiosarcoma	15–76 yr	RA, pericardium	Valve obstruction, effusion, "pleuritic" pain

SD, sudden death; RV, right ventricle; LV, left ventricle; VF, ventricular fibrillation.

Atrial Myxoma

The atrial myxoma, despite its rarity, assumes importance because it is "dramatically curable."[6] Furthermore, if a myxoma is present but the diagnosis is not made, the patient remains exposed to the risks of potentially lethal embolization and sudden death. If myxoma is not suspected and invasive studies are undertaken, embolization may be precipitated.[7] For all these reasons, we should make every effort not to overlook it. Secondary tumors, though about 20 times more common,[8] are far less important because they are incurable.

The myxoma is usually not diagnosed clinically, and before the advent of echocardiography it was generally a surprise at catheterization, surgery or autopsy[6,9]; in the Mayo series of 40 patients encountered over a span of two decades,[10] the diagnosis was made clinically in only five. Nevertheless, there are circumstances in which you should especially consider myxoma in the differential diagnosis (Table 39–2): In any patient thought to have mitral disease who is in congestive heart failure but in sinus rhythm; in any patient whose cardiac symptoms or signs vary unduly with change in posture; in any patient whose dyspnea improves with lying down or following an embolus[11]; or in any young individual with embolic manifestations. Thinking of the diagnosis and then suspecting it are major steps along the diagnostic trail.

Although myxomas may present at any age, patients are almost always adults, and the mean age in most series is between 40 and 50 years. Of the 42 myxomas found in the 40 Mayo patients, 34 (81%) were in the left and eight in the right atrium. The patients' ages ranged from 17 to 73 years (mean 44.5 years), and two-thirds of the patients were women. Nineteen of the 40 were initially diagnosed as having mitral valvular disease.[10]

Symptoms

Patients with left atrial myxoma may present with the "classic triad of obstructive, constitutional, and embolic effects."[2] The pendulous tumor may intermittently occlude either the mitral orifice or one of the pulmonary veins, and so cause symptoms from either impaired left ventricular output with syncope, or from pulmonary congestion, or from both.[12]

Table 39–2
Special Circumstances Suggestive of Atrial Myxoma

1. Apparent cardiac dyspnea improved by lying down
2. Mitral disease in congestive heart failure but in sinus rhythm
3. Cardiac symptoms or signs that vary unduly with change of position or from exam to exam
4. Mitral regurgitation with accentuated S1
5. Mitral regurgitation with unusually early "S3"
6. Mitral stenosis with unusually late and low-pitched "opening snap"
7. Any young patient with embolic manifestations
8. Dyspnea that improves following embolism

Table 39–3
Symptoms and Signs in Atrial Myxoma

	Nasser[9] (1972)	Peters[2] (1974)	Bulkley[13] (1979)	Sutton[10] (1980)
Number of patients	9	17	24	40
Left:Right	7:2	15:2	22:2	34:8
Syncope/dizziness	3	9	–	9
Emboli in SA rhythm	4	3	5	13
Pyrexia	–	–	–	12
Chest pain	6	–	7	–
Dyspnea/CHF	8	–	13	28
Edema	8	8	–	–
Weight loss	–	–	–	11

SA, sinus; CHF, congestive heart faiure.

In the Mayo series, the most common presentation was heart failure in the context of suspected mitral disease. Next most common was embolism to the brain or limb. Weight loss, pyrexia, and syncope were found in 10% to 17% of their patients, but the rest had one or two of a motley array of symptoms, including weakness, fatigability, chest pain, arthralgia, and anemia.

The frequency of various symptoms, as reported in several series over the past two decades, is listed in Table 39-3.

Physical Signs

Mitral stenosis may be faithfully mimicked. An accentuated apical first sound, sometimes widely split—the second component signalling the systolic uncorking of the mitral orifice as the errant tumor is dispatched into the left atrium—and a loud pulmonic closure sound are not uncommon.[5] "Tumor plops," readily mistaken for opening snaps, were heard in 15% of the Mayo series. Systolic murmurs were reported in almost half the patients, and were more than twice as common as diastolic murmurs. A pansystolic murmur at the left lower sternal border, varying with respiration and presumably due to tricuspid regurgitation, was present in three of the 40 patients; and more than a quarter of their patients had signs of serious embolization.[10]

Particularly suggestive clues are auscultatory findings of mitral disease that vary more than would be expected with change of position or in successive examinations; the unexpected association of a mitral regurgitant murmur with an accentuated first sound or supposed opening snap (in reality a "tumor plop"); mitral regurgitation with an unusually early "third sound"; or mitral stenosis with an unusually late "opening snap."

The *right atrial myxoma* may produce right ventricular failure with cyanosis, syncope, or abrupt dyspnea. A prominent "a" wave may dominate the jugular pulse. Signs of tricuspid regurgitation may be prominent, and both systolic and diastolic tricuspid murmurs may louden with inspiration. Repeated pulmonary emboli may occur and result in pulmonary hypertension. The clinical picture may be one of persistent fever, changing murmurs, and progressive congestive failure.[4]

In the differential diagnosis of right atrial myxoma, one should consider rheumatic tricuspid involvement, constrictive pericarditis, Ebstein's anomaly, infective endocarditis, obstructive cardiomyopathy, pulmonary emboli from peripheral venous sources, and the malignant carcinoid syndrome.

MESOTHELIOMA OF THE A-V NODE

This rare neoplasm affects women more than men. Complete A-V block and Adams–Stokes attacks in young subjects suggests the possibility of this diagnosis.[14] It may be the cause of unexpected death, especially in youth, and it has been characterized as "the smallest tumor capable of producing sudden death"!

ANGIOSARCOMA

This is the most common malignant tumor of the heart, and, thanks to its extreme vascularity, may produce an audible continuous murmur.[5] It often affects the right heart and therefore produces right ventricular failure; pericardial involvement may lead to tamponade, or a superior vena caval syndrome may develop.[15]

SECONDARY TUMORS

The most common sites from which tumors spread to the heart are breast, bronchus, esophagus, pancreas, kidney, and testis[3]; the heart may also be secondarily invaded by leukemia, lymphoma, and melanoma.[8] Carcinomas of the breast and lung produce the largest number of cardiac metastases, but the tumor most likely to metastasize to the myocardium is the less common melanoma.[16] You suspect metastatic involvement of the heart when a patient with known malignancy develops unexplained symptoms or signs of cardiac involvement: These may include chest pain, pericardial rub, tamponade, or atrial arrhythmias. When the right atrium is involved, constrictive pericarditis and tricuspid stenosis may be mimicked and therefore suspected. Most secondaries are relatively silent, and the diagnosis of myocardial metastasis is made before death in less than 10%.[16]

CARCINOID SYNDROME

Although this is not caused by a cardiac tumor, it is the result of a remote tumor that affects cardiac anatomy and performance. Carcinoid tumors (argentaffinomas) of the small intestine—less often of the ovary—secrete serotonin (5-hyroxytryptamine), which plays havoc with the cardiac valves. Serotonin is inactivated in the lungs and so its destructive effect is confined to the right heart; tricuspid regurgitation—less often stenosis—and pulmonic stenosis result.[17,18]

The clinical diagnosis is easy for anyone familiar with the syndrome's unique constellation of features. There may be a history of diarrhea, asthma, and flushing, and attacks may be brought on by meals so that the patient becomes afraid to eat.[19]

On physical examination one finds an enlarged liver (from metastases), peculiar blotchy, reddish-blue ("violaceous") cyanosis of the face, and right-sided valvular lesions. A few patients develop pellagra.[18]

REFERENCES

1. Goodwin, JF. The spectrum of cardiac tumors. Am J Cardiol 1968;21:307.
2. Peters MN, et al. The clinical syndrome of atrial myxoma. JAMA 1974;230:695.
3. Bloor CM, O'Rourke RA. Cardiac tumors: clinical presentations and pathologic correlations. Curr Probl Cardiol 1984;9:7.
4. McAllister HA. Primary tumors and cysts of the heart and pericardium. Curr Probl Cardiol 1979;4:8.
5. Hall RJ, et al. Neoplastic heart disease. In: Hurst JW, ed. The heart, ed 7. New York: McGraw Hill, 1990: 1382.
6. Marpole DGF, et al. Atrial myxoma, a continuing diagnostic challenge. Am J Cardiol 1969;23:597.
7. Pindyck F, et al. Embolization of left atrial myxoma after transseptal cardiac catheterization. Am J Cardiol 1972;30: 569.
8. DeCock KM, et al. Metastatic tumor of right atrium mimicking constrictive pericarditis and tricuspid stenosis. Br Med J 1982;285:1314.
9. Nasser WK, et al. Atrial myxoma: I. clinical and pathological features in nine cases. Am Heart J 1972;83:694.
10. Sutton MGStJ, et al. Atrial myxomas: a review of clinical experience in 40 patients. Mayo Clin Proc 1980;55:371.
11. Greenwood WF. Profile of atrial myxoma. Am J Cardiol 1968;21:367.
12. Zitnik RS, Giuliani ER. Clinical recognition of atrial myxoma. Am Heart J 1970;80:689.
13. Bulkley BH, Hutchins GM. Atrial myxomas: a fifty year review. Am Heart J 1979;97:639.
14. Manion WC, et al. Benign tumor of the heart causing complete heart block. Am Heart J 1972;83:535.
15. Glancy DL, et al. Angiosarcoma of the heart. Am J Cardiol Am J Cardiol 1968;21:413.
16. Applefeld MM, Pollock SH. Cardiac disease in patients who have malignancies. Curr Probl Cardiol 1980;4: 5.
17. Grahame-Smith DG. The carcinoid syndrome. Am J Cardiol 1968;21:376.
18. Strickman NE, et al. Carcinoid heart disease: a clinical, pathologic and therapeutic update. Curr Probl Cardiol 1982;6:11.
19. Wood P. Diseases of the heart and circulation, ed 3. Philadelphia: JB Lippincott, 1982:737.

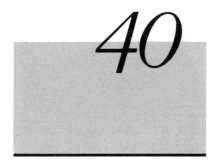

Disturbances of Rhythm and Conduction

The diagnosis of arrhythmias by physical examination alone is fun—and it can attain a gratifying degree of accuracy. Moreover, there are times when the physical examination reveals detail that the electrocardiogram (ECG) fails to show. Six simple signposts point the way:

1. The pattern of the rhythm disturbance,
2. Pulsations in the neck veins,
3. The intensity of the first heart sound,
4. Splitting of the heart sounds,
5. The effect of vagal stimulation, and
6. The effect of atropine or exercise.

As in all other approaches to diagnosis, the first and biggest stride is to *think of it*. So with the arrhythmias at the bedside, the first step is to know and think of the possibilities for the pattern of rhythm disorder you face. It is therefore imperative to know the causes of the basic deviations from the normal, regular rhythm that are listed in Table 40-1, and we will consider each of them in turn.

The best visual aid to learning the physical signs of arrhythmias is the corresponding ECG, so keep your eye on the tracing while you visualize the time relationships of atrial and ventricular contractions and their telltale hemodynamic consequences. When tackling an arrhythmia at the bedside, *keep your eye on the neck veins while you listen to the heart.*

THE PREMATURE BEAT (EXTRASYSTOLE)

The most common form of rhythm disturbance is the premature beat or extrasystole,[1] and of these the ventricular variety (VPB) is much the most common. In differentiating extrasystoles at the bedside:

1. Observe the neck veins for *cannon waves,*
2. Listen for *splitting* of heart sounds, and
3. Note length of *postextrasystolic pause.*

Table 40–1
The Seven Basic Disturbances of Rhythm

1. The premature beat
2. The pause
3. The regular tachycardias
4. The regular bradycardias
5. Bigeminal rhythms
6. Group beating
7. Chaotic irregularity

The VPB is recognized by three features: Wide splitting of heart sounds (due to asynchrony of ventricular contraction); cannon waves in the neck (due to atrial contraction against closed A-V valves) (Fig. 40-1); and a compensatory postextrasystolic pause (since the sinus discharge is uninterrupted; Fig. 40-2A). The pause following an extrasystole is "compensatory" if the interval between the beat immediately preceding the extrasystole and that immediately following it is exactly two full regular cycles (in Fig. 40-2A, a = b), indicating that the sinus pacemaker has been undisturbed. If the pause following the extrasystole is less than compensatory (in Fig. 40-2B, a < b), the sinus rhythm has presumably been disturbed by an atrial impulse of ectopic origin. With a sense of rhythm and a little practice, the length of the postextrasystolic cycle can be judged quite accurately; but if you need a metronome, a tapping finger or foot that maintains the preceding sinus

rhythm will decide whether the beat following the ectopic beat was on time or early.

Exceptions: The above are good general rules about the postectopic cycle—to which there are so many exceptions that one must never depend on the length of the postextrasystolic cycle alone. In fact, there are six circumstances in which the VPB is followed by a less than compensatory pause, and three circumstances in which atrial premature beats (APB) are followed by fully compensatory pauses.[2] Most of them are relatively uncommon, so that the above rules provide about 90% probability.

In contrast with the VPB, the APB has normally split or unsplit sounds, is not followed but may be preceded (if atrial contraction occurs before the tricuspid valve has reopened) by a cannon wave in the neck (Fig. 40-3); and is usually followed by a less than compensatory cycle.

Junctional premature beats are indistinguishable from atrial if atrial contraction precedes ventricular. Cannon waves distinguish them if atrial contraction coincides with or follows ventricular.

If ectopic ventricular beats occur frequently enough—as in persistent ventricular bigeminy, or idioventricular rhythm (Fig. 40-4)—so that you can appraise their sounds in both phases of respiration, you can often tell which ventricle they come from: The *left* ventricular beat looks more like *right* bundle-branch block (BBB) *and behaves like it*, that is, the already wide splitting of S2 widens with inspiration (persistent splitting, as in Fig. 40-4); the *right* ventricular beat looks more like *left* BBB *and behaves like it*, that is, S2 splits

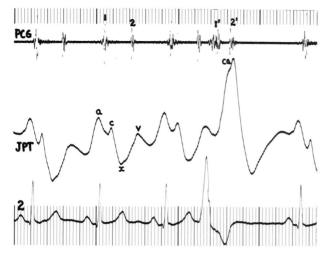

Figure 40–1. Sinus rhythm is interrupted by a ventricular extrasystole (VPB) followed by a cannon wave (ca) in the jugular pulse (JPT). In the phonocardiogram (PCG), 1 and 2 are first and second sounds of the sinus beat; 1' and 2' are first and second sounds of the VPB.

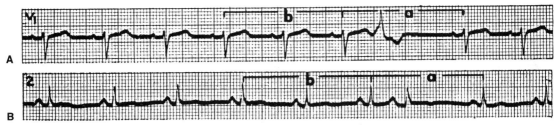

Figure 40–2. **(A)** Ventricular extrasystole followed by compensatory cycle (ie, "a" = "b"). **(B)** Atrial extrasystole followed by less-than-compensatory cycle (ie, "a" is less than "b").

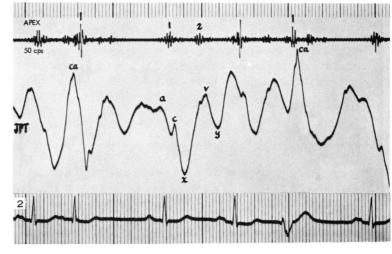

Figure 40–3. Atrial and ventricular extrasystoles producing cannon waves (ca). Note that the cannon wave of the atrial extrasystole peaks *before* the first sound (1) of the premature beat, whereas the cannon wave of the ventricular extrasystole peaks *after* the first sound (1) of the premature beat.

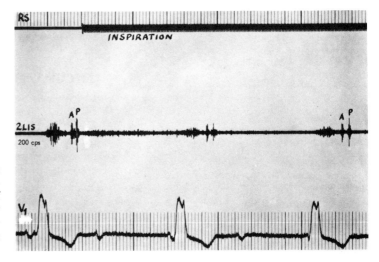

Figure 40–4. Complete A-V block with left idioventricular rhythm. Persistent splitting of S2, characteristic of left ventricular ectopy: S2 is widely split (0.06 second) at the end of expiration, but even more widely split in inspiration (0.08 second).

Table 40–2
Characteristics of Ventricular and Supraventricular Premature Beats

Cannon Waves		Splitting		Postextrasystolic Pause	
Present	*Not Present*	*Present*	*Not Present*	*Compensatory*	*Non-compensatory*
Ventricular	Most atrial*	Ventricular	Supraventricular	Ventricular	Atrial
Most junctional		SV with aberration		Atrial with SAN suppression	Junctional
				Junctional with SAN suppression	Ventricular with retrograde conduction

SAN, sinus nodal.
*If early enough, cannon wave precedes first sound of APB.

with expiration and closes with inspiration (reversed or paradoxical splitting).[3]

The diagnostic value of cannon waves, S2 splitting, and the postextrasystolic cycle is summarized in Table 40-2.

OTHER EARLY BEATS

There are several nonextrasystolic causes of early beats (Table 40-3). Each individual *parasystolic beat* has the characteristics of a VPB; you may suspect parasystole clinically if you can recognize that the arrhythmia is due to premature beats with varying coupling.

You can recognize the *capture beat* (Fig. 40-5) if it is preceded by the sequence of signs typical of A-V dissociation: S1 getting louder with successive beats (as the P–R shortens); then a cannon wave or two (as atrial contraction now coincides with or follows ventricular); and then the early beat. It is impossible to distinguish this clinically from a reciprocal beat, because this same sequence of events precedes both.

One of the most important factors determining the intensity of the first sound is the time relationship of atrial to ventricular contraction (Fig. 40-6). The loudest sound usually occurs when the P–R interval is 0.08 to 0.10 second, when the inflow of blood from the atria has opened the A-V valves to their fullest extent. When the P–R is much longer or shorter than this, the first sound as a rule is relatively soft.[4] This A-V relationship, however, varies in different hearts, and in some the loudest first sound occurs when the P wave is almost superimposed on the QRS (P–R = 0.02–0.04 second).

You may suspect that a captured beat is due to supernormal conduction if you have already diagnosed a high grade of A-V block from its characteristic signs (see below).

Table 40–3
Early Beats

1. Extrasystoles
   Ventricular
   Atrial
   Junctional
2. Parasystole
3. Capture beats, including supernormal conduction during A-V block
4. Better conduction interrupting poorer conduction, eg, 3:2 interrupting 2:1
5. Reciprocal beats

THE PAUSE
(TABLE 40-4)

Much the most common cause of an unexpected pause interrupting an otherwise regular rhythm is the *nonconducted APB* (Fig. 40-7**A**, and see Fig. 40-9). Its hallmarks are a cannon wave at the beginning of the pause (occurring earlier than the next expected "a" wave), and the pause itself is almost always less than two of the regular cycles.

Next most common is the dropped beat completing an *A-V Wenckebach* (Fig. 40-7**B**). Here,

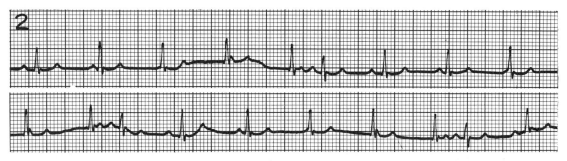

Figure 40–5. A-V dissociation, due to accelerated junctional rhythm, with ventricular captures. Follow the sequence of beats in the ECG as you read the descriptive text.

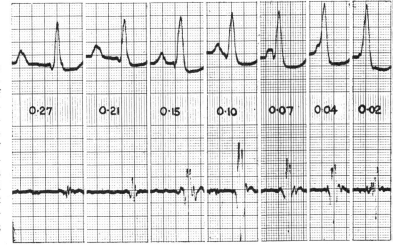

Figure 40–6. Selected cycles from a continuous ECG strip (paper speed = 50 mm/second) of complete A-V block with accompanying phonocardiogram illustrating how the first sound increases in intensity as the A-V (P-R) interval shortens. The loudest S1 occurs when the interval is about 0.10 second. (Reproduced with permission from Marriott HJL. Bedside recognition of cardiac arrhythmias. Geriatrics 1975; 30:55.)

by contrast, the "a" waves preserve an undisturbed regularity, but the pause itself is again less than two of the shorter cycles. The first sound may become progressively softer as the A-V interval increases before the dropped beat. In the much less common form of second degree *A-V block type II* (Fig. 40-7**C**), an "a" wave is similarly seen during the pause, but the pause is equal to two of the

Table 40–4
Causes of Pauses

1. Nonconducted atrial premature beats
2. Dropped beats in A-V block
   Type I
   Type II
3. S-A block
4. Concealed conduction

regular cycles—unless there is an interfering sinus arrhythmia.

Another uncommon pause is that due to *S-A block* (Fig. 40-7**D**). Again, the dropped beat may conclude a Wenckebach phenomenon, in which case the pause is less than two regular cycles; or it may be dropped without benefit of Wenckebach conduction so that the pause is equal to two shorter cycles. Such pauses are distinguishable from those due to second degree A-V block only by the absence of "a" waves during the long cycle.

Finally, the pause may result from *concealed conduction* interrupting a run of A-V dissociation (Fig. 40-7**E**): The atrial impulse penetrates to the A-V pacemaker and discharges it (junctional capture), thus delaying its next beat, but fails to reach the ventricles and achieve ventricular capture. Such a pause is recognizable because it is preceded by exactly the same train of signs described above as preceding a ventricular capture beat.

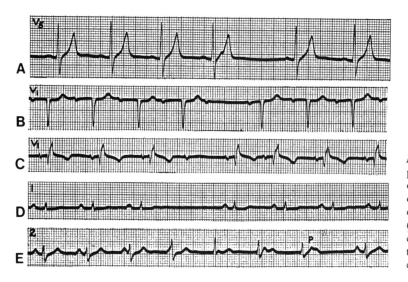

Figure 40–7. Some causes of pauses. **(A)** Nonconducted atrial extrasystole. **(B)** Dropped beat concluding A-V Wenckebach sequence. **(C)** Type II A-V block. **(D)** S-A block. **(E)** Concealed conduction into junction ("junctional capture") interrupting A-V dissociation.

THE REGULAR TACHYCARDIAS

Although the philosophy "Why diagnose when you can convert?" still has its adherents, the careful therapist prefers, if possible, to know what he or she is dealing with. The differential diagnosis of the regular tachycardias therefore remains an important, though at times difficult, exercise. Since ventricular aberration in the ECG can closely mimic an ectopic ventricular mechanism, the greatest difficulty, both at the bedside and in the ECG, is in those tachycardias that present widened, bizarre ventricular complexes due to asynchronous activation of the two ventricles.

SUPRAVENTRICULAR TACHYCARDIAS

In the absence of aberration, supraventricular tachycardia—including sinus, ectopic atrial, ectopic junctional, A-V nodal reentrant, and orthodromic tachycardia—presents with unsplit heart sounds, a first sound of constant intensity, and either no cannon waves or one with every beat. The presence or absence of cannon waves depends on the relationship of atrial to ventricular contraction (Table 40-5).

Cannon Waves

In A-V nodal reentrant tachycardia in which atrial and ventricular contractions are more or less si-

multaneous, and in orthodromic tachycardia in which atrial contraction follows ventricular but occurs before the A-V valves have opened, there are regular cannon waves. Regular cannon waves are also present in the rare ectopic junctional tachycardia, and in either sinus or ectopic atrial tachycardia if the rate is fast enough or the P–R interval enough prolonged for atrial contraction to occur before the A-V valves have opened.

Splitting of Sounds

If aberrant ventricular conduction complicates any of the above tachycardias, the findings will be similar except that the heart sounds will be split.

Table 40–5
Cannon Waves in Supraventricular Tachycardia

No Cannon Waves

Sinus tachycardia	
Ectopic atrial tachycardia	} If P–R normal and rate moderate
Atrial flutter	

Regular Cannon Waves

A-V nodal reentrant tachycardia	
Orthodromic tachycardia	
Ectopic junctional tachycardia	
Sinus tachycardia	} If fast or if first-degree A-V block
Ectopic atrial tachycardia	

Intensity of S1

In the rare situation of an ectopic junctional tachycardia, without retrograde conduction and therefore with independent atrial activity, the first sound will vary in intensity from beat to beat.

Atrial flutter, as long as the A-V conduction ratio is 2:1, produces signs that are indistinguishable from the other supraventricular tachycardias—except that the rate is usually 140 to 160/minute, whereas with the other SVTs, the rate is more often over 160/minute. Vagal stimulation may exactly halve the ventricular rate by doubling the A-V conduction ratio; conversely, if the ratio is 4:1, exercise may exactly double the ventricular rate. With the ratio at 4:1 or greater, rippling flutter waves may be visible in the jugular pulses (Fig. 40-8), and the frenetic atrial activity may be audible.[5,6]

VENTRICULAR TACHYCARDIA

Ventricular tachycardia presents with wide splitting of the heart sounds, sometimes producing a quadruple or multiple-sound cadence.[7] If the atria are beating independently, as they do in about half the cases, signs of A-V dissociation are present: Variation in intensity of S1 and irregular cannon waves. When these signs of dissociation are present in the company of widely split sounds, the evidence in favor of ventricular tachycardia is strong but not conclusive; there is always the remote possibility of a junctional tachycardia with ventricular aberration (producing split sounds),

without retrograde conduction and therefore with independent atrial activity.

If there is retrograde 1:1 conduction to the atria—a not infrequent occurrence—the first sound has constant intensity, and there may be a cannon wave with every beat.[8,9] If the atria are fibrillating, the first sound is constant but there are no cannon waves.

Since respiratory movements alone can cause alterations in the intensity of the heart sounds, and also produce an ebb and flow in the neck veins that makes their waves more difficult to interpret, you should always evaluate these while the patient holds her breath.

Variation in peak ventricular pressure, as determined at the bedside by intermittent Korotkoff sounds,[10] merely affords a further method of detecting independent atrial activity, and is no more specific for ventricular tachycardia than any other sign of A-V dissociation. Vagal stimulation has no effect on ventricular tachycardia.

To recapitulate:

1. If the heart sounds are single (or normally split), if the intensity of S1 is constant, and there are regular or no cannon waves in the neck, it is a supraventricular tachycardia.
2. If the heart sounds are widely split, the intensity of S1 is constant, and there are regular or no cannon waves in the neck, it is a ventricular tachycardia with 1:1 retrograde conduction, or a supraventricular tachycardia with ventricular aberration.
3. If the heart sounds are widely split, the intensity of S1 varies, and there are irregular cannon waves, it is almost certainly ventricular tachycar-

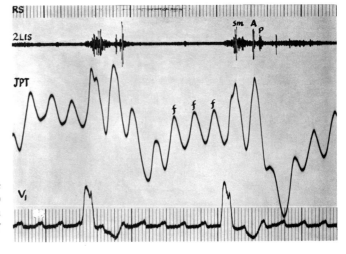

Figure 40–8. Atrial flutter with complete A-V block leaving its flickering imprint (f,f,f) on the jugular tracing. The PCG records an ejection systolic murmur (sm) and a widely split second sound (A,P).

dia, or (possibly, and very rarely) junctional tachycardia with both independent atrial activity and aberrant ventricular conduction.

THE BRADYCARDIAS

The causes of bradycardia are listed in Table 40-6.

Sinus bradycardia is recognized by its completely normal venous and auscultatory findings—except for the slow rate.

Nonconducted atrial bigeminy is recognized by the cannon waves in the jugular pulse following every ventricular beat of the seeming sinus bradycardia (Fig. 40-9).

Junctional rhythm with antecedent atrial activation may be indistinguishable from sinus bradycardia, except that the short A-V interval is likely to generate a louder than normal S1, and this may awaken your suspicion. When atrial contraction follows ventricular, a cannon wave follows every ventricular beat (Fig. 40-10). Junctional rhythm, of course, is not a *cause* of bradycardia; it can hold sway only if the sinus node abdicates (sick sinus) or the sinus impulses are blocked (A-V block).

Complete A-V block is one of the easiest bedside diagnoses. First the bradycardia alerts you. Then the presence of independent "a" waves in the jugular pulse with occasional cannon waves; palpable independent atrial impulses at the apex

Table 40–6
Causes of Bradycardia

1. Sinus bradycardia
2. Nonconducted atrial bigeminy
3. S-A block
4. A-V block
   Fixed ratio, eg, 2:1
   Complete

(Fig. 40-11); palpable atrial impulses in the peripheral arterial pulse[11]; variation in intensity of S1 (because of varying relationship of atrial to ventricular contractions—Fig. 40-11), with occasional explosive first sound ("bruit de canon") when atrial contraction shortly precedes ventricular; and sometimes audible atrial sounds correlatable with the "a" waves (Fig. 40-11). Some or all of these compose a picture so unmistakable that the diagnosis can hardly be missed.

In *fixed ratio* (2:1, 4:1, etc.) *A-V block*, the extra "a" waves between the ventricular beats indicate the block; and then the number and constant relationship of the "a" waves to the ventricular contractions, being an exact multiple of the ventricular rate, identifies the A-V ratio.

Even first-degree A-V block may be recognized at the bedside: In normal sinus rhythm, the "x" descent occurs during ventricular systole (ie, after

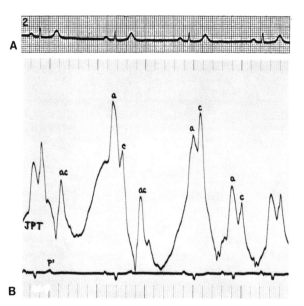

Figure 40–9. From an otherwise healthy 10-year-old boy. **(A)** Rhythm strip of lead 2, from which it is impossible to recognize the nonconducted atrial bigeminy masquerading as sinus bradycardia. **(B)** Nonconducted APBs follow the first two sinus beats, after which normal sinus rhythm prevails. Note in the jugular pulse tracing (JPT) the cannon waves (ac) following each of the first two beats and attesting to premature atrial activity.

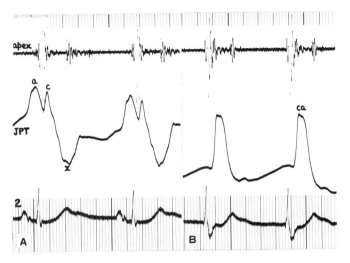

Figure 40–10. Jugular pulse tracing (JPT) before **(A)** and after **(B)** development of junctional rhythm with retrograde conduction to atria. In **(B)**, the jugular pulse is dominated by a cannon wave in systole.

S1); if the jugular "x" descent takes place before a soft S1 (Fig. 40-12), there must be an abnormally prolonged A-V conduction interval (ie, first-degree A-V block).

Although "a" waves, cannon or otherwise, are the bedside standard for recognizing atrial activity, notice in passing that there are no less than five other ways in which you may, on occasion, recognize mechanical atrial activity at the bedside:

1. Presystolic hepatic pulsation,
2. Palpable precordial atrial impulses (Fig. 40-11),
3. Palpable atrial waves in peripheral arterial pulses,
4. Atrial sounds (Fig. 40-11), and
5. Atriosystolic phase of pericardial friction (Fig. 40-13).

It is not uncommon for atrial fibrillation to accompany the higher grades of A-V block. If the block is not complete, a slight irregularity in the

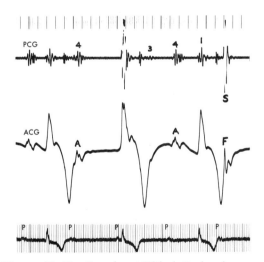

Figure 40–11. Complete A-V block. In the phonocardiogram (PCG), note the independent atrial sounds (4), and variation in the intensity of the first sound (1), including an explosive *bruit de canon* when the independent P wave is close to the QRS (short P-R interval, about 0.10 second). In the apexcardiogram (ACG) there are independent, easily palpable "a" waves. S, summation sound, when third and fourth sounds coincide; F, peak of rapid filling wave. (Reproduced with permission from Marriott HJL. Bedside recognition of cardiac arrhythmias. Geriatrics 1975;30:55.)

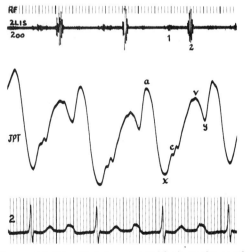

Figure 40–12. First-degree A-V block: In the jugular pulse, the "x" descent, instead of normally occupying systole, is completed before the first sound.

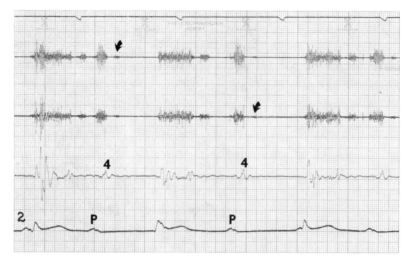

Figure 40–13. A-V block producing A-V dissociation in a patient with acute inferior infarction and associated pericarditis. The independent atrial sounds are recorded in the low-frequency PCG (4), whereas the high-frequency tracings record both systolic and diastolic (arrows) atrial rubs. (Reproduced with permission from Spodick DH, Marriott HJL. Atrial diastolic friction. Chest 1975;68:122.)

slow ventricular rhythm may give a clue to the underlying fibrillation, and this can be readily confirmed by noting the characteristic wave form in the jugular pulse (Fig. 40-14). Since in atrial fibrillation there is no effective atrial contraction, there can be no relaxation; therefore, since there is no "a" wave, there can be no "x" descent either, and this results in an easily spotted systolic venous pulse similar to that seen in tricuspid regurgitation. In addition, you may see fibrillary waves in the jugular pulse. If the ventricular rhythm is perfectly regular and there is no fibrillary motion in the neck veins, the mechanism is indistinguishable from complete S-A block with idiojunctional or idioventricular rhythm. If not only the rhythm is regular but the rate is normal, *unless you study the neck veins* the situation may easily be mistaken for normal sinus rhythm. And this can be serious, for you may be missing an important sign of digitalis intoxication.

Rarely *atrial flutter* is complicated by high-grade (eg, 8:1) or complete A-V block (Fig. 40-8). These can be distinguished only if the flutter waves can be seen in the jugulars, or if atrial sounds are audible.[5] These are most likely to be heard toward the ends of the longer diastoles, and best in the 3rd *right* interspace.[6]

In complete block, A-V or S-A, you can attempt to identify the location of the ventricular pacemaker. Unsplit or narrowly split sounds in-

IF SPLITTING IS:	THE MECHANISM IS:
Persistent	Either idioventricular from a left ventricular focus or idiojunctional with RBBB
Paradoxical	Either idioventricular from a right ventricular focus or idiojunctional with LBBB

dicate a center situated above the bifurcation (idiojunctional rhythm), whereas widely split sounds indicate either an idioventricular pacemaker or an idiojunctional rhythm with bundle-branch block. By noting the effect of respiration on the splitting—persistent or paradoxical—one can further narrow the mechanism down:

In Figure 40-4, the idioventricular rhythm was from the left ventricle and the splitting was persistent.

One of the more common forms of "bradycardia" encountered in the hospital is a pseudobradycardia—reported by the pulse-taking attendant, but in reality a sinus rhythm with ventricular bigeminy due to digitalis intoxication, the extrasystoles being too premature to raise a pulse. Cannon waves following each of the palpable beats, and careful auscultation for the thud of the early coupled beat quickly reveal the true situation.

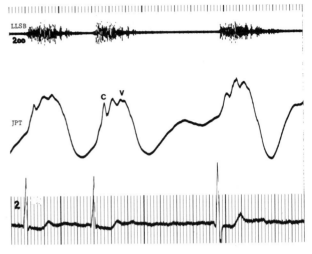

Figure 40–14. Atrial fibrillation in a patient with tricuspid regurgitation; note the pansystolic murmur recorded at the left lower sternal border. The jugular pulse contains no "a" wave and no "x" descent: the normal jugular pulse is replaced by a systolic surge consisting of merged "c" and "v" waves.

BIGEMINAL RHYTHM

When the beats are paired, obviously the most likely mechanism is extrasystolic bigeminy, usually ventricular; atrial and junctional bigeminy are much less likely, and the features that distinguish them during bigeminy are no different than the criteria applied to single premature beats (Table 40-7).

There are, however, several other not uncommon causes of bigeminal rhythm, of which perhaps the most common is a repeated 3:2 A-V Wenckebach (Fig. 40-15A). With or without the Wenckebach, the 3:2 mechanism is recognized by the occurrence of a normal "a" wave in the jugular pulse (unless it occurs early enough to produce a cannon wave) following the second of each pair of beats, itself not followed by another ventricular response. You suspect the Wenckebach if you can recognize

that the A-V (jugular "a" to carotid pulse) interval is longer in the second ventricular cycle than the first; and if your sense of rhythm permits you to recognize that the longer ventricular interval is not quite twice as long as the shorter. Without the Wenckebach phenomenon, the longer interval will be exactly twice the shorter (type II A-V block).

Another fairly common pairing mechanism is *atrial flutter with alternating 2:1 and 4:1 conduction* (Fig. 40-15**B**). In this situation there is almost always a Wenckebach at work, and this again can be suspected if the longer ventricular interval is less than twice the shorter. You can spot the underlying flutter only if flutter waves are visible in the jugular pulse, as in Figure 40-8.

Less common mechanisms of bigeminal rhythm are *escape-capture* sequences—of which there are many forms. The mechanism illustrated in Figure 40-15**C** consists of an undisturbed sinus discharge, but only one in every three sinus impulses is conducted. The blocked sinus impulse would produce an "a" wave not followed by a ventricular response, and then the A-V escape beat would not be preceded by an "a" wave at a conductible interval; a cannon wave might appear, depending on whether the dissociated atrial contraction was just before, with, or just after the escaped beat. The form seen in Figure 40-15**D**—the pairs consisting of junctional escape beats followed by conducted sinus beats—would easily be mistaken for a 3:2 A-V Wenckebach, since atrial contractions resulting from sinus or A-V activation produce identical jugular "a" waves. But there would be no "a" wave following the second beat of each pair as

---

Table 40–7
Some Causes of Bigeminal Rhythm

1. Extrasystolic
2. 3:2 block
   S-A
   A-V
      Type I
      Type II
3. Alternating 4:1 & 2:1 A-V conduction
4. Reciprocal
5. Escape-capture sequences

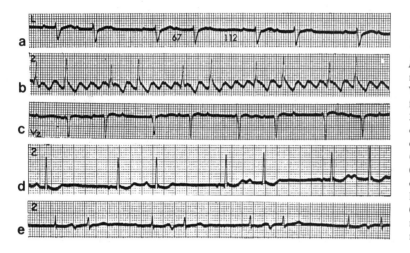

Figure 40–15. Some mechanisms of bigeminy. **(A)** 3:2 A-V Wenckebach periods. **(B)** Atrial flutter with alternating 4:1 and 2:1 A-V conduction. **(C)** Escape–capture bigeminy (junctional escape, ventricular capture). **(D)** Escape–capture bigeminy (ectopic atrial or junctional escape, sinus beat with prolonged P-R). **(E)** Reciprocal bigeminy (junctional rhythm with delayed retrograde conduction and reciprocal beating).

there would in any form of 3:2 A-V block, and so the rhythm would simulate 3:2 S-A block.

The rare reciprocal bigeminy (Fig. 40-15**E**) has no "a" wave preceding the first beat of each pair, but has one—which may assume "cannonized" proportions—sandwiched between each pair. The mechanism may be suspected, but it cannot be distinguished from an escape-capture bigeminy at the bedside.

Occasionally, during atrial fibrillation, the ventricular beats tend to arrange themselves in pairs—"fortuitous pairing." This can usually be spotted at the bedside by the absence of "a" wave and "x" descent in the jugular pulse; and by the irregularity of the pairs, both in the longer intervals separating them and in their own "coupling" intervals.

Bigeminal rhythm due to 3:2 sinus Wenckebachs can be suspected if the rate is relatively slow and if each beat presents the normal hemodynamic findings; obviously the longer interval separating the pairs must be less than twice the shorter interval. This may be quite indistinguishable from atrial bigeminy due to atrial extrasystoles, except that the coupling interval of the premature beats is usually considerably shorter than the shorter sinus cycles in 3:2 S-A block—but this of course depends on the prevailing sinus rate.

Finally, a form of bigeminy may result from alternating A-V conduction times, presumably due to concealed junctional extrasystoles occurring every third beat. This could be suspected if the alternating A-V relationship could be accurately pinpointed, and if the atrial contraction earlier in the cycle (P wave landing before end of T wave)

produced a cannon wave followed by a ventricular response.

GROUP BEATING

When beats occur in intermittent short spurts separated by longer intervals, the term "group beating" is applicable, and one of two mechanisms is almost certainly at work: Either short bursts of "repetitive paroxysmal tachycardia," ventricular or supraventricular; or supraventricular tachycardia with repeated Wenckebach periods. When repetitive tachycardia occurs, the paroxysms are almost always separated by one or two sinus beats (Fig. 40-16**A**), the first beat of each paroxysm being coupled to the preceding sinus beat.

At the bedside, these two mechanisms may be indistinguishable. In each, the interval between the groups may be less than twice the short cycles; in each, the rate may accelerate within the group of beats—because of "warm-up" in the paroxysms of ectopic tachycardia, and because of the classic structure of Wenckebach periods in the other case. Always remember the propensity of the Wenckebach type of conduction to leave beats grouped in pairs, threes, and fours—all the pairs, trios and quartets in Figure 40-16 (**B** to **D**) are the result of Wenckebachian whimsy. The three examples are selected in order of decreasing transparency. In the first (Fig. 40-16**B**), the mechanism is undoubted because the P waves are plain to see. In Figure 40-16**C**, the mechanism is immediately suspected because of the trio-grouping, and then a careful search reveals the P waves (arrows) and confirms

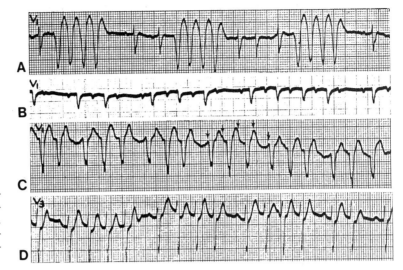

Figure 40–16. Some mechanisms of group beating. **(A)** Repetitive ventricular tachycardia. **(B–D)** Supraventricular tachycardia with 4:3 and 5:4 Wenckebach periods.

the mechanism. In Figure 40-16**D**, again one's suspicions are immediately aroused, but then the P wave search is less revealing, and one cannot prove the Wenckebach mechanism, which nevertheless remains most likely. Some causes of trigeminy—the prototype of group beating—are listed in Table 40-8.

CHAOS

Careful attention to the neck veins will unravel most of the mechanisms of chaotic irregularity (Table 40-9). Undoubtedly *atrial fibrillation* is the most common, and is readily recognized by the combination of patternless ventricular irregularity with absence of both "a" wave and "x" descent in the jugular pulse (Fig. 40-14). There is no repe-

tition of the irregular pattern, and it is usually obvious to the ear that the arrhythmia is due to longer than average cycles as well as shorter cycles—this distinguishes it from the irregularity produced by multiple prematurities. And, of course, the intensity of S1 varies.

Atrial flutter, when it is associated with unpredictably variable A-V conduction, is a good mimic of fibrillation. It can be differentiated only if regular flutter waves are visible in the jugular pulse during the longer cycles—and even then, remember that coarse atrial fibrillation may make a similar flickering imprint on the jugular pulse. A grossly *wandering atrial pacemaker*, often associated with atrial premature beats, can be identified by the presence of "a" waves before each ventricular beat despite the gross irregularity. If APBs are associated, some may be early enough to produce cannon waves.

You may suspect a *chaotic (or multifocal) atrial tachycardia* if you can make out "a" waves pre-

Table 40–8
Some Causes of Trigeminal Rhythm

1. Extrasystolic
   a. Two extrasystoles coupled to sinus beat
   b. Extrasystole every third beat
   c. Extrasystole interpolated between two sinus beats
2. 4:3 block
   S-A
   A-V
     Type I
     Type II
3. Group beating of ventricular tachycardia

Table 40–9
Causes of Chaotic Irregularity

1. Atrial fibrillation
2. Atrial flutter with varying A-V conduction
3. Shifting pacemaker, often with APBs
4. Multifocal atrial tachycardia
5. Multifocal extrasystoles
6. Mixed arrhythmias

Table 40–10
Jugular Clues in Arrhythmias and Blocks

The Clue	Hemodynamic Significance	Condition Where Seen
Independent "a" waves	Atria beating independently	High-grade A-V block Complete A-V block A-V dissociation
Regular cannon "a" waves with every beat	Atria regularly contracting with or just after ventricles	Junctional rhythm Supraventricular tachycardia Ventricular tachycardia with 1:1 retroconduction
Intermittent cannon "a" waves	Atria intermittently contracting with or just after ventricles	Ventricular premature beats Atrial premature beats Junctional premature beats A-V dissociation Ventricular tachycardia Complete A-V block
Absent "a" waves	Absent or ineffective atrial contraction	S-A block Atrial fibrillation
Absent "x" descent	No contraction, no relaxation	Atrial fibrillation
Rapid rippling waves		Atrial flutter or fibrillation
"x" descent before S1	Delayed ventricular contraction	First-degree A-V block

ceding the irregular ventricular beats; and again, if any of the ectopic atrial impulses is early enough, it will generate a cannon wave. *Multifocal ventricular prematurities* with varying coupling intervals, occurring frequently but irregularly, can be partially identified if some of the beats can be taken for sinus (preceding "a" wave), and if some of the premature beats can be recognized for what they are by the wide splitting of their sounds and trailing cannon waves. Obviously, combinations of these chaotic mechanisms can and do occur, and may successfully defy all attempts at bedside identification.

The various clues in the jugular pulse that may help to identify an arrhythmia are summarized in Table 40-10.

THE ARTERIAL PULSE

Although an arrhythmia is often first detected in the peripheral arterial pulse, the pulse itself adds nothing to the diagnosis that auscultation of the heart cannot provide. *Pulse deficit*, often thought of as rather specific for atrial fibrillation, is purely a function of prematurity, and does not help us to determine the mechanisms of the prematurity. Any

of the causes of "chaos" can be associated with a pulse deficit, as indeed can any arrhythmia containing premature systoles.

A final word of caution: Although the signs described are classic and common, there are times when the expected hemodynamic expression of an arrhythmia fails to appear. For example, the atrium contracting just after the ventricle may fail to create a recognizable cannon wave; or the ventricular extrasystole may occur so early that only a first sound is produced as a single thud that does not seem split. The presence of one of the clinical signposts may be of greater value in confirming the mechanism than the validity of its absence in excluding it.

REFERENCES

1. Marriott HJL. Depolarization, contraction, systole, complex, or beat? Take your choice, but may my sinus node go on *beating*! Heart Lung 1987;16:117.
2. Marriott HJL. Pearls and pitfalls in the electrocardiogram. Philadelphia: Lea and Febiger, 1990:48–51.
3. Haber E, Leatham A. Splitting of the heart sounds from ventricular asynchrony in bundle branch block, ventricular ectopic beats and artificial pacing. Br Heart J 1965; 27:691.

4. Beard OW, Decherd GM. Variations in the first heart sound in complete A-V block. Am Heart J 1947;34:809.

5. Neporent LM. Atrial heart sounds in atrial fibrillation and flutter. Circulation 1964;30:893.

6. Massumi RA, et al. The audible sounds of atrial tachyarrhythmia (flutter?): a note on their genesis. Circulation 1966;33:607.

7. Harvey WP, Corrado MA. Multiple sounds in paroxysmal ventricular tachycardia. N Engl J Med 1957;257:325.

8. Kistin AD. Retrograde conduction to the atria in ventricular tachycardia. Circulation 1961;24:236.

9. Kistin AD. Problems in the differentiation of ventricular arrhythmia from supraventricular arrhythmia with abnormal QRS. Prog Cardiovasc Dis 1966;9:1.

10. Wilson WS, et al. A simple diagnostic sign in ventricular tachycardia. N Engl J Med 1964;270:446.

11. Harvey WP, Ronan JA. Bedside diagnosis of arrhythmias. Prog Cardiovasc Dis 1966;8:419.

Index

Page numbers in boldface indicate a major discussion of a topic. Page numbers followed by *f* indicate illustrations; *t* following a page number indicates tabular material; *n* following a page number indicates a note.

ISBN 0-397-51085-3

90000

9 780397 510856